The Treatment

MARTHA STEPHENS

The

The Story of Those Who Died

in the Cincinnati Radiation Tests

Treatment

DUKE UNIVERSITY PRESS   DURHAM AND LONDON 2002

© 2002 Duke University Press   All rights reserved
Printed in the United States of America on acid-free paper ∞
Typeset in Quadraat by Tseng Information Systems, Inc.
Library of Congress Cataloging-in-Publication Data
appear on the last printed page of this book.

Tyger! Tyger! burning bright

In the forests of the night,

What immortal hand or eye

Dare frame thy fearful symmetry?

—WILLIAM BLAKE

This book is dedicated to the ninety victims of the human
radiation experiments in Cincinnati General Hospital (1960–1972);
it has been written so that history may remember their injuries and
afflictions, and their unwitting sacrifice in a project sponsored by
the U.S. Department of Defense and carried out by researchers in
the College of Medicine of the University of Cincinnati.

Contents

This book is the story of one tragedy of medical research that stretched over eleven years and affected the lives of hundreds of people in one Ohio town. A word might be said about the way it came to be written.

As I explain in the opening chapters of the narrative, I had known, for over two decades, about the tragic train of events that had taken place in our public hospital in Cincinnati, but for all those years a conspiracy of silence on this subject reigned and I did not think it could ever be broken. My life proceeded in other directions, and it was not until new circumstances in 1994–95 that I began to feel I might be able to relate the full story of the experiments and the injuries and deaths that had occurred. In 1994 new information emerged that had been hidden away for many years—a mass of private correspondence, for instance, within the University of Cincinnati College of Medicine. I learned for the first time the identities of the victims and met their surviving families. I could examine the full hospital records.

Since I was myself involved in the efforts, both in the seventies and again in the nineties, to open the case to the public at large, my own story of study and detection and eventual cooperation with the press, forms part of this account. Whether this is for good or ill, others will have to judge; but it would have seemed to me disingenuous, to say the least, to have approached the subject any other way.

The primal tale, nevertheless, must lie in the details of the experiments themselves, and in what exactly happened to the victims as new groups of people ill with cancer were brought into the study year by year.

Readers not greatly interested in the step-by-step unmasking of the case in the press in 1994–95, may find what concerns them most in the final two parts of this book. What I have termed "the medical story" and then "the legal story" are recounted as human dramas in themselves, but as for factual accuracy and completeness, I wrote with the hope that they would withstand the scrutiny of scholars in medicine, law, and human experimentation. I am not an expert in any of these fields, nor in the deliberate exposures of the Cold War. My aim was to recreate the full anatomy of one major medical project gone badly wrong.

BUT SUCH A BOOK as this can hardly be the work of one person. Many people helped make the telling of this story possible, and their endeavors were critical and indispensable.

From the beginning of the legal action in 1994, Jennifer Thomas, in the offices of Cincinnati attorneys Kircher, Robinson, Newman, and Welch, and then of the firm Newman and Meeks, sent me all the documents I asked for and more as the suit progressed, and answered endless questions on the telephone. Thanks to her work on this case, it became one of the best-organized lawsuits known; this book is one of the beneficiaries of her labors and of the generous cooperation of the two firms named above.

The early chapters of this volume, recounting the at times day-by-day evolution of the story in the press, could not have been written without the assiduous work of David Logan, today the director of a well-known alcohol program for low-income people, but once my colleague in the English Department of the University of Cincinnati and president of the UC Junior Faculty Association at the time we issued our critique of the experiments in 1972. Beginning in 1994, Logan kept a superb anthology of the ever-spreading mass of news reports. He accompanied me to hearings around the case and was always ready to advise and consent, consider and consult in late-night, exploring conversations that helped me settle my own views about what was taking place. He helped bring about the congressional hearing in Cincinnati in 1994.

In that same year Laura Schneider was a graduate student in English at UC, and she went to work on this case with unflagging energy and nerve, and succeeded in finding the four surviving families who made possible the filing of the lawsuit by Robert Newman. Schneider also kept detailed tables of data on the full list of victims as to what we were learning about each one; this record I constantly referred to as I wrote, and it still hangs, in a greatly enlarged version, on the wall of my study. Schneider read the early drafts of this book and made copious notes for my elucidation. In due time she also located a Kentucky family who would otherwise not have become known and who became the subject of feature reports in the *Lexington Herald-Leader*. An undergraduate student, Bridget Marion, was also a valued coworker on this book for over a year, as was my student assistant, Mary Ann Thomas.

I must also offer special thanks to Doris Baker, an individual of unusual penetration whose grandmother was irradiated in 1962. Baker became the founder and leader of a Cincinnati organization of surviving families. She remained alert to everything happening around this story for over five years, and was thus a flooding fount of knowledge about the perspectives of family members and the workings of journalists, attorneys, and official Washington.

All the families I came to know I have regarded as partners in the unveiling of this long-suppressed story; the crucial information they supplied can be read in the pages of this narrative. I am especially grateful for the many important conversations I had not only with Doris Baker but with Lilian Pagano and family, Barb Tatterson, Barbara Ann Mathis, and Joseph P. Larkins, each of whom had close family members irradiated.

A number of reporters also became *compadres* in this mission to render the darkness in which this case had been enveloped penetrable at last, and their stories, too, are recounted in this narrative. I was happy to be able to work with two talented British journalists, Julian O'Halloran and John Slater. They made extended visits to Cincinnati and featured the UC tests in documentaries for the BBC. It was a pleasure to work with reporters who go about their tasks in an open, inclusive spirit without screens and distances; they furthered my own understanding of how this project would be regarded outside the United States. The 1994 program O'Halloran created, with producer Barbara Want, was titled "The Sacrifice Zone" and aired on the Panorama Show. John Slater, with producer Peter Hoare, made a comprehensive three-part radio program on U.S. Cold War experiments titled "Atomica America," the opening segment of which spotlighted the Cincinnati tests.

I must mention, too, the careful and exhaustive work of another enterprising journalist described in this book, Akira Tashiro, senior staff writer of the daily paper of Hiroshima City, Japan, the *Chugoku Shimbun*.

I am most grateful to Scott Simon and senior editor Gwen Tompkins at *Weekend Edition* of National Public Radio for allowing me to give on the air a detailed account of the Cincinnati tests and to present facts of the case that most national media were not prepared to acknowledge.

Peg Rusconi and her editors at Cincinnati's WKRC made the comprehensive and accurate television reports in early 1994 that gave this story its first public life, and a few weeks later, Nick Miller broke the print story in exhaustive detail in the *Cincinnati Post*. At the *Cincinnati Enquirer*, Linda Reeves pursued this case, once she engaged with it, with dogged accuracy and precision, giving us an expressive parade of front-page interviews with families that effectually settled the question of consent. Dilva Henry made contributions of several important kinds on Cincinnati's WCPO.

At the *Enquirer*, Tim Bonfield, who is known in Cincinnati for studious medical reporting, eventually took up the technical side of this issue in a long series of crucial reports. He and reporter Steve Bennish played out their parts in the best journalistic style, as did an editor at the same paper, Tony Lang, who brought to this story an open mind and a disturbed conscience and was a steady ally in the attempt to keep the publicity accurate and up-to-date.

As to the media world, I was more than happy to make the acquaintance in 1994 of a peerless raker of muck of old-time habits of mind and conscience, Eileen Welsome, now of Denver, Colorado. It was Welsome's uncovering of the identities of the plutonium victims and her series of articles in the *Albuquerque Tribune* in 1993 that led to the sudden explosion of interest in other Cold War tests. I met Welsome when she visited Cincinnati in 1994, and she and I later explored in long and discursive telephone conversations the history of U.S. deliberate exposures. In a sense, her work on this early period was the progenitor of all the rest, and her comprehensive account, in *The Plutonium Files*, of the historical roots of the Cold War radiations is a work of lasting importance. Welsome read my completed manuscript and responded, most generously, with chapter-by-chapter questions and annotations.

My talks in 1994 with David Egilman, a physician in Braintree, Massachusetts, whose findings about the UC project are described in this book, were always interesting. Carl Gandola, a clinician in the Cincinnati Health Department and one of the very few doctors in Cincinnati willing to discuss this subject with me, read with great care and perspicuity two drafts of this work and twice gave me splendid notes and suggestions.

As to readers of manuscript, I must also thank not only Eileen Welsome and Carl Gandola, but Jennifer Thomas, Herb and Judy Shapiro, Robert Newman, and my husband, Jerone Stephens.

Herbert Shapiro, my long-time friend and colleague in the History Department at UC, known especially for his scholarly work in African American history, was a trusted consultant all along, and Judy Shapiro as well. They have had for some years a deep personal interest in the victims of the Cincinnati tests, and Herb Shapiro served with distinction on the radiation panel appointed by Cincinnati City Council in 1994.

Many friends in Cincinnati progressive movements could be counted on for encouragement in the pursuit of this story, including the late Maurice McCracken and the late Buddy Gray, loved and respected warriors for peace and justice in the downtown neighborhoods of Cincinnati where many of the test subjects had lived.

I would like to thank Gary Stern of the Advisory Committee on Human Radiation for many frank exchanges about the experiments and his willingness to confront facts of the case that were not being otherwise acknowledged. Stern waged a good fight within the Committee, and in spite of this group's determination not to examine any record of actual injuries and deaths, was able to help bring about a generally accurate, if limited, account of the Cincinnati tests in the Committee's Final Report of 1995. I am grateful, too, for the encouragement of Committee member Jay Katz, retired professor of law and medicine at Yale, whose distinguished work on human experimentation is described in these pages.

The enterprising work of attorneys Robert Newman and Lisa Meeks is the subject of many scenes of this book; they played crucial roles in the legal action that helped bring the case before the public, an action that led to a landmark federal ruling on dangerous human research and the citing of the Nuremberg Code. Their fellow attorneys David Thompson, Robert Nelson, Gary Lewis, and David Kamp, and each of the office staffs involved, must also be remembered with appreciation.

I would like to thank David Sterling of the UC History Department, Carol Rainey in English Studies, ex-City-Councilman Tyrone Yates, and Judy Daniels, medical director of the Cincinnati Health Department, for their steady interest and encouragement. My friend Donna Kopp, a nurse and paralegal, provided invaluable help with medical terminology. UC archivist Kevin Grace was always willing to assist. My literary agent, David Hendin, has been active on behalf of this story and a true believer in the need for it to be made known.

On the campus of UC, my daughters Paige and Shelley Stephens and their fellow activists in the peace and justice brigade were stalwart public defenders of the rights of the families to be granted complete information about what had taken place.

Back in the seventies, political scientist Henry Anna was an intrepid and ingenuous colleague during the endeavors of the UC Junior Faculty Association to bring these experiments to light.

My husband, Jerone Stephens, has labored in an infinite number of ways to help make the events in our hospital better understood. In the seventies he wrote incisive political analyses of what had taken place, and as for my own work, he continued to believe that in spite of a marked visual limitation, I would be able to compose this account. He and I discussed in detail almost every facet of this story, and he not only read manuscript but found footnotes, keyed in complex passages, and read for me directly or onto tape many documents, books, and other materials not available from libraries for the blind and impaired.

The adaptive equipment and student reading assistants provided me by the UC Department of English and the College of Arts and Sciences helped make it possible for me to continue teaching for some years and to complete this study and other writings.

Mary Beth Lukco, a volunteer from the Hamilton County Library for the Blind, provided most generous assistance in the final stage of this project.

Last, I must mention Reynolds Smith, Executive Editor at Duke University Press and my editor for this book, an individual of courage and insight. I realized early on that most presses were not going to want to engage with a narrative as severe in its critique of U.S. medicine as this one. But Reynolds Smith, when he read this story, was disturbed by what he learned about our public hospital of the sixties and its military experiments. He felt that the facts were the facts and needed to be made known. His associate Rebecca Johns-Danes was also a warm and always encouraging partner in this project and the kind of exacting editor every book needs. Lynn Walterick's careful copyediting was a valuable contribution. All citizens interested in humane medicine and humane government, common justice and respect for all people, will be comforted, I hope, in these sometimes dark days, in what Duke University Press has been willing to set before us.

In 1953 a woman named Lula Tarlton was working as a domestic for a family in Cincinnati. One day, waiting for a bus to go to work and straightening the blouse of her white uniform, she felt a lump under her collar bone. She realized at once that she might have breast cancer and instead of going to work, she made her way to Cincinnati General Hospital.

Tarlton did have breast cancer, and a few weeks later she had a right mastectomy, then the following year a mastectomy on the left. For over five years Tarlton lived a normal life, but then complications and more treatments ensued.

In the spring of 1960, unbeknown to Tarlton and other cancer patients, a new research project had begun within Cincinnati General Hospital for the U.S. military. This project needed subjects who could be irradiated over their whole bodies as if for treatment for cancer. On December 4, 1960, Lula Tarlton was exposed to a large dose of total body radiation in a specially built room in the basement of the hospital. The radiation was given in one continuous dose in an effort to simulate the exposure of soldiers in nuclear war.

Tarlton's niece, Barbara Ann Mathis, remembers well her aunt's last illness and her radioactive treatment. In the hospital a two-inch-thick metal shield was placed at the foot of her bed and the family told to stand behind it when they came to visit, not to approach the patient.

Lula Tarlton and her niece both lived in a small African American enclave in Cincinnati's East End, a long corridor of lower-income neighborhoods that runs outward from the city along the eastern stretch of the Ohio River. Over that Christmas, Mathis took her aunt home with her to the East End. Tarlton was vomiting profusely and becoming more and more ill. A bucket was kept upstairs for her to vomit in. She was soon returned to the hospital and fell into convulsions. No treatment availed — in time the doctors noted that she was "totally unresponsive," and on January 22 Tarlton died.

No one in Tarlton's family knew that she had been used in an experiment, nor that she had had radiation over her whole body. No consent form had been offered her. According to the doctors, patients were being told "they were being treated for their disease."

Many years passed, and in 1994 Barbara Ann Mathis was working as an information clerk in the same hospital where her aunt had died. She was reading the morning paper during a break at her desk one day when she saw her aunt's name and began to weep. She wept because the paper reported that her aunt had been experimented on, and also because her name was printed among the names of those who had no relations. To think that her aunt had had no one to claim her, as if she had been all alone in the world, was the most sorrowful thing of all, Mathis said. Tarlton was sixty-six when she died, those many years ago, and the youngsters in the family had known her only as "Aunt Lula." Mathis felt that she herself might be the only living person who could still recognize her aunt's full name.

In time Mathis spoke to a coworker that day. "I wish you would look at this," she said. "This is my aunt — here is her name. And look at this that happened to her."

Barbara Ann Mathis had known her aunt well and remembered her as a strong woman who could do anything she made up her mind to. She loved to travel. She had come to Cincinnati from Bryson, North Carolina, and she often went back there to visit. Once she took a young grandchild by the hand and got on a train to California, just for the fun of it, and though she didn't know a soul out there to call on.

"She just loved to *go*," Mathis said.

Mathis read in the papers that a legal action had been filed on behalf of the families of the victims of the experiments, and she contacted the attorney whose name she saw. Many patients, she learned, had been less ill than her Aunt Lula when they were exposed and yet had died within weeks of their radiations.

Mathis became part of the legal action, and in 1999, after many bitter disputes among the contending parties, thirteen researchers and their institutions agreed on a settlement of over five million dollars with their accusers. A memorial plaque in honor of the ninety victims of the experiments was placed in a yard of the hospital.

In time the surviving families began to learn the full story of these strange events — how it was they had come to pass, and why so few had ever known of them.

I

The Story of the Press and the Public Campaign

1

The First Public Knowledge of the Tests

It is clearer and clearer to me that life is not held sacred in this country; it is cheap. — SENATOR MIKE GRAVEL, 1972

Life, we all know, does not run a true course; it twists and turns on us and brings us up against the most unexpected circumstances.

In the fall of 1971, ten years after the death of Lula Tarlton, new radiations were still taking place in our public hospital in Cincinnati. But the first tentative explorations were being made by the press, and that October a small story appeared in the *Village Voice* that would restructure my own life for a full year and more, and affect my thinking deeply for many years to come.

I was a teacher of English, but the research I undertook that winter had nothing to do with literature—I took up the study of radiology.

What I learned about this science made me so respectful of radiation that I began to refuse to have even a chest x-ray or x-rays at the dentist. My husband and I decided that our children were not going to be irradiated at all except in a genuine medical crisis, and for years we had running disputes on this issue with our doctors and dentists.

Over that fall of 1971 I acquired—in a curious way which I shall presently describe—certain critical documents on the experiments, and during the December holidays that year, I sat up late at our dining room table, after children were put to bed, amidst a sea of books and papers on radiation, including reports sent to the Department of Defense from the medical school at my university. I was learning that, just as the *Village Voice* had suggested, medical professors on my campus were conducting experiments on radiation injury, using human subjects, and the experiments were being funded by the Defense Atomic Support Agency of the Department of Defense.[1]

The trouble was that the researchers were not looking for subjects to study who had been exposed to high radiation *accidentally*, but were exposing people directly right in the hospital.

I was studying the case histories of eighty-seven individuals who had already been part of the experiments. Many of these people were coming to a tumor clinic at the hospital run by our College of Medicine at the University of Cincinnati. They were being irradiated over their whole bodies—or sometimes half their bodies—in one fell stream of radiation. The great majority knew nothing about the team's study of radiation injury or being part of any research whatever, and thought they were simply being treated for their cancers. But I was learning that the military radiation they were being given had virtually no chance of improving their health.

Indeed, twenty-one of these eighty-seven people had died within about a month of being irradiated.

Very few of these individuals had been acutely ill or lying close to death, and those who survived the severe short-term effects of the radiation, the crucial first month or so when bone marrow is most likely to fail, often lived a long time. A number of patients were still active at home or at work when they were brought in for this treatment; some had only recently been diagnosed with cancer and were in the hospital to be evaluated.[2]

I was examining closely certain case histories, including that of the domestic worker "L. T.," our "Lula Tarlton," as we would know her in later years—the "Aunt Lula" who loved to ride trains.

A patient we would eventually know as "Maude Jacobs" was another case that drew my rapt attention. "M. J." was forty-nine, the doctors wrote, when she was irradiated, and she had breast cancer that had apparently spread to her bones.

But Jacobs had been at home caring on her own for three young daughters, keeping house and cooking supper and so on, when she was called in one day for a "treatment." She had no one to take her to the hospital and had put on her hat and called herself a taxi. Her oldest daughter, from an earlier set of children born to her when she was very young and still living in the Kentucky hills, came in that day to take care of the smaller ones. Jacobs was given a large dose of radiation over her whole body. She went home again, but the next day was so violently ill that she was taken back to Cincinnati General Hospital. She died there twenty-five days later, desperately ill and mostly out of her mind.

Jacobs's medical profile in the doctors' reports records her white blood cell counts and platelet counts, two classic indexes of radiation injury to the bone marrow. These two blood scores started falling seven days after radiation and went down to almost nothing the day before she died.[3]

When the bone marrow fails and no new white blood cells can be made by the body, infection swoops in and there is nothing to fight it with.

Death will ensue.

I HAD LONG BEEN used to reading in plays and novels of tragic deaths, full of pity and sorrow, but as I wrote for a newspaper years later, I had not been used to this pity, this sorrow . . . of people sick and confused coming for help and then being brutally abused. It was clear that these tests would have to be brought to an end and that any of us on campus who could help must do so.

The report I wrote after Christmas that year was issued at a press conference on January 25, 1972, by a group of untenured professors called the Junior Faculty Association.

Though the experiments had been going on for eleven years, I was the first person, as far as I knew, in Cincinnati or indeed in most of the country, to read as I had the actual case histories. I had been shown the small piece in the *Village Voice* by a colleague, and did not know at the time that the first person to have unearthed the UC project and to have referred, at least, to possible patient deaths—was an independent journalist named Roger Rapoport, and that the work he was doing on a book called *The Great American Bomb Machine* had become known among certain writers in the eastern press and was the reason we had been able to read what we had in the *Village Voice*.

The Vietnam struggle was still ablaze, and like many other citizens around the country, those of us in the Junior Faculty Association were involved in resistance to that war. In the spring of 1970 there had been the bombing of Cambodia, and then in our own state of Ohio, the killing of four student protesters at Kent State by the Ohio National Guard. Thus, the report we had read in 1971 about Defense Department activity at UC had been discouraging, to be sure, since we would have been happier not to have had *any* military research on our campus. Still, the details had not seemed extremely alarming. We had read that cancer patients were being irradiated in a project funded by the DOD and that some had been made "ill" by the radiation. They had had "nausea and vomiting" afterward, and the writer questioned whether or not they knew they were part of an experiment, and whether this kind of radiation could reasonably be considered "treatment," even of an experimental kind.[4]

We had thought about this for a time, and we began to feel we ought at least to look into the matter. We reasoned that, after all, this was *our* university, and that all of us working there were responsible for what took place and accountable to the citizens of our town who paid our salaries. Surely, we felt, we ought not to have to rely on reporters outside to tell us what was happening; we ourselves should find out and let people know.

That may sound like perfectly straightforward thinking and just common sense, but of course within universities, and most other institutions, such an attitude is regarded as provocative in the extreme, and above all unprofessional. Nothing is worse than snooping about in your colleagues' activities, in work that is none of your business, especially in departments or colleges other than your own, where—this reasoning goes—you can't possibly understand what is taking place.

ONE DAY, NEVERTHELESS, I had gone over to the medical school looking for information about the DOD project. I had very little to go on but the account in the *Village Voice*. I met with the director of the medical center, Edward Gall, a large, shy, diffident man with crew-cut gray hair. I recall that in spite of what he told me that day I rather liked Dr. Gall and that later I even regarded him as a little bit of a hero because he had eventually caved in and given us the doctors' reports.

But what Gall told me, confidentially, that first day, was that he did not feel he had the right to ask the researchers to give him copies of their work for outsiders, and that—besides—these were scientific documents, and English professors would not be able to make head or tail of them. And after all, he said, they were bulky, extensive papers— surely no one would want them *all*. "We do, though," I remember saying. "We would like to see them all, Dr. Gall." He would look into the matter, he said.

I bided my time. I went back several times and used several different arguments on Dr. Gall. "We don't know whether the reports we've heard about these experiments have any truth in them," I would say. "We certainly hope they don't, Dr. Gall. We *assume* they don't. We certainly assume that researchers in your college would not do anything that was not in the best interest of their patients." But people outside were discussing our affairs, I pointed out, and seemed to think we were up to something, so I wondered if some faculty organization should look into the matter and possibly clear it up. He would do what he could, he said.

One afternoon I drove over from main campus to the College of Medicine to call once more on Edward Gall. When I walked in, I saw a stack of documents on his desk, and that day he simply handed over to me the doctors' reports to the DOD. He said, "Here they are if you really want them." I was surprised, and I thought, "I wonder if I *can* read this work." I later wondered, and I still wonder, why Gall gave these papers to me, or the research team agreed to it—if in fact they *did* agree—considering the profoundly serious things they described.

Gall handed me that day about six hundred pages of double-spaced transcript in several dark brown folders.

These were the papers I would study over the holidays that year and on which I would base my report for the Junior Faculty Association, but that first day I drove back to main campus and parked way up on the round drive in front of my home building, McMicken Hall. I was so anxious to see what I had that I pushed my car seat back and opened the folders onto my lap. Once I began to read, I read and read and could not stop, and I forgot everything else; when I finally got out of the car, I remember that it was as if I hardly recognized the drive I was parked on or knew where I was.

I looked away at the sloping lawn of green stretching way down to the city street below, and it was as if I did not know that I had ever seen it before. I felt very, very odd and everything around me looked new and strange to me. The red bricks, the white tower, of McMicken Hall looked strange and as if I had never encountered them before.

I realized I did not know much about things. I had grown up in a small town in Georgia among uneducated people who knew nothing of the world. My mother and father had never seen a university; it was a concept that meant nothing to us. My mother had taken a business course and gone to work as a secretary in our one office building so I could go to college, and I went to a country college only a few hours away, where still the wider world only barely peeped through; and though of course I read about things, and read, for instance, about life in universities, it was not the same as knowing about them. Then I myself had gone to a university in Georgia, and then to another one in the midwest; at Indiana University I had earned a doctorate degree (what a fine thing to do!), and yet it seemed that it was only then, reading what I was reading in my car on the drive that day, that I began fully to understand what universities are and that there may be no reason to admire or respect a university, that universities do not necessarily intend any good to the human race.

Now I had not been present in those narrow chambers into which the sick people I had read about had been rolled to be irradiated. I had not seen the attendants composing their limbs and adjusting the dials and beams. I had not seen all that—and it is strange to think that during some of those years I had been getting in and out of my car on McMicken Drive, just as I was on this day when I was reading about those lives. Yet what had happened I felt touched me directly. I was a teacher in the same university, this was my university, and around the corner of McMicken Hall I could see the towers of the hospital buildings where these events had taken place.

I recall that when I did get out of my car that afternoon, I walked around the corner of the hall where I worked to look over the cityscape of hills and glassy peaks toward the medical towers across the way. I gazed at them in confusion for a long time, and I remember pacing slowly back and forth on the walk, thinking rather chaotically, no doubt, about the awesome things I had been reading about.

It seemed to me then, and it seems to me now, that we had become a secret slaughterhouse, we had become a death camp. The doctors appended to each of their annual reports profiles for each person exposed, and I could readily see, that first day, that one patient had died six days after radiation, and others on day seven, day nine, day ten, fifteen, twenty, twenty-two, and so on. In the winter and spring of 1969, all but one of the seven patients used in the tests had been given the higher doses of radiation and had died shortly afterwards.

In this 1969 brigade, a woman of eighty—whom we knew then only as "M. B.," case number 090—had, like certain other individuals, been experimented on *twice*: not just with a total body exposure of 150 rads, roughly the equivalent of three or four hundred mammograms, but with an operation to remove bone marrow from her chest for later reinfusion—in a crude attempt to keep her blood from being destroyed by radiation. It was she who had died on the sixth day after exposure, of a stroke related to the anesthesia for her bone marrow operation, the shortest survivor of all. Today we know her family and that she was an African American schoolteacher in Hillsboro, Ohio, named Margaret Bacon, and was not acutely ill when she entered the hospital that spring for tests.

I assume that I went in that day to teach my afternoon class, but of course I don't remember the class, and I expect it passed for me in a rather dreamlike way.

I had been learning about radiation, and as it turned out I could read well enough the doctors' reports and their case histories. I knew what radiation death was, and in fact, if you are not a medical investigator trying desperately to camouflage and cover up a rite of human sacrifice, such deaths are not difficult to explain. I assume that children are taught about radiation injury in science class or in the study of the U.S. nuclear attacks on Japan at the end of World War II.

The report I went on to write, over that December, was to spell out the details of the eleven years of these tests. It spared nothing. It told the simple truth about these citizens' lives and deaths. Yet it also looked at every possible way in which the doctors could attempt to justify what had been done. The record it compiled was accurate, and though it has been hidden and suppressed, mocked and reproved by the researchers and their coconspirators in every way these things can be done, the *facts* that it records have never been replied to by these investigators, and the point is—they cannot be replied to; and that is why so very few of the researchers have ever spoken of these matters to the public at large, and why we had, in time, a lawsuit and a settlement for the surviving families.

The report I have been speaking of, seven typescript pages addressed originally to "the campus community," told people that there had been no consent forms of any kind for the first five years of the project, and that according to the doctors themselves the patients were told simply that they were being treated for their disease. "The patient is told that he is to receive treatment to help his sickness," says the first report to the DOD in 1961; and the report for 1963 puts it this way: "The patient is told that he is to receive treatment for his disease." In the 1963 report the doctors say that having now irradiated eighteen people, they are totting up the scores on people's deaths, calculating, they say, in their matter-of-fact, textlike language, with the chill of the sterile laboratory about it, the "importance of radiation in precipitating demise." In 1966 they matter-of-factly refer to the "severe hematologic depression"—the damage, that is, to blood cells—they have found "in most patients who expired."

The report we issued also registered these crucial facts: that when the project began, no design could be discovered for a study of cancer, and that no patient had been irradiated before the start-up of funds from the DOD for the study of radiation sickness. There was not a single extended publication by the doctors on wide field radiation as cancer treatment during the eleven years of the project, but on radiation injury we found a long series of papers and publications. One could say this, I believe: there were so many smoking guns left behind in these original papers for the DOD that one could hardly make out the papers through the smoke that enveloped them.[5]

THE PRESS CONFERENCE of the Junior Faculty Association in 1972 was held one winter afternoon in the UC student union. Not many people came. After all, no one in Cincinnati could have expected so somber a tale. A year later, one of the doctors, Edward Silberstein, wrote me the only letter—a very brief one—I have received from the team of investigators since the day we released our report. Beforehand Silberstein had been cordial enough and had granted me an interview down in the basement corridors where those specially built radiation rooms were located—he had thought, it seems, that cordiality was all that was required—but in his note to me afterwards, Silberstein attached a letter announcing that the radiation team's colleagues at the University of Texas had awarded them a prize for their work on whole body radiation, and he signed his note to me, penned on December 24, 1973, *Yours for bigger and better press conferences*.

Indeed our report had been almost completely suppressed in Cincinnati, where of course it would have posed the grave danger to the researchers of alerting victims and their families to what had happened to them. My colleague in the political science department, Henry Anna, had arranged for publicity, and a television team had appeared in town from CBS, to cover our press conference, but that afternoon, just as the team was finishing up a film on the experiments for that night's evening news, a fire broke out at a nearby nursing home; the team dropped the radiation story like a shot and rushed to the site of the fire. The news that night was of fire, not of the deliberate exposures by our government. (And so it goes, all too often, with American journalism.)

Still, a stringer from the *Washington Post* did come to hear us that day and to carry away a copy of our paper, and the tale we told was printed almost entire the next morning by the *Post* and then entered into the *Congressional Record* by Senator Edward Kennedy. A number of other papers followed suit, and for a day, at least, some knowledge of the Cincinnati tests winked through the heavy ether of the normal daily news of natural disasters, official government releases, interesting crimes, and so on.

Kennedy was preparing for hearings on medical experimentation around the country, had become interested in the UC case, and was making a strong effort to force the College of Medicine to let his staff interview their subjects. We know now, in fact, that a great deal of the adrenalin pouring off the doctors' desks during those early months of somewhat scattered publicity in 1971 and '72 was directed at blocking this most hazardous of all moves against them—the gaining by anyone of direct access to living victims of the tests or their families.

From the day of the JFA press conference, Kennedy's aide Ellis Mottur was in daily contact with us—there seemed to be the feeling on his part that these doctors had been penned irrevocably in a very tight corral by our report. "Do you *believe* what we have said?" I remember asking him. Did his office regard our findings as an accurate measure of what had taken place? Mottur said that the Kennedy office had determined that we were more than credible. "We have sent the JFA report out to our medical sources and they have told us that it makes a very damaging case against these doctors."

But that is not politics, is it? After our report, the medical school doubled its efforts to block access to the patients and privately hired special counsel in Washington to fortify the legal wall between patients and potential interviewers. Silberstein and Eugene Saenger, the lead investigators, constantly urged noncompliance with all such requests and claimed ever-mounting evidence that the patients themselves did not want to be known.[6]

The school stepped up its efforts with their political friends to get them off what was now a very sharp hook. Why not get the various "liberals" together, they reasoned, including the new progressive president of the university, Warren Bennis, and talk sense to them about this unfortunate affair? Would it make sense to punish the entire medical school and all the local citizens it served because of the poor judgment of a few doctors in accepting money for their work from the U.S. military—their only misdeed? In time Bennis met with Kennedy and with Kennedy's fellow liberal and friend, Ohio governor John Gilligan, and the three of them made a pact: Kennedy would agree to no interviews with patients and no congressional investigation into the basement chambers, in exchange for the halting of the project by UC, or at least the refusal of any further funds from the DOD.[7]

This is how it came to pass that the Cincinnati case was slipped, finally, very softly away into a deep secret drawer of history . . . meant never to be opened again. The rest would be silence.

And indeed no word was spoken of those subterranean chambers at UC in the congressional hearings that followed on human experimentation as it existed at that time in these United States.

New subjects had ceased to be irradiated, and this was, of course, a major victory. Lives would be saved. It was not a full resolution, but those of us who had fought the tests had to be content with that. The Cincinnati papers would not print any of the facts we had outlined about patient deaths, or anything from the individual case histories, so the victims and their families had no way of knowing what had happened to them. At that time, a small number of victims did, in fact, still live, but the UC College of Medicine was not compelled to notify them that they had been used as human guinea pigs.

The team of doctors lost their project and their funds, and that was bitter for them indeed, as we shall see, but beyond that, they paid no price for what had been done, were not investigated by a congressional committee, by the local Academy of Medicine, or by the state medical board.

EARLIER THAT SAME FALL, the anguished interest of Senator Mike Gravel had been evoked by the work on Cincinnati by Roger Rapoport, and when the Junior Faculty report was issued in January, Gravel became the only elected official who would write to us. In a letter I received from him on February 2, 1972, he said, "It is clearer and clearer to me that life is not held sacred in this country; it is cheap." Dr. Saenger's experiments, he went on, "seem to be a symptom of a very much larger barbarism."

Gravel had asked the American College of Radiology to examine the UC project for him, but he had been deeply dissatisfied with the clearly unserious report he had been sent. He said it was "evasive, disorganized, and deficient in almost every piece of relevant information," and that the report by the JFA was "extremely well-organized and to-the-point." But it is easier, after all, to bring forth the simple truth than to invent an elaborate disguise for that truth.

In March of that year, Gravel asked once more for information from the ACR and they ignored him this time completely. "It does not surprise me," he said on March 14 to a publication called *Drug Research Reports*, and then he made a prophetic statement: "*I believe in due time, Dr. Saenger will have to answer all these questions and more.*"[8]

That time was indeed to arrive in the winter of 1994.

IN 1972 A HANDFUL of medical writers and other researchers got in touch with us and studied our report. Our findings held up. We know now that there was a time early on when the founder of the project, Eugene Saenger, had wanted badly to respond to us, but that his friends in medicine had advised him not to do so. Then in 1975 he and Edward

Silberstein authored an article—never to be published—titled "Ethics on Trial: Medical, Congressional and Journalistic," in which they struck out at their critics in the press and in Congress, but as the *Cincinnati Enquirer* would observe in 1994, "saved their sharpest comments" for the JFA.

"On adding up the result of the multiple investigations," they wrote, "the *only* unfavorable comments had come from a handful of local, and non-medical junior faculty members." In a related letter, a friend of the team in La Jolla, California, Dr. William Crosby of the Scripps Clinic, wrote Edward Silberstein that the charges of the JFA were "ridiculous" and that he had been "on the receiving end of one custard pie after another, pitched by a pack of sly, self-seeking, savage clowns." [9]

During all those blanketed years, the UC College of Medicine never acknowledged any wrongdoing, and the cover-up was assisted strenuously by the local press and politicians.

Thus the full names of the victims were never known. We had only their initials . . . and our guilty knowledge of the way in which they had passed from the earth, these Cold War warriors who did not know they *were* warriors, this invisible army, as I came in time to think of them, that fought by night—that is, in ignorance of all that was taking place and the battle being waged over their lives and deaths.

2

1994 and a Secret Drawer Reopened

This is not just evil . . . it is beyond evil. —ELISE FELDSTRUP of the radiation of her mother, Rose Strohm, case study #107.

Years went by and I expected to hear no more of this affair; I went on with my teaching and writing and with other forms of political work, and in time it came to pass that most of the people who knew me did not know I had ever been involved in such a campaign. The records I had acquired rested for years in an old rusty filing cabinet down in my basement.

Still, what I knew to have taken place, in my own university, would always be a sore wound in my memory. It would affect all my thinking about my profession and every other profession, and as these memories mixed and moiled about in my mind with many other apperceptions about the way we live in the United States, they led me to feel that it takes an enormous nerve for a society like ours to try to convince itself that it has arrived at true "democracy." *If we say we are trying to build a democracy*—I would sometimes reflect—*that is another matter; let us hope we are still trying to do such a thing.*

But what is important is that in the winter of 1994, twenty-two years after the events I have described, the grave of all this history suddenly opened again.

In November a tiny woman reporter in Albuquerque with amazing enterprise and nerve had succeeded in finding families of people who had been injected with plutonium for military researches of the 1940s. This reporter, Eileen Welsome, had begun by hunting through old papers at Los Alamos and gone on to write a complex chronicle of the whole mostly secret project, a story published in three installments in the *Albuquerque Tribune*, circulation 35,000.[1] From there a government department seized the initiative—the Department of Energy under Hazel O'Leary—and other Cold War tragedies such as ours at the University of Cincinnati suddenly began to bloom out over the public consciousness like dark and fascinating flowers.

On January 4 my winter quarter was starting up and I was about to go to school for my first class when I received a call from a local television station. A caller asked if I knew who had written a report on radiation for a group called the Junior Faculty Association. I told her that I had this information and that I would be glad to tell someone all about it the next day, after I got my classes started, but when I finished class that afternoon, a cameraman and a young woman reporter were waiting at my office. The reporter was Peg Rusconi from Cincinnati's WKRC, Channel 12, an ABC affiliate, and she had brought with her a yellowed copy of the original JFA typescript report we had once circulated on campus. She said it had been left off at her newsroom that day by some unknown person.

Rusconi had read this report and understood it. She waited while I read it myself—I had not looked at it in a good many years—and then she asked me the crucial questions it raised and let me answer them on her film. That seemed to me amazing, since I had never been able to speak this truth before in my hometown, where, after all, most of the victims of the tests had lived.

The local press of the past had been a watchdog, to be sure, but what it had watched over with tender care had been our business leaders and their friends in all our city institutions, including the university, at that time a city-owned school. Although our review of the doctors had been known to many on campus, and had been covered in one fast flurry of reports in national papers, its primary assertions had never been made public in Cincinnati. No one in the local press of that day had broached the term "radiation death," and indeed there had been a determined effort to keep our basic charges from ever being widely known in the city where they would pose the greatest danger, where living victims and their families, that is, might learn what had happened to them and take action against the offenders.

But on the night of January 4, 1994, I was able to explain on WKRC the issue of consent. "No consent form would have been valid for these experiments," I said, "unless it had said, 'You may die of radiation sickness within forty days if you accept this treatment' . . . and of course no form said that—or there would not have been any subjects." That night Peg Rusconi also set up on the screen in large-print type other basic assertions of the Junior Faculty report: that no consent form at all had been attained for the first five years of the project; that twenty-one of the subjects had died within thirty-eight days of being irradiated; that there had been no publications by the team on cancer during the eleven years of the project and no cancer grants. I felt it was a very good job of work on the part of this young reporter.

WKRC, I learned, had, on the previous evening, broadcast interviews with a doctor from the medical school, Bernard Aron, and with a local congressman, David Mann, and these two had calmly and confidently assured all and sundry that nothing had gone wrong in our medical school back in the sixties and that the ethical standards of the day had been scrupulously adhered to.

In a few days the station called me back. They wanted me to appear the following Sunday morning on a show called Newsmakers. The host of the show, Brad Johansen, would talk with David Mann and me about the radiation project; the woman I spoke to, producer Kelly Leon, clearly felt it would be a dramatic confrontation.

I thought about it, and I was not enthusiastic. I am not a viewer of the network shows; I did not know whether this one would provide a forum where I could defend my charges against the researchers. The producer called me back to say that WKRC wanted me to feel welcome and would make things as convenient for me as possible—they would send a car to collect me on the morning of the taping.

I felt rather tense about all this. The old Junior Faculty friends who had backed me up most strongly in the past were no longer at the university. My husband, who had once studied the political context of the tests, was away on a sabbatical year in Central America. My children had no memory of this part of my past life, and few of my present-day peace-and-justice friends knew anything at all about it.

But on that Friday morning a company car from Channel 12 arrived at my house, and I did go over and tape the show with Mann and Johansen, and, as it turned out, to have joined this contest with David Mann was a step, at least, toward the uncovering of the facts of the case.

Congressman Mann, I think one could say, made quite a spectacle of himself trying to defend the doctors and the College of Medicine, endlessly repeating certain not very compelling phrases. "Since nothing new has come out about these experiments, I don't see what the problem is," he said. "Since there's nothing new. . . ." "But there's nothing *new*," he kept repeating. Mann had another favorite phrase that day: "Well, since I'm not a physician . . . just not a physician . . . when you're not a physician. . . ."

That was directed of course, not very subtly, at me; if I was not a physician but an English professor, how could I presume to say whether physicians had taken people's lives or not—no matter *what* they did? But—I asked myself—where does responsibility for physicians lie, in the minds of public men like Mann? What if the doctors had bludgeoned people to death in parking lots, let us say, studying "urban assault"? Would that be all right too?

On *Newsmakers* Mann tried hard to filibuster me out of the conversation, and a small, now-white-haired woman with an incorrigible southern accent must have seemed at first easy to rout, and yet I believe something he could hardly understand went badly against him that day, and it was obvious that he felt extremely distressed about the show after it was over. I had brought some of the case histories with me, and the consent forms, such as they were, and had succeeded in flashing these papers more or less squarely in Mann's face, as it were—with their fundamental implications of death by radiation.

The host of the show pitched in too by reading from a book that had appeared in 1972 and had also presented in detail the original findings of the JFA. The book was a study of radiation risks called *Silent Slaughter* by medical writers John Griffiths and Richard Ballantine.[2] I was glad to see this volume brought out; I had once corresponded with Griffiths and been sent a draft of what he was composing. The book in those days had the working title of *The Invisible Killer* and had helped me understand the risks posed by x-rays and other medical radiation, risks that very few radiologists would concede—then or now.

After the show, in a glassed-in conference room of the studio, I attempted to show David Mann more copies of patient histories. I said, "David, this can't be covered up this time. Look at what these papers tell us. I'm giving them to the newsrooms here, and I intend to give them if I can to reporters out of town, and the whole story will be known this time. People *died* in these tests." I felt that day as disturbed as I had ever been about these events and about what I felt was yet another instance of grotesque complicity in these deeds, and actually I had no idea whether I could spread, even now, this gospel I was threatening to spread, and indeed it seemed, in the weeks to come, that I could not.

I remember that Peg Rusconi told me afterward that it was entertaining to watch the pantomime of David and me behind the glass. Mann is a large individual, and he would stand up heavily, said Rusconi, as I spoke and the papers were brought forth, and then suddenly sit back down, stand up and then lapse heavily into his chair again.

Weeks later, when the doctors' reports had made their way into the Cincinnati newsrooms, and the story had finally broken in waves and cycles of ever-burgeoning detail in the local print media, Congressman Mann had no choice but to turn around in his tracks and try, not just to recover a little credibility on the issue, but to make it work *for* him in the upcoming Democratic primary, where he was running against a strong African American contender and needing to cut into this man's black and working-class support. Mann would win the primary over his opponent Bill Bowen, but only by four hundred votes. The following November he would lose his seat to a Republican challenger, Steve Chabot.

By the time the local papers were flying ahead with the radiation story, they were also, needless to say, favoring in this Democratic primary business-backed Mann over the more dissident Bill Bowen, who had little money to run on and no corporate support, and they played up Mann's severe distress over the UC tests. No one was more pained than Mann by the travails of the radiation families, it now seemed, and Mann ended up calling for compensation for the families and a congressional hearing right here in town—before the primary, of course.

But in any case, there eventually followed, after these early stories on Channel 12, a tumbling avalanche of press—over five hundred local reports on television and in the papers on UC radiation; and the doctors suddenly found themselves swept hurly-burly down a raging stream of revelations about what had been done.

BUT FOR SOME WEEKS after those first reports on WKRC, the story had died, and it certainly appeared that it would never wake up again. When it did, such a phenomenon was only possible, it would seem, because of those dirty and dog-eared and much-scratched-on papers in my basement. Peg Rusconi was the first of the reporters to want to copy them, and it took me some days to find them down there—in a warped filing drawer in a rusted metal cabinet; it seemed at first they had been thrown away. But eventually, four newsrooms in town would come to get them, and in due time a copy of the same tattered batch would arrive as well at the *New York Times*.

Rusconi, I began to see, was going to follow this story all the way. She had grown up in the east, among Italian and Irish immigrants who had once worked as laborers on the Boston docks, and it seemed to me she had a little bit of the dissenter's zeal for such a tale.

But what she felt she needed, for the next stage of the Channel 12 inquiries, was to find local physicians who would study for themselves the Department of Defense reports and consent to be interviewed. She was a little astonished that none could be found—*not one*. With this I told her I could not help. I knew it was impossible. No doctors we had ever known had been willing to deliver, openly, a blow to their local medical establishment and its medical school. I knew that we were up against professionalism in its most severe guise, and that medical collusion around this case would probably be no different in 1994 than it was in the sixties when the project took place or in the early seventies when it first came to light. Doctors and scientists had not spoken out against what was happening to the Cincinnati victims then, and I did not think they would speak out now.

One medical doctor practicing not in Cincinnati but in Massachusetts was an exception to the above. David Egilman, who had once worked in Cincinnati for the National Institute of Occupational Safety and Health, was willing and anxious to speak. Rusconi arranged for a crew from an ABC affiliate to talk to Egilman in a town near Boston and send back a film that she could use on WKRC.

Egilman had learned about the tests, originally, from the JFA report, while working in Cincinnati, and had found what we had said credible. He had once paid me a visit to examine the documents. With the reopening of the case in the winter of 1994, his interest was evoked again, and he began working up a study of the status of whole body radiation for cancer at the time the doctors began the tests. He testified about our case in a brief early hearing led in the House of Representatives by Representative Phil Sharp. "The medical purpose of this study," said Egilman on January 18, "was suspect and disguised, and as a result the research resulted in the deaths of at least eight, and probably more than twenty-two of the participants."[3]

Egilman went on to explain in a detailed written statement the history of whole body radiation as medical treatment, from its beginnings near the turn of the century. It had once been tried in a variety of maladies, including asthma, migraine, and arthritis, he said, then eventually narrowed to cancer. But even applying it in slow doses on several different days, the conclusion by 1942 was that it was not useful for solid tumors. He quoted scholars Medinger and Craver, writing in 1942: "The reason for this is quickly apparent. Carcinomas are much more radioresistant than lymphomatoid tumors, and by total body irradiation the dose cannot be nearly large enough to alter these tumors appreciably." A dose that is large enough to kill the tumor, Egilman explained, "will also kill the patient."[4]

Other physicians, though, did not emerge to follow Egilman in protest against the UC project, in Cincinnati or elsewhere. The one Cincinnati doctor who would eventually agree to speak at a local hearing, and was expected to speak—Judy Daniels, the medical director of the Cincinnati Health Department—did not appear and answered no calls that day.[5]

But if we did not have doctors, we were soon to have others whose testimony was indispensable.

During the early weeks of the publicity, I came to feel that it would not make sense to let another siege against the project be played out without finding the families of the victims, the people who had been invisible to us all these years. I knew that they could, after all, be found, and I tried to interest the reporters one by one in this search. For reasons I probably do not perfectly understand, their editors felt this was a task that could not be taken on in any organized way—as avid as the reporters were to talk to such people.

But a graduate student friend in my department, Laura Schneider, became interested in this affair and turned out to be a natural detective, with an eagle eye for the kinds of clues we needed. One night at my house we talked about the dramatic unfolding of the case in the papers.

I said, "The trouble is, though—we don't know the people who were experimented on. The reporters are not looking for them and I don't believe they're going to."

We sat brooding about this. "I can't do it," I said. We knew it would be very nearly a comic task for one with my low vision. "Poring over a mass of old records and micro-film . . . all that small print. . . . I can't do that."

Laura sat thinking, and then she said, "Well. Do you want me to find these families for you?"

I couldn't take this seriously at first. "No, no," I said. "You're writing your dissertation."

"But I don't *like* my dissertation," said Laura. She thought about it again. "I'd rather do *this*."

A few days later, Laura Schneider set about to study certain public records: obituaries, court bulletins, funeral archives, street directories, and so on, in the way we had learned they could be studied, and she soon came up with a list of eighteen names of people who seemed to match our patient histories. When we had also succeeded in finding some of their surviving families, I contacted a human rights attorney, Bob Newman, whose work I knew, a lawyer of conscience with a background in legal aid, and within a week he had filed a federal lawsuit on behalf of four surviving families.[6]

I remember, especially, one particular night during this adventure of finding the families. Laura Schneider had come back to my home after a day-long search of newspaper obituaries and of death notices in the Cincinnati Court Index downtown, breathless, a little white, with the first positive identification. "We *have* one—we have 'I. S.'"

"My god," I said. "We do? What is her name?"

Laura could hardly speak. "Her-name-is-*Irene-Shuff*."

"My god . . . ," I said again, ridiculously, as if it was an utterly remarkable name, and yet of course any name we had found would have seemed to us remarkable that night.

"Her sister is still living in the same house and here is her phone number. You could call her tonight."

"I don't know . . . perhaps I will but—I don't know. . . ."

"Well you wanted—"

"Yes I *wanted*—but . . . I may call tomorrow."

It had always seemed to me an awesome thing to do. Would the families really want to have this news I would bring them? Would *I* have wanted to know it if my mother had been used in that way, had been one of those who had lost her life in her own hometown hospital, in a crusade of her government she had not even known about?

I DID IN TIME reach Irene Shuff's sister, Mary Seiter, a woman of eighty, and then through Seiter the deceased woman's son Greg, and Greg came, stern and astonished, to my home one night, and we sat over my living-room coffee table and looked at his mom's two-page history together and spoke rather quietly about her illness and death. I said, "Of course, Greg, your mom was sick, she had cancer, we don't know how long she would have lived if this had not happened to her . . . but as you see, she had this whole body radiation only three weeks before she died, and so—even though her records are not as full as some we have, you may want to ask why they would subject her to this and make her more ill than she was and put her through it all . . . and possibly take her life." [7]

Greg was to become the "Shuff" of *Shuff v. Eugene Saenger* and fourteen other defendants.

The Greg Shuff I met that evening in 1994 was a tall, strong-looking man of about forty, a courteous person who thought things over before he spoke and did not say very much; I remember him in western boots and plaid shirt that night. I felt it was good of him to lend his name to the suit, and then to be so loyal a presence at our hearings and family meetings. He told me that Sunday night that he had recently lost his own wife to cancer and was raising two kids on his own.

Cincinnati is a German town—for every two Smiths there is a Schmidt—and when we were able to match a name with a set of initials on our patient histories, from death notices of various kinds, it was then sometimes possible to find survivors by that name. Laura had found the families of Irene Shuff and a woman named Rose Strohm rather quickly—there aren't many Shuffs and Strohms—and the Larkinses and Websters we also managed to talk to in time.

We had looked especially for the families of short survivors, the most damaged subjects of the tests—often damaged to death, in fact—and of these four families, not only Irene Shuff but also John Edgar Webster, a country musician and a caretaker for many years at a Catholic elementary school on the west side of town, had died within a few weeks of being irradiated. Webster's autopsy told us he had died of infection and "leukopenia," or failing white blood cells.

I left a telephone message one night for a man named "Steve Strohm," who we hoped was Rose Strohm's son, but he never returned the call, and I assumed we had not found the right "R. S." A week later, though, a call came from a woman named Elise Feldstrup, Steve Strohm's sister. She had been reading the papers and felt she already knew what news I would give her about her mother, who had been irradiated in 1970 at the highest dose generally given (two hundred rads), and had died a painful, isolated death in a public hospital for incurables a few months later. Her mind had been badly affected, I learned, and I was not greatly surprised to hear it, since mental derangement as an effect of radiation was a topic the doctors had been studying for the Department of Defense. Would a pilot exposed to radiation be able to land his plane? How long would he continue to function? What would happen to "combat effectiveness," the researchers had asked in one of the early reports to the Pentagon, among soldiers who had been exposed to a nuclear bomb?

Elise Feldstrup and her brother were in high school when their mother had died. They had once lived a normal life in a normal neighborhood and had regular doctors, but when their father had died and their mother then became ill with cancer a year later, the house had been lost, and they had had to resort to public medicine. There was no one but the two youngsters to watch over the mother in her illness. "We did not know what to do and we let this happen to her," said Feldstrup. "But how could anyone do what they did to Mom? How could they do it? It's not just evil—it's *beyond* evil!"[8]

Feldstrup too came to my home one night and was accompanied, as Shuff had been, by a supportive friend; she had brought a picture of her mother Rose, and I saw a slender, dark-haired woman with a lively expression standing in the yard of the modest home the family had owned before their troubles had descended on them.

Rose Strohm was what we came to call a perfect match; there could be no doubt, once we had heard from her children, that she was the person we sought, and so it was with our other families.

These first families were told about attorney Robert Newman, who had quickly agreed that he wanted to work on this case, and they went to see him. A press conference was called, and Greg Shuff and Newman and I, sitting under bright lights at a long table in the offices of Kirchner Robinson Newman and Welch, who mostly did labor law, attempted to answer the questions of the press.

There were newspeople there I had not met before, and to me they said, with natural suspicion, with some sarcasm even, "Has this been a personal crusade of yours all these years?"

No, I explained.

"Why didn't these charges you're making come out back then, when all this first happened?"

I described what had taken place back in the seventies. I knew what had happened in our medical school, yes, and certain independent journalists around the country had known even earlier than I had, but the revelations that came out of the early scattered press reports and then from the press conference of the JFA had been mostly in vain. There had been, and would probably be again, a nearly united front within the medical community of the country to disarm all such critiques, and a new defense of the doctors would probably be led by the craft guild of the radiologists, the American College of Radiology, which back in 1971 had called Eugene Saenger a hero for doing what he had done.[9] The UC doctors, in other words, had simply called in their colleagues in the ACR, and then their political friends, to get them off the hook. And off the hook they had come.

So then the whole case had passed unresolved into the famous wastecan of history, I told them, where I for one had thought it would always remain. But at least, I reminded them that day, the radiations had been stopped.

I don't know if all this history was made clear that day, but in the Cincinnati papers, at least, the suit was more front-page news; Laura

Schneider's names of victims were circulated and eventually printed in the *Enquirer*, and people called in to be matched with the patient histories, copies of which were by this time being kept out on the various newsdesks. More and more families were found and photographed and interviewed; a local panel of experts was set up by an African American councilman, Tyrone Yates, who had been in the WKRC studio the day Mann and I had had our dialogue. In April the congressional hearing developed by David Mann took place in the federal courthouse in Cincinnati. I was able to give a bit of my own account, not only in the local press, but for the BBC, on National Public Radio, and for daily papers in Japan.

But I have not described the *way* this story broke through in our local papers and became one of the most written-up stories of many decades in Cincinnati—and yet almost did not break through, even after the initial reports on Channel 12.

This is a segment of the tale that has queer twists of its own that are worth the telling, and the point is that we missed only by the skin of our teeth having the story buried once more and for good this time— no families, no hearings, no lawsuit, and with medical history none the wiser for these rites of human sacrifice once practiced in our public hospital.

3

The Press in Full Flower

She had no idea as she suffered, that researchers observed her agony, made careful notes, and wrote reports for eventual delivery to the Pentagon's Defense Atomic Support Agency. Ten days after the treatment, Study Number 022 died. — NICK MILLER in the *Cincinnati Post*, January 29, 1994

The radiation story was almost lost once more, and yet it was saved at the last minute in a rather curious way.

Among the many images I have of the mass publicity around the Cincinnati case in 1994 is one of a young woman reporter who felt she had dropped the story when it first came to her desk at the *Cincinnati Enquirer*, standing in a small anteroom of McMicken Hall one day asking for help, and saying in a low, trailing voice, "I know I blew this . . . but it may be the most important story I'll ever have."

This reporter, Linda Dono Reeves, had had the telltale documents on her desk for some weeks, unread, and then one day had had to read the whole startling tale they contained on the front page of "the other paper." In due time, Reeves would recover the initiative rather dramatically, but on that day she had been greatly oppressed by the fact that it was a reporter named Nick Miller who had broken the print story in Cincinnati on January 29, 1994. From his report the case spun off to other services and caught the attention, for instance, of the BBC, which a few weeks later brought to town a production team to develop a documentary.

Miller works for an afternoon paper owned by Scripps Howard, the *Cincinnati Post*. He had come over to my office at UC one afternoon, packed up my documents to copy, and examined with me the patient profiles. It had been three weeks since the television reports on WKRC, and I felt the story had died.

Miller and I stood over my desk in my small office in McMicken Hall that day and looked soberly and with pondering seriousness at certain profiles drawn from the set. "I hope you will study this one," I said, as we looked together at the two sheets that told the life and death of "E. J.," an African American woman in her forties with lung cancer who in 1962 had lived only ten days after receiving a treatment of 150 rads—the equivalent of over a hundred and fifty chest x-rays—over her whole body. The radiation had been given her in one continuous dose in a matter of hours.

"E. J." (case 022) was not one of those for whom we had been provided blood counts, and so we could not say for sure how exactly she had died. There was no autopsy. But could she have lain so close to death that she could have died—coincidentally—simply of the ravages of her disease one week after receiving this shock to her weakened system? A month before her total body radiation she had been given local radiation to ease the secondary trauma to her right pelvis and hip—"with considerable diminution of pain," the doctors had said. But where, we may ask, in the case of "E. J.," was the "increased well-being" the investigators say the patients experienced from the whole body form of radiation?[1]

These are the doctors' words in the paragraph that ends the original history of "E. J." under their care:

> May 11, 1962, the patient received 150 rad midline absorbed tissue dose . . . total body radiation. She experienced anorexia, vomiting and nausea immediately following therapy but they cleared. She became very lethargic and increasingly weak with mental confusion and hallucinations. Her course was progressively downhill and she expired May 21, 1962 (10 days post TBR).[2]

Nick Miller and I stood long reflecting on this sorrowful story that afternoon; I believe we both were feeling that here was a fellow citizen who had needed our tenderest care, and yet — this was what we had given her. We looked together at several other patient profiles, but Miller did not forget "E. J."

During the weeks that had elapsed since the Channel 12 shows, I had already struck out with the Enquirer, our major daily. I had not succeeded in interesting them in what I had to say, and the only reason I had agreed to meet with Miller of the Post that day was that he had told me on the phone that he had a copy of the Junior Faculty Report, had used it to write two small stories I had not seen, and felt he had made a start in getting out the facts of the case.

He had been in touch with David Logan, who directs an alcohol treatment center in Cincinnati, Prospect House, but had once taught English at UC and served as president of the Junior Faculty Association. Logan had delivered our report on radiation at our press conference back in 1972. He had told Miller about my work on the project, but when Miller called, I had told him I didn't think it was worth our while to get together, that I felt the story was too much, too serious somehow, for any local paper to handle. Miller told me what he had already done and was not surprised that I hadn't even known about it. "I work for a dying paper," he said.

I thought about it. I felt I was about to be engulfed by other chores; I did not want to devote time to a lost crusade. Still, Miller seemed to be on the right track. I said, "Nick — you come over and bring me your stories. I will read them and if I see any reason to think you're serious about this, I'll work with you — and I'll give you everything I have."

Miller came over, rather nervously; he wanted very badly, as it turned out, to get out in front with this story, and indeed he had the cunning to see the whole affair for what it was. (Later I learned what Miller had originally thought about this scrutiny of his work I was going to make, and he and I both smiled to think back on this odd misconnection. He had said to himself, "My lord, I'm going to take my work over to an English professor and she's going to assess my style to see if I can write well enough to work on this story with her.")

I saw that day that Miller's early reports were on a good straight track; he had certainly made a decent start on the facts of the case. He assured me he *was* serious, he was going to do this, but still, I wondered if he would, if he could, because, again, the whole truth had never been told in print.

During the weeks after the WKRC reports on Channel 12, the *Enquirer*, our large-circulation morning paper, owned by Gannett, had worked with me on the story off and on but had not decided to run it. I assumed they saw it as a case of one strange little nonconforming individual against a whole school of prestigious researchers and virtually the whole medical community, and they weren't quite sure what to do with me or whether I had any of the facts on my side, or whether, in any case, it was a fight they wanted to wage.

They had pulled up their reports from back in the seventies and tended to believe that old derelict copy of theirs, in which the researchers had had *their* say, along with all the public officials involved, but we had never had ours. Their published reports on the JFA back then had centered on the statements of the dissenter in our group, our vice president, a fellow named Dodd Bogart of the Sociology Department, who had at the last minute taken fright and come out against us, had walked around the edges of our press conference telling reporters we were—to use a literary term—unreliable narrators. The local reporters had wanted *his* story, not ours. Bogart had handed out a statement saying that the three of us leading the press conference were acting as individuals, that what we were saying about the tests wasn't authorized by our organization. In fact it *was* authorized; a vote had been held and carried almost unanimously on the releasing of the report.[3] The next day Bogart would write to President Bennis, saying, "I would like you to be aware of problems I have had with the current leadership of the JFA." He described several actions of ours that he felt he had been excluded from and wrote in closing, "I hope that we can move the JFA to a more representative and responsible group of young faculty members."[4]

In any case, in 1994 the *Enquirer* had pulled up this old copy of theirs about Bogart and so on and weren't too impressed with it. Their reporter Linda Reeves later told me that she was the sixth reporter who had been tossed this bit of news (if it *was* news), and for one reason or another not one of the others had followed up on it and apparently no one at the *Enquirer* much cared.

Reeves does her job though; she is fastidious about assignments, and so she did write up the story of David Mann and Dr. Bernard Aron sitting amicably and comfortably down together over at the medical school one day and saying, in effect, what Mann had said a few days beforehand on Channel 12: *Citizens, rest assured—your medical school would never do you any wrong and loves you very much.*

Most of the "facts" given out to Reeves by Aron on that January day—"60s Radiation Experiments Reviewed"—were the same casual misstatements given out by the school in the past. The number he cited of individuals irradiated was wrong, the doses were wrong, the information originally given to patients was clearly wrong, the effects they suffered were wrong, as Aron cited them—all these were wrong, according to the doctors' own reports to the Defense Department, which the school was still assuming, apparently, no one but the dismissible JFA would ever read.

"The patients were never radioactive," Reeves quotes Aron as saying. "The effect of the study was a short prolongation of their lives." [5]

Aron was presenting himself as simply a "spokesman" for the school, as he had on Channel 12, and Reeves did not know, as far as one could tell from what she wrote, that he himself had been a member of the radiation team. When I later was able to make this known to the reporters, to show them Aron's name as an author of each of the last three DOD reports, the medical center quickly snatched him back in and he was a spokesman no longer. After this, they really had no physician at all for comment and rebuttal. Once the lawsuit was filed, Eugene Saenger's attorney became the chief defender of the researchers and their tests.

But when I saw this *Enquirer* report on Aron and Mann, I had sighed, *Oh well . . . here we go again.* And though it seemed like the most futile gesture one could make, I did pick up the phone that day. I called the *Enquirer,* I asked for this Linda Dono Reeves, and thus began, strangely, what would turn out to be a long collaboration with this reporter that I came to value very much. But Reeves and I didn't start out very well at all. Reeves's "balance" for her report on Mann and Aron, full of officialese, had been this one sentence: "A 1972 statement from UC's Junior Faculty Association criticized the program."

But how "criticized"? Why? What had we said? Nothing, apparently. We had just "criticized." So I said to Reeves on the phone that day, "Well, you know some people *died* in those tests. And that's there, in this JFA report. Don't you even have a copy of it?" Reeves fussed and fluttered through her papers and said well no, she didn't, and she would like to have one.

Reeves came out that day to my house to get the report. She is a friendly, talkative young woman, and she was not in a hurry that afternoon. We had a rather discursive talk in my living room. We discussed the tests, and she began to cogitate, and she said that well, wasn't it possible that though some people did suffer from the radiation, the doctors had been trying to help them? trying to give them a chance against their cancers? I said, "Well—read the report, and then we'll see what you make of it . . . okay?" We talked about other things, about the way of life in this country and what she thought about it and what I thought about it, and she walked around in my living room and noted the dissident posters on the walls, and it seems she thought, "Umm . . . I don't know about this person." Linda Reeves took away my report, but she did not write it up that day or on any of the days that followed. There was nothing in the Enquirer to follow her piece on Congressman Mann's assurance that there was "nothing new" on UC radiation and no reason for anyone to fret.

So it had certainly seemed that Mann was winning this contest after all, was sticking up very admirably, very loyally, for his friends at the medical school, who had been special allies of his in his past tenure as a Cincinnati councilman.

Yet Linda Reeves did come back to my home one day to get the DOD documents to copy; but unlike Peg Rusconi, and later Nick Miller, Reeves felt she had to read all this backup even to report (not endorse, after all) what had been charged by the JFA. (I suppose it is obvious that as newspapers see it, for congressmen, for officials of major institutions, no backup is needed. What they say is what they say; it's news on its own, and that's that. But others have to work very hard for the right to have any view of anything.)

Still, maybe this was a step, I felt—the Enquirer's acquisition, at long last, of the doctors' reports. Reeves had the JFA report as a guide to these documents and now she had the mass of documents themselves, including the patient histories. She had my lists and compilations about the patients—how many units of radiation each one had received, how soon they had died afterward, their racial make-up, and so on.

But time passed . . . *nothing in the paper.* Two weeks went by, and I considered the story dead.

Then Nick Miller of the *Post* came over.

THE DAY MILLER broke the story on the front page of the *Post*, four days after he had come to copy my materials, I found the *Post* in my mailbox that afternoon, placed there by a friend, and I stood for a long time in twilight in my dining room looking at it in wonder, and a deep calm came over me; I remember a great slow letting go of something that had lain tight around some piston of my heart for almost half my lifetime.

For several days I felt very calm, very quiet inside. I went to school, but at night I came home and took the phones off the hook and sat rather sleepily in the cool winter rooms of the house, my family mostly away, and looked desultorily at science documentaries and nature films on public TV, or made casual notes for school the next day.

I felt that a small miracle had happened in my life and that I needed a lot of time to think about it, deeply, and try to see what its meaning was.

THE STORY NICK MILLER composed was abundant and thorough. It was intelligent, it seemed to me, and—most thankfully—almost entirely accurate. It did not withhold any of the crucial facts of the case. I thought it was a tour de force of journalistic study and composition. It would have had to be done in a whipping whirlwind of intense reading and analysis, and yet Miller had also made important inquiries of his own.

He had continued to rely on the framework provided by the JFA report, but he studied the DOD documents themselves, along with the original internal review still being given out by the College of Medicine, and a recent statement of David Egilman's. He made a chain of inquiries of radiology departments in various towns and succeeded in talking with a radiology professor at Stanford, Herbert Abrams, about the issue of total body radiation as cancer treatment. He spoke to the local head of the Physicians for Social Responsibility. He also had in hand, of course, the highly generalized recent statements of the College of Medicine and the biographical materials they supplied for Eugene Saenger, who "declined to be interviewed"—just as he would decline, along with all the other investigators, throughout virtually the entire campaign.

For "balance," then, Miller's article encompassed a long boxed column about Saenger's professional work and distinctions: graduate of Harvard, medical consultant to the Air Force surgeon general and to the Atomic Energy Commission, winner of national prizes in radiology, and so on. It must have seemed discouraging to some to learn that this doctor was the director of the local chapter of the American Cancer Society.

Miller's lead was this: a recounting of the short history of the patient "E. J." we had looked at in my office: "She is known as Study Number 022, a 46-year-old woman fighting lung and spinal cancer," he wrote. "In 1962, doctors at University of Cincinnati General Hospital exposed her entire body to radiation."

There followed five bulleted items of information about the project, and then these paragraphs, as Miller returned to "E. J." (whom we should now dignify with the name we know her by, *Evelyn Jackson*):

> After Study Number 022 was treated with whole body radiation from Cobalt 60, she became nauseous and vomited. According to her clinical evaluation—which identified her only by sex, age, race, study number, chart number and initials—she also became weak, lethargic and began to hallucinate.
>
> She had no idea as she suffered, that researchers observed her agony, made careful notes, and wrote reports for eventual delivery to the Pentagon's Defense Atomic Support Agency.
>
> Ten days after the treatment, Study Number 022 died.

This account of Evelyn Jackson is the only patient profile sketched in Miller's report, and it should be made clear that the article is not one that focuses too heavily, without sufficient scientific back-up, on individual lives and suffering; it is not in this or any other way of a tabloid-like character.

In Miller's piece Abrams and David Egilman both attacked the research team's claim that they had construed total body radiation as treatment for cancer, and Miller cited Egilman's statement before the House Subcommittee on Energy and Power, chaired by Representative Phil Sharp (D-Indiana), to the effect that the purpose of the study was "suspect and disguised," and that "the research resulted in the deaths of at least eight, and probably more than twenty-two of the participants." The researchers, Egilman said, "had intended to mimic the effects of nuclear war on soldiers."[6]

Miller had exploded into print an account that would shake and stir the pages of both daily papers for many months, and he followed this initial report with a number of others, notably one which unearthed some cogent testimony of Eugene Saenger's during a Cincinnati workmen's compensation trial in 1993. The trial concerned the death of an employee at Fernald, a uranium-processing plant on the outskirts of Cincinnati.

During his testimony, Saenger was asked what he had observed during his whole body studies for the Defense Department, and Miller cited a number of Saenger's statements about the project. Speaking of 10 percent of the patients irradiated, Saenger said, "People who observe the results of these studies could say that it seemed possible that maybe the treatment [itself] was the cause of death." He went on to say that "in this ten percent" he thought that "the combination of the therapy and of the cancer was responsible for the terminal event."

Of the DOD project as a whole, Saenger said, "This was the first and only group of patients who have been studied in this fashion, and these studies are still used today within the Department of Defense to study the reaction of people to radiation, and its effect on their cognitive abilities." About what the Pentagon had wanted to learn, he said this: "What they were interested in is when a person was exposed under these circumstances would it affect the judgment which they would have . . . a pilot going through a nuclear cloud, or a commander of a troop or a squad. . . ." Of the subjects of the DOD experiments he said, "These people were sick. They had far advanced cancer and we gave them this treatment to see whether we could improve their condition. It was not intended to be curative therapy. And we simply analyzed what their treatments showed."[7]

Miller then added this paragraph: "Critics of the U.C. program say Saenger and his fellow researchers should have known medical science already had established that whole body radiation was ineffective for the types of 'radio-resistant' cancers that afflicted most patients in the study. One critic, Boston-area physician Dr. David Egilman, told a congressional subcommittee last month that cancer therapy was used to cover the project's main goal, military experimentation."

Nick Miller's work on the Cincinnati tests was accurate, studious, and resourceful, altogether extremely valuable for public understanding of the case. Within a week of the original story, David Mann had accomplished his reversal of position and called for congressional hearings on the project, and the senior vice president of the UC Medical Center, Donald Harrison, was setting up a team of people to respond to the press, as well as a hot line for families who felt they might have had a relative irradiated. The hot line, though, did not seem to most inquirers even warm to the touch, since those staffing it were not given a list of the victims, or even the patient summaries the newsrooms had, with initials and dates of death. Another reflex of Miller's story, reported in the Post on February 5, was that the Hamilton County prosecutor was meeting with the U.S. Attorney's office to — as he termed it to the Post — "explore the possibility of a criminal investigation." [8]

Besides all this, the Post's fellow daily, the Enquirer, was in a state of considerable turbulence, and publishing a penitent editorial apologizing for having downplayed and defended the tests and for attacking individuals like Senator John Glenn who had wanted investigations. [9]

Nick Miller had been on the cops-and-courts beat at the Post that January and was starting work at 5:30 A.M. When he took up the radiation story, he was not relieved of this beat but was still being sent out before dawn to look for people who had witnessed killings on dark city streets. But in his "afternoons," which began in his case at 10 A.M., he was given time for radiation.

"I worked like hell," he said later on. "I was a madman. I went on three or four hours sleep and wasn't even tired — there was so much adrenalin in it." Miller is a tall sturdy fellow from a small town in Indiana named Brazil. He has said that during those days before his story was filed, he would go home to his apartment around two o'clock, taking the documents with him, then set off first for a hard bicycle ride to clear his head. He would then settle in by his front window, which faced the Ohio River from the Kentucky side, and read the reports, looking out over the river from time to time, his mind racing over the whole problem.

At some point, Miller says, a reporter realizes, in certain stories, that he has reached a juncture where his own mind and moral sense is engaged, and he asks himself what he actually *believes* about what he is reporting. "What do I feel and think about this—as a human being?" he says he would ask himself, and he later traced for me the points in the story that helped convince him that the radiations had been wrong.

I was learning that Miller had attended, as I had, Indiana University and then worked for small papers in Indiana before arriving at the *Post* in 1988. He remembers well a story he was proud of which explored the causes of poisoned wells in Shelbyville and the eventual relocation of these wells, which his story helped bring about. He also took on a child-abuse case against a citizen of Winnimac. "They wanted to drum me out of town, but we sold more papers that week than we ever had before," he says. In those days he would take on almost anything. "I was just out of college and I had ideas—it was total idealism." [10]

SOME OF US in Cincinnati, pondering all these events in the months that followed, wondered at times whether or not major publicity around the Cincinnati case was bound to have been set in motion sooner or later, no matter what happened at the *Post* and the *Enquirer*, as Clinton's advisory commission on radiation took up our case that spring. But in fact we came to realize that there was no reason to assume such a thing, and we looked, for instance, at the example of Houston, Texas.

Not long after the onset of our campaign, we became aware, through the Energy Department disclosures, that in this Texas town a massive total body project had been carried out during the years 1951–56 at M. D. Anderson Hospital for Cancer Research in association with the University of Texas Medical School. These tests were sponsored by the U.S. Air Force. Two hundred and sixty-three individuals were irradiated over the five years of the tests, and at least thirty of these patients were given the kinds of large doses that took the lives of certain subjects in Cincinnati. In parallel experiments at Baylor University in the same town, another 112 people were irradiated from 1954 to 1963—with what individual outcomes we do not know even now.

No community or university group monitored this Cold War research, and even when the national Advisory Committee was taking up these cases—after its fashion—in 1994, no Texas paper fell upon the story and developed the publicity that would rake up from the local roots all the hidden and half-hidden facts of the case and the identities of victims and surviving families. No lawsuit has been launched in Houston that would lead to the further disclosures we have had in Cincinnati, and the final report of the Advisory Committee in 1995 added little to what had been known. The reporter who in 1993 found the families of those injected with plutonium, Eileen Welsome, was able to enlarge somewhat on the bare facts of the Houston exposures in her book *The Plutonium Files* in 1999, and to identify the lead investigator at M. D. Anderson as one of the German "paper-clip" scientists, Herbert Gerstner.[11]

But little more than that has become known of these projects, almost nothing of the fate of the victims; in short, very few citizens of the city have any idea to this day that cancer treatments that may not have *been* treatments once took place in their hospitals.

IN CINCINNATI Nick Miller's story at the *Post* on January 29 had a jolting effect not only on the College of Medicine and local officials, but on another city newsroom a few blocks away.

It is not difficult to imagine what happened at the *Enquirer* when the *Post* broke—in such dramatic form—the story the *Enquirer* had tossed aside. The *Enquirer* newsroom burst into a tumult of activity and within a few hours of the *Post* early edition on that Saturday, three *Enquirer* reporters were working on the story full time.

As for myself, the *Enquirer* was anxious, those first days, to reclaim my attention, and I was walking around in my living room listening to them on my answering machine and being more than a little bemused. Given the long cover-up they had helped keep in place, it was gratifying to know that they had had to read the story on the front page of the *Post*—*The Secret History of U. C.'s Radiation Tests*—with the whole tale sitting right there on the desk of Linda Reeves.

Reeves of course was broken, distraught, full of entreaties, abjectly apologetic. She had *wanted* to do the story, I heard her saying on my machine, but had been sent out of town on a murder case. "A college guy killed his girlfriend in Berea!" she began. She had been sent to this town in Kentucky for two days, she said, even though she had told her editors repeatedly that she needed to read—she *had* to read—the documents on her desk. And of course we know that the personal violence among us—sexual violence, whenever it can be found—is, in fact, the news matter our media seem to value most. After a while Reeves would call again. She just wanted to explain, she said.

I did not talk to Reeves again for some days, and so she and I started out, in a way, as antagonists. I felt she had helped bury this tragic story, been willing to see it slide back down into the Ohio River once and for all, no one the wiser.

The following week, though, I came out of class one day to find Linda Reeves outside my office. I wasn't prepared to discuss the case any further, but Reeves followed me inside. It seemed to me, I told her, that she had not cared about the people who had been irradiated. She had believed the doctors, had *automatically* believed the doctors. I didn't feel she cared about common people but only about important people. She told me again about Berea, but after a time I sat down to some work on my desk. Reeves did not take her leave—she sat down too, rather timidly. For a time she sat thinking, and then she said, "I *do* care." Didn't I remember what she had told me when we had first met? I had asked her about her family, how she grew up, how she felt about working for papers that gave no news of the struggles of ordinary people, on their jobs, for instance, as they were systematically reduced, deskilled, sped up, laid off—their wages and benefits cut and cut again, their fragile strikes ignored and ruined—with no one to tell people what they were even about. Until recently, Reeves had been a business reporter, she had told me, and she had liked that, but she had felt there should be labor news too. . . . She had said that one of her grandfathers had died of black lung in the coal mines and the other of silicosis working in a rubber plant in Pennsylvania.

So now she reminded me of all that, and of course it was something one had to listen to. But shouldn't we keep the faith, I asked her, with our grandfathers?

Reeves looked very pale and unhappy that afternoon. Perhaps some editor had told her, "You go over there and you get that woman to say something—and don't come back till you do." Linda Reeves was thirty-two, had grown up in Nashville; on the phone, especially, she had that fussy, fluttery manner certain women in the south do have, and yet one liked, somehow, her rather soft feathery style of expressing herself. She was not cut out for confrontations, that was clear, she needed to get on with people—with her editors, with me, with the public people she seemed to like reporting on. In her work you don't *have* to confront the business world she was writing up—or the officials of government who represent that world. Not confronting them is what newswriting is mostly about these days. Linda had told me, during the one long talk we had had, that there had been a certain individual in her past she had not confronted about a matter of personal importance—and explained what this had led to in her life.

No, she was not a confronter of things, and perhaps that was both a limitation and a strength for her as a reporter. Her friendly, nonconfrontational southern style would eventually stand her in good stead with the radiation families; they trusted her and talked freely to her, considered her a friend, as I would too in time. That afternoon, I came to realize what I should have known all along—that the national press in the United States would still be wary of the severe charges being made and that with eleven years of radiation afflictions to try to place on the public record, we needed all the assistance anyone was willing to provide.

"Can't I at least get out my notebook?" Reeves was asking. I had drawn up a statement for the scattered newspeople inquiring from out of town, and I found a copy of this piece in my book-bag. I felt there would be something there Reeves could use. But she was not much encouraged by this offering; written statements are not much prized in the news writing world, and somehow to me it was all very strange. It felt very odd to be able to command and subdue, even for a day—for I felt sure that I would be forgotten again quite soon—someone from the great mean *Enquirer*, which had, all through my years in Cincinnati I felt, commanded and subdued *me*, turned back almost all the efforts I had ever made, and those of all the other reform-minded people I knew, to communicate with it. The *Enquirer* would seldom print columns or letters of serious dissent or cover any progressive event, not even the Cincinnati opposition to Desert Storm.

Once the U.S. bombing had started in Iraq, a curtain had dropped down on all dissent. I remembered all too well that on a certain evening in the winter of 1992, bus loads of Cincinnati peace activists had departed for the march on Washington and that the *Enquirer* had run a story about this departure. It was not, though, a story about the protest but about the counter-protest, interviews, that is, with the much smaller group of citizens coming out to deride the departing marchers.

Later on, in fact, in this winter of 1994 I'm writing of, when street protests sprang up downtown by groups challenging various policies of the city, I would ask my new friend Linda Reeves why there was no notice of such things in the paper. But didn't I know the policy? she asked. "Well, you won't like this a little bit," she said, "but street actions and demonstrations are not to be covered at all—unless there's violence." Was it really manifest policy at the paper that unless those of us who demonstrated could arrange for some violence, we couldn't expect anyone to know about us? [12]

Reeves said she too found this puzzling and ridiculous. "I just work there," she said.

Still, the Enquirer is the major paper in Cincinnati, printing almost a quarter of a million copies every day, and so you have to work with it whenever it will let you, no matter how galling it is. In 1994 the Gannett Company would do a business of 3.8 billion dollars and turn a profit of 23 percent, as I would read in the Enquirer itself on July 25, 1995. That July the company had signed a merger agreement with Multi-Media of Greenville, South Carolina, for 1.71 billion dollars, and would embark on the television trade with fifteen TV stations (including a major station in Cincinnati, WLWT) and over twenty-five cable and TV franchises. It would add eleven new daily papers (and forty-nine nondailies) to the eighty-two dailies it already owned and up its daily circulation around the country to 6.4 million.

IN NOVEMBER OF 2000, the paper would have its hands full, so to speak, when Cincinnati became host to the TransAtlantic Business Dialogue (TABD). More than a hundred executives arrived in town from around the world, probably expecting to find safe harbor among the staid burghers of Cincinnati. Mass protest, however, evolved. Though the action was certainly passionate and aggressive, it was mostly quite peaceful, but was met by an enormous brigade of police on horse and foot, and armed to the teeth, a force which helped to create the disorder that ensued in some quarters.

The Enquirer covered in detail both the conference and the protests and ran a front-page color photo of a mass march on Friday, November 17, that could later be seen on the placards of rebellious groups. Cincinnati had become a rallying point for dissident young people from around the country. The *Post*, too, along with the electronic media and an African American weekly, the *Cincinnati Herald*, ran large graphic stories. In recent years the two daily papers have had to contend with a new local rival, a thick progressive weekly called *CityBeat*, which has become home-base for Cincinnati dissidents of all kinds and provides vivid and voluminous coverage of action on the streets.

As many people know, the 2000 TABD protests in Cincinnati were mild compared to the volcanic eruptions in the spring of 2001, when a young black man, Timothy Thomas, who had committed no serious offense, was shot to death by a Cincinnati policeman in a downtown alleyway. This death, which followed a number of other such shootings, all of young African American men, led to a long period of mass protest on city streets and in the halls of council—mostly, again, of a nonviolent character though on some days and in some areas there was serious damage to property. Hundreds of arrests were made, many for quite minor offenses, and severe penalties exacted. (As of the summer of 2001, sixty-two individuals still wait in the county jail for resolution of these charges.) The new violence by the police seemed truly to astonish people—the unexplained firing of buckshot, for instance, into small groups of peaceful mourners randomly gathered on sidewalks on the day of Thomas's funeral. A week of historic eight o'clock curfews throughout the city was ordered by Mayor Charles Luken.

As of this writing, the rebellion of African Americans and their supporters seems to be moving toward a long-term campaign of resistance. Local ministers have led the way, including downtown activist Damon Lynch, and Donald Jones, who made a succinct analysis of the economic issues at a large solidarity rally and march on June 2. As in most U.S. cities, the poor in Cincinnati are getting poorer no matter how hard they work, and in this town of old-line wealth and privilege, the income gap is savage indeed.

Business in Cincinnati is clearly fearful of the economic consequences of the "days of rioting and unrest," as this period is often termed. The *Enquirer* reported on June 15, 2001, that Great Britain had issued a warning to those traveling to Cincinnati. "Cincinnati is on the same level as Libya and Afghanistan as far as the government of Great Britain is concerned," wrote the *Enquirer*. Visitors had been advised, it said, "to stay off the streets after the close of the normal working day." The business interests of the city seem to be devising their own agenda for addressing the problems of unrest. They want to neutralize downtown poverty and police conflict by bringing in more developers and removing more low-income residents—to upgrade housing, that is, not for the neighborhoods as they exist, but for new residents who can pay "market" prices.

The recent protests stemmed largely from the same neighborhoods where many of the radiation victims had once lived and worked—and been unable to find respectful health care—and we can hardly doubt but that some of their grandchildren and other relations played out their parts in the lines of rebellion and resistance that formed in 2001. The language of the new protest often echoed the defiance of an African American movement around General Hospital in 1972–73, during the year following the first public knowledge of the radiations, when aggrieved hospital employees attempted to change the make-up of the hospital board. (The People's Health Movement of those years is discussed in chapter 10 of this volume.)

In 1995, another campaign of resistance developed among hospital workers and concerned citizens over the privatization of the hospital and the assault this move represented on people's health care and on workers' wages and unions. Four public hearings were held in a large auditorium on the medical campus, and these meetings, coordinated by downtown activist Lorry Swain, were marked by an unusually combative spirit among the opponents of the plan. When UC President Joseph Steger attempted to take his turn at the speaker's podium, he was silenced by the crowd in the hall and unable to deliver his remarks. (In 1997 four hospital unions filed charges with the State Employee Relations Board and in court, claiming that with the official privatization of University Hospital in late 1996, 2,075 workers had been terminated and collective bargaining weakened.)

BUT ON THAT February afternoon in 1994, I pulled up my chair to that of Linda Reeves of the *Enquirer*. The *Post* had given her a nasty kick—all right—but she could catch up, I said. "Did it occur to you that no one has named the other doctors on this team? It wasn't really one man, you know. . . ." Reeves was not altogether cheerful when she left that day, but she did file a story, pulling together for her piece a few scraps of the talk we had had when we first met, the names of books and music on the shelves of my small office, and highlighting the dusty cabinet in my basement where the DOD documents had lain for so many years.

In time Reeves did make a comeback on the story, and would do a lot of the major work on it, eventually matching up, in her methodical, almost fanatically careful way, surviving families — from among the hundreds that called in — with the patient summaries, then going right out to interview them day after day. She made very few mistakes on any aspect of the tale, and as to the proper identification of the victims and survivors, none at all as I recall.

She would print nothing about these families until five conditions could be met as to the deceased victim: the name had to match the initials on the patient history, and then there had to be matches as well of the individual's age, race, type of cancer, and date of death. Thus she felt she needed in each case not just the family's own information, usually not fully documented, but a death certificate, which generally they did not possess and which she had to go over to the courthouse to find — and could find once she had a name to ask for.

Reeves, I came to see, was, if not a bold reporter, nevertheless a good clear intelligent one in her way, with a talent for accuracy and for the clear representation of technical detail. I had in fact already begun to learn that about her through work she had done on the environment, which at the time the UC story broke had been made her new beat. (In most towns it's not much of a beat, of course, and on the whole the less said of the environment the better, where our mass media are concerned.)

It was, to be sure, Rusconi of WKRC and Miller of the *Post*, and their editors, who took the early risks, sized up the UC story correctly and decided it could be run — because for one thing, the President of the United States was now on the side of disclosure. It had been Rusconi and Miller who went out on their limbs, as it were, but the massive back-up study needed to complete the task was done not just by Miller and his associates at the *Post* but in due time more and more by Reeves and her fellow reporters Tim Bonfield and Steve Bennish at the Enquirer, with its larger resources and staff.

Though I felt Linda Reeves had helped keep the UC story out of sight, still, once she took hold of it, I came to respect her work and we spent time together almost daily for many weeks—on the phone or in my office, or sitting sometimes late at night at my thickly papered dining room table, sorting through the technicalities of this evolving tale. I gave her things and she gave me things—her database, for instance, for the eighty-eight known subjects of the tests, somewhat different from any database I'd had, and after a time, as to certain lines, more up to date. Everything I could tell her or help her with I did, though I usually didn't withhold anything from other reporters either, and they too traded with me at times. Excited phone calls would sometimes come from them after events they didn't fully understand—the enunciation of the lawsuit, for instance, and the often confusing symptomology of the families calling in to see if they had been irradiated ("here's a woman who says her aunt had bad burns on her chest"), the first disclosures by UC.

After the lawsuit press conference, I remember urgent messages on my machine from Reeves as she banged out her story and talked on the phone at the same time and also fumbled with one hand through her papers on the plaintiffs. She was looking for the history of John Edgar Webster, who had been a custodian at a Catholic elementary school on the west side of town and had died thirty-six days after being irradiated, his immune system clearly destroyed. "Where is he? I can't find him . . . I'm looking everywhere . . . my god . . . I see a J. W. but it doesn't look like him . . . no . . . my god . . . it doesn't match." I called back to her machine. "Linda . . . look for 021 . . . don't get Webster mixed up with 025." ("J. W." case 025 we now know was an African American man named John Henry Wells, who lived only thirty-three days after his exposure; no family has appeared for him.)

But Reeves didn't mix things up, as occasionally happened elsewhere, and the dogged accuracy of her work and that of the rest of the Enquirer staff, including the editorial writers, along with the very canny labors of Miller at the Post, was a splendid gift to this campaign.

What almost frightened Linda Reeves about the new bond between us was that I was not a buyer of the *Enquirer* and had not been for years, though I often managed to examine it down at the coffee shop I frequent. I am one of those who buys alternative papers and newsletters but not the papers or magazines of major companies. I was buying our *StreetVibes*, a paper about the homeless, and *Everybody's News*, an alternative weekly operating at that time. (I have had low vision most of my life, and like other impaired people, I listen to daily news on the radio, and to volunteers reading local publications through a telephone service for the blind and impaired.) I had said, at first, about not being interviewed, "If you do write a little puffy piece on me, I won't see it . . . I don't buy your paper and don't plan to help keep it in business." *My god*, Linda Reeves had murmured; and then she had thought of the answer. *I'll bring it to you*, she said, and indeed she did bring it, not just that day, but every day she worked for many weeks to come.

Even in the great ice storms of that punishing winter, Reeves's bootprints appeared on my glassy steps and the paper materialized in my mailbox day after day. I asked her to desist. Please stop this, I said. But somehow it was important to her to come every day, a painful act that she had chosen, it seemed, as a kind of penance for a dereliction of duty early on.

On some mornings Reeves would come inside and read me the day's story on radiation, or with the papers would come a note in her meticulous hand about stories in progress. "Dear Dr. Stephens: Tomorrow we'll look at Dr. Saenger and his career, and our political reporter will look at the wheeling and dealing that went on back then, as well as problems at the *Enquirer*—today you'll see that we are mentioning the [*Enquirer's* own] whitewash! Tim [Bonfield] and I are seeking out the co-researchers. . . ."

I find a lot of these notes from Reeves in a large scrappy file from those early weeks, and I note this one in particular: "We found the family of Maude Jacobs today. . . ." Jacobs was the forty-nine-year-old mother who had died twenty-five days after her exposure. Her name had been turned up by Laura Schneider and then printed in the *Enquirer*, and family members had called in to say, "This is our mom."

When Reeves spoke to Jacobs's oldest child, Lilian Pagano, Pagano said at once, "This is like Hitler. This is like the Holocaust." In due time I would meet Pagano and exchange views about the whole tragedy with a number of Jacobs's children and grandchildren, unpretentious, uncalculating people with a great fund of common sense and easy to talk to. The case of "M. J." was one I had always brooded about, and her case became increasingly important to me.

Within two weeks of Nick Miller's base story there were eighteen reports in the *Enquirer*, many of them authored or coauthored by Reeves; and after another month, when she had to take temporary leave for foot surgery, Reeves had signed thirteen stories on radiation, some of them massive reports, and written up over twenty-five interviews with the emerging families. She would sometimes group these interviews in one large multisectioned piece, and the leads to these reports were often very satisfying to read.

A long article on March 7 included interviews with eight new families, and it began this way:

> One by one, their case numbers take on identities: a cook, a homemaker, a railway worker—all leaving a legacy of bitterness among loved ones seeking to learn more about the way they died.
>
> Relatives of the newest patients identified said their loved ones were ill but did not know they were part of a Pentagon experiment to determine the effects of radiation on soldiers in nuclear battle. . . .
>
> Researchers have said they informed them generally of the experiments and obtained consent.[13]

An article of February 20 introduced the families of nine victims:

> A janitor, a housewife, a bartender. A beautician, a bricklayer, a cook. A porter, a maid, a dry cleaning spotter.
>
> They are ordinary people who took the most extraordinary risks, men and women who made sacrifices for Cold War radiation experiments. . . .[14]

Through these interviews, Reeves was helping to build up rich new layers of information about the exposures. (For the details of what we were learning about individual lives and deaths, see chapters 8 and 9 of this narrative.) I enjoyed the emphasis on the working lives of victims and families, for as I wrote that month in a statement of my own printed in the same paper, the subjects of the tests whose families we were meeting were turning out to have been not "indigents," as they were often termed, but people with regular jobs, citizens keeping the city running and helping to pay the taxes that ran the hospital. They were paying the salaries of those of us in the JFA, I wrote, and the salaries of the doctors who irradiated them. They helped fund not only the hospital but the war machine of those days that sponsored the tests (just as they were funding the U.S. bombing machine of the nineties). They had been helping to cover the paycheck of John Gilligan, the governor of Ohio, who had convinced Senator Kennedy to remove UC from the Senate hearings on human experimentation. Representative David Mann, I wrote, had attempted to play the same role in 1994 and seemed to regard the UC doctors "as important constituents of his, but not the working people of his town who use this hospital and were abused."

I pointed out that many of us in the JFA had grown up among common working people—my own father had worked for the railroads, my mother in a low-paid clerical job—and that we tended to identify with such workers rather than with "leaders and experts who want to control everything." People like ourselves were still hoping that "the U.S. could grow into a true democracy and that common people would take the lead and learn to control their own society."

This statement of mine was printed entire in the *Enquirer* on February 16. In view of all the difficulties of the past, the printing of this piece seemed to me as amazing as the other developments of these early weeks. This was the "written statement" I had given to Linda Reeves when she and I first talked—and quarreled—in my office. I certainly never expected to see the entire seven-page narrative in print, with no editorial changes or cuts, and with a title taken from the piece itself: "A Tragic and Terrible Tale."

A boxed quote in this article concluded with the sentence I had least expected to see recorded. "Many of these deaths seemed to me to be executions, and they still do today."

In those days I liked to teach my classes in the afternoons and sometimes stayed at school until eight or nine o'clock in the evening. In the mornings I took it easy, and most mornings I walked down through the wooded streets of our neighborhood to a coffee shop on the main street at the bottom of our hill.

During that winter it would often be there in the coffee shop that I would first see the morning's Enquirer, and at other times I would meet, on my walk, Linda Reeves driving up our hill to take the paper to my mailbox. We met up this way on the morning my narrative on the radiation project was printed, and I remember how cheerful Reeves was that day, how pleased to be handing me so much of my own prose.

I had protested about the printing of it, but had then spoken to one of the paper's editors, Ray Cooklis, and been reassured that what I had written would not be altered or even reduced. Still, that morning I stood at Linda's car window and looked this piece over rather cautiously. Didn't I like it? she asked. Didn't I think it was a wonderful idea? It did look as if the whole piece was there and just as I had written it—occupying most of a whole page of newsprint—exactly what I had wanted to say years ago.

But I wondered how such a state of affairs could possibly continue. Surely this tide too would turn—one day when we least expected it to.

ONCE THE ENQUIRER had been backed into the story by Nick Miller of the Post, their regular medical reporter, Tim Bonfield, had taken over the science and Reeves the human side of things. Steve Bennish and others helped with various topics, the political angles for instance, and the documents eventually disclosed by UC, as did a Gannett correspondent in Washington, Paul Barton.

Miller's story had appeared on a Saturday; by the following Tuesday sets of small stories began to follow each day in the Enquirer, and on Friday we read a big spread titled in 48-point letters, "Radiation Records Revealed." Like many papers, the Enquirer has no shame about such matters, and it brazened out the pretense that with this dramatic report it was breaking the radiation story. "In the heat of the Cold War thirty years ago," the report began, "eighty-nine people with terminal cancer—mostly African-American, mostly poor—suffered the nausea and pain of radiation-induced injury in Cincinnati. Some died painful, premature deaths. As families hunt today for answers, and Congress debates whether to compensate the unwitting guinea pigs of the Cold War experiments, documents from the University of Cincinnati to the Department of Defense obtained by the Enquirer begin to reveal what happened in the basement of General Hospital from 1960 to 1971."

A boxed insert titled "Survival time: 173.9 days" attempted to assess the life spans of patients after radiation, but the data arrived at was incorrect; Steve Bennish had failed to note that for many subjects the date of death was unrecorded or unknown and that one subject, for instance, was known to have lived at least five years—no one knew how much longer. We would later find, as I have already explained, the niece of a patient who had lived, unbeknown to the researchers, over *twelve* years.

The long series of stories the *Enquirer* would then print on the case ranged from the present into the past and back again; they detailed, for instance, the Kennedy investigations of the early seventies and the deal finally struck with Governor Gilligan and the university, which eliminated Cincinnati from the senate hearings on experimentation and left these meetings to focus on the Tuskegee syphilis case and the use of children, prisoners, and the mentally ill.

I remembered very well that the tragedy of Tuskegee had surfaced during the summer following the partial revelations about Cincinnati. In the Tuskegee Study it was not the Defense Department but the U.S. Public Health Service that had conducted the research. In July 1972 over four decades of secret studies on four hundred black men with advanced syphilis had finally been forced into public consciousness by a young specialist in venereal disease, Peter Buxtun, working with a reporter from the Associated Press, Jean Heller. The Tuskegee research focused on "untreated syphilis," and treatment was consistently withheld from the men brought in for study, even when penicillin became available in the 1940s.[15] Back in the seventies some of us at UC had noted the many intriguing similarities in these two major medical disasters, Tuskegee and Cincinnati, and especially in the ways they were justified by the researchers.

Over the early months of the radiation campaign, the *Enquirer* printed a number of full-page and even double-page stories on our case. Tim Bonfield collected, for more "balance," and in the face of the definitive silence of the investigators, a lot of random information and comment on the career of Eugene Saenger, with kindly quotes about him, for instance, from old schoolmates. When such pieces appeared, I would hear a number of harsh remarks about them. *It's the way all serial killers seem to be described*, one caller said to me.

I did not of course reply to such remarks, and indeed I often heard, from acquaintances of the doctors in town and on campus, viewpoints entirely different from these, from individuals, that is, who felt there would eventually be good and reasonable explanations for all that had taken place.

4

African Americans Lost and Found

They wouldn't have done it to their pets. — The great-niece of
Louise Richmond, case study 082, at a "big tent meetin'" at UC,
February 21, 1994

The unexpected exposure of the experiments in the press, spun off by
the series of curious happenstances we have been examining and then
by Nick Miller of the *Post*, can be rounded out in the pages that follow.

In February of 1994 certain compelling themes still remained to be
explored by local newsrooms, and it was also during this month that
the BBC would start in Cincinnati its documentary on U.S. radiation and
that National Public Radio would become involved in our story.

Most people in Cincinnati seemed to be learning through one me-
dium or another about the events in our hospital and following the
emergence of the surviving families. Hundreds of calls were coming in
from people who thought their relatives had been irradiated.

One day a young African American reporter I had not met before,
from Cincinnati's Channel 9, a CBS affiliate, came out with a cameraman to talk to me about the experiments. I told the story once again,
rather murmurously that afternoon, sitting at my dining room table
looking out my big windows onto the subdued winter lawn, and I remember that when I finished speaking and looked back up at the reporter, she had quite a blanched and stricken look on her face. I felt this

young woman, Dilva Henry, might prove to be a good person to have on this beat, and indeed it was she who turned up, a few weeks later, an artifact of considerable interest to the case.

Henry would work, she would actually *dig*, and she had gone over to the medical school library one day just to see what she could turn up. On the back shelves she found a 1986 promotional film about Eugene Saenger's radioisotope laboratory; it did not look all that promising, but Henry took it back with her to the station and put it on a spool. She saw Saenger and two other eminent UC radiologists sitting around a table talking informally and rather inconsequentially, on the whole, about the lab, but after a time their conversation turned to the long-suspended radiation project, and she heard Eugene Saenger saying that while those opposed to the project had claimed, in the seventies, that the subjects would not have wanted to participate had they known the military was involved, he wished to make it clear that these critics were quite wrong, and that many patients had told him that if there was any way they could be helpful to "our soldiers abroad," they hoped he would let them do so.[1] This segment of the film was hastened onto the WCPO evening news, Cincinnati's Channel 9 — and it was a deed well done for Dilva Henry.

Channel 9 seemed to give their reporters more space for reportorial activism than most newsrooms, but also to be somewhat less watchful about the accuracy of what was aired. Lawyers at Peg Rusconi's Channel 12 were consulted with some frequency about the radiation stories there, but this did not seem to be happening at Channel 9. As for myself, this station once referred to me on film as a "local physician," and another lapse occurred in the second year of the campaign when a new reporter replacing Henry on this beat — she had by this time moved to a new job in St. Louis — had shown a dramatic report on an elderly woman said to be a living victim of the tests. This individual said she had had radiation from the team on her leg and after that could hardly walk. But clearly she was not part of the radiation project for the DOD.

A member of the family organization alerted me to this film, and I contacted the Channel 9 reporter to ask that they set the story straight the next day — and check Henry's patient summaries for any callers who thought they had been irradiated. We agreed we'd had a good clear story and wouldn't want to see it down the drain, and that after all there was now a lawsuit in progress. No correction of the story was announced, as far as I know, but at least we had no more new "victims" of this kind.

When Dilva Henry had first become involved, she had also gone to work and found on her own a surviving family—the first African American family to be located.[2]

By mid-February we had located a quarter of the families of those irradiated, but one fact about these families was discouraging and strange: none of them were African Americans. Laura Schneider had found a number of names of minority victims but we had no families for them, and no minority families had called in to the papers. Yet two-thirds of the victims had been African Americans.

One Friday morning in February I received a call from Henry about coming out to my house to make another film. I could not meet her that day, but I told her about the African American problem I felt we had and asked her to come by and take from my mailbox a sheet I had made up on a group of African American victims whose families we were looking for. I had collected the data that Laura Schneider and I had fetched up on these individuals from old funeral home records, and I had drawn up a one-page flier on what we knew. One of the profiles read this way:

Thompson Funeral Home buried *Louise Richmond*. Lists her as African-American. Age 49. Died 3–11–68. Charges paid by Viola Mackland. Originally lived in Cleveland, Ohio, but had moved in with Mackland. Father was Frank Spear, mother's maiden name Roxie Rainey. Born Ocilla, Georgia. Buried in Hillcrest Cemetery, lot 60, grave 1, section 5. Services at funeral home with Reverend Robert Hairston Jr. (unknown). Died at Cincinnati General Hospital.

I had attached a note below this paragraph: *No doubt Louise Richmond is our "L. R."*

On the phone I had suggested that Henry, if she could find none of these families, go out to one of the cemeteries named and simply take a picture of one of their gravestones and show it on the evening news. Henry did come by that day to get the information sheet, and two days later, on a Sunday, she called to ask me to watch her evening news. "You'll be so happy!" she said. And on the news that evening I saw Henry sitting in the living room of an attractive dark-skinned woman of middle years, Katie Crews, niece of Louise Richmond.

Crews was one of the relatives who had been present with Richmond in a large cancer ward of General Hospital during her final days. Her Aunt Louise was, as our information had suggested, only forty-nine when she was irradiated in 1968. She had colon cancer, was given three hundred rads of lower-body radiation and lived only thirty-four days afterward. Richmond was not living in Cincinnati when she became ill, but her sister, Crews's mother, had felt she should come to town and be treated at General Hospital. "We had confidence in the hospital," Crews says; "we went there for everything." Crews and her nine sisters were all born there.

Crews's mother knew many of the doctors because she did their laundry. A number of them lived in apartments at Cleveland and Reading Road, a major street a mile or so from the hospital, and the Crews family lived in a neighborhood nearby. Crews remembers carrying large baskets of shirts and pants and other items of clothing down to the doctors, two kids hefting a big basket between them, and bringing back what was dirty. She says she feels that many of the hospital doctors were good people but that the radiation team made the serious mistake of not telling people what they wanted to do to them.

Shortly after the identification of Katie Crews on Channel 9, this station also played a part in a large public meeting held on campus. A student group at UC, the local chapter of the International Socialist Organization, was strongly supporting the radiation inquiries and lawsuit, and they called an informational meeting on the case for the evening of February 21. They put out a flier titled Killer Radiation at U. C.—the Real Story and asked Dave Logan and myself to speak, along with a longtime ISO member, Bill Roberts. Logan was the English Department instructor who had been president of the Junior Faculty Association when we had issued our report back in 1972; he had read the report at our press conference. In 1994 Logan had been helping out in a number of ways and had succeeded in interesting one of our local congressmen in the case, Representative Rob Portman. The ISO flier cited the fact that—at this somewhat early time in the events—the hospital was claiming to have lost or discarded the original records of the victims. We decided that one purpose of the meeting would be to provide all comers a chance to see if their family members could be located on the DOD patient summaries.

That night I brought copies of eighty-eight summaries and simply spread them out on a table up in front of the hall. The ISO had contacted the local media, and Channel 9 had aired several prominent announcements about the meeting, and this meant a large turnout. The room that had originally been reserved in the student union had to be canceled, and signs directed people to a much larger room, a vast raked lecture hall in one of the science buildings nearby. We had hundreds of people, including many who seemed to be ill or half-lame or very poor, struggling up great dark stairways into the lighted lecture hall. No doubt some families came because they were in bad straits and *hoped* to be part of a lawsuit. Attorneys came, looking for clients.

My friend Dave Logan gave a dignified, composed talk about the reasons why the JFA had first looked into the experiments years ago, and at the end of the meeting Roberts attempted to examine what had happened from a historical perspective. But the crowd was clearly restive about all this, and I saw that my own remarks had better be quite sharp and to the point, and that the sooner people could file up to look at the patient records, the better. But I remember saying that I thought that what had been done to people in the experiments was only possible because of the class conflict we have in this country. "I'm not sure these researchers would have done what they did to people of their own class," I said, wondering how the others might feel about this; and in reply a woman's sardonic voice spoke out as clear as ice from a seat down in front of the hall: *"They wouldn't have done it to their pets."*

For a moment the whole hall was silent, stunned, as the weight of what had been said seemed to break slowly over the throng.

People were asked to help us find the minority families named on the sheet of victims, and I read off the six names. When I mentioned "Louise Richmond," forgetting, I think, for the moment that Richmond's family had already been found, two women down in front said, "That's us—that's our aunt," and there was quite a commotion. The younger woman, Carmelita Russell, was the one who had spoken up. They were the family we had just seen on TV. Katie Crews and her daughter Carmelita then spoke to the hall about their Aunt Louise and the way she died. She had had a lot of pain in the days following her radiation.

"When we came into the ward in the evenings," said Katie Crews, "she would be crying aloud. She would be gripping the metal rails of the bed-post with all her might. We didn't know what to do and there was no one to help . . . no one did *anything*."

At the end of the meeting people massed up front and rummaged through the loose sheets of patient records until they were an unsightly mess all over the front of the room — but no one found a matching history for a relative with cancer that night.

Two weeks later the same student organization staged a picket line at the entrance to the hospital. They gave out an aggressive flier. "We demand," it said, "that the university Open the Books — Tell the Truth! Make a Public Apology — NOW! Compensate Family Members. Reveal all current contracts with the Department of Defense. Stop Unethical Testing." One of the family members joined the picket line that afternoon. This was Katie Crews, and the UC student paper, *The News-Record*, showed a picture of her on its front page holding in a stately and somber way a large picket sign.

Some weeks later, when I spoke to Crews on the telephone, she said that she had developed high blood pressure for the first time, high enough to need medication. I told her that I had never known whether the families should be told about these tests or not. I had wondered if it *would* make them ill, or if they would just feel *Why do we want to know this — now that it's too late?* I said I had never known how I would have felt to be told such a thing. But Katie Crews was quick with an answer to that. "Why, Martha, you know this," she said, "the hospital would not have told us a thing. Not one thing! They would *never* have divulged those records. We would never have known about it," she said, as if this would have been a great pity.[3]

I was never sure all the families felt that way, but on the whole, it seemed that they did.

THE NEWSPEOPLE out on the beat who covered the radiation story not only did some strong new work on it, but at times they grew quite thoughtful about what had taken place.

I remember speaking to the *Enquirer's* Steve Bennish on the phone one day as he was going over the DOD reports and reflecting on the whole project. What he said reminded me of a sorrowful line by one of the critics of the Tuskegee project, who said that nothing learned from the long years of this study, during which hundreds of men became more and more ill with untreated syphilis, "would prevent, find or cure a single case of the disease."[4]

Bennish, thinking over the Cincinnati tests, was reflecting on the search the researchers had made for a urine or blood test that would measure the dose of radiation an individual had been exposed to.

"You know," he said, "the worst thing is—as bad as these experiments were, they didn't even find out anything. This *dosimeter* they were looking for, for instance—they never found one." He seemed very rueful about this.

"They never even found it," he said.

AT ABOUT THE SAME TIME as the early *Enquirer* stories, the film crew arrived from the BBC.

Even before Nick Miller's first report in the *Post*, I had begun to receive calls from a journalist in London named Julian O'Halloran, working for the BBC show *Panorama*. He had acquired a copy of the Junior Faculty Report. O'Halloran and I debated, I recall, whether he needed to read the DOD documents for himself and if I should mail him a carton of them, but since he was not getting any convincing replies to his inquiries from the College of Medicine, that step did not seem altogether necessary. He seemed to have learned nothing that had led him to question the findings of the JFA. Of course he wanted and needed to cover both sides of the issue, and that would eventually have a curious sequel.

When Miller's story broke, O'Halloran made rapid plans to fly to Cincinnati, and he and his producer and two technical staff people came in on a Sunday afternoon in early February. The team had decided on a radiation tour that would take them to four other sites as well. From Cincinnati they would go to Oak Ridge, where a certain number of whole body radiations had also taken place, though not on people with solid tumors as at UC, and from there to Vanderbilt University in Nashville, where as many as eight hundred pregnant women had been given "radioactive cocktails." A suit was being launched there and the possible injuries to the children of these mothers investigated. O'Halloran and his associates would then travel to the fallout fields of the Nevada test sites and to the cancer-ridden areas around the Hanford nuclear plant in the state of Washington.

In Cincinnati the group spent some difficult hours at the Greater

Cincinnati Airport, complaining of our customs department and the handling there of their rather sensitive equipment. They checked into a downtown hotel, and later in the evening I met them at a Chinese restaurant near my home in an older suburb of the city. I would meet, in due time, a number of my "radiation friends" at this eatery, the Blue Gibbon, just around the corner from my house. "Shall we meet at your Green Monkey—or your Blue something-or-other . . . you know?" John Slater would ask, I recall, on his trips to town for British radio. There came to be a little bit of humor about this place of assignation—and after all, there was little enough about this story one could smile about.

The Sunday I met Julian O'Halloran had been an unreal kind of day, because earlier that same evening I had met Greg Shuff, the first living relative of a radiation victim in whose presence I had ever found myself and whose hand I could actually take. I had been speaking on the phone for almost two weeks to the four families Laura Schneider and I had located, but I had not met any of them yet, and indeed the first family whose faces I could examine had appeared a few days before on the front page of the Enquirer.

THE HAGERS had called in when they read the early radiation stories and were matched by Linda Reeves with one of our patient histories. I found the paper in my mailbox one morning, left there by Reeves, and of course it was the last thing I expected to see that day—a huge portraitlike close-up in living color of two individuals looking forward into the camera with almost strange composure: a petite pretty woman with fluffy curly hair and her rather muscular husband in a working man's T-shirt.[5] This had been a good break for the Enquirer during the week following Miller's base story—this couple, that is, calling in to say, "We've read the papers and we think Dad was one of those irradiated." This was Catherine Hager and her husband Bob. Catherine's dad was a man named Joseph Mitchell, who had been irradiated over his whole body for lung cancer in 1965 and lived afterward for seventy-four days. The Hagers proved to have plenty to tell, had been Mitchell's primary caregivers back in 1965, and were quite ready to discuss every aspect of his illness, treatment, and death. They would later testify at all the major hearings.

The emergence of the Hagers was the good news I was able to share with Julian O'Halloran that Sunday night. I felt sure this couple would talk to him on camera, whereas none of the four families with whom I was privately developing the lawsuit were yet prepared to become public. (Greg Shuff would shortly consent to be the named plaintiff of the suit as it was first filed, and to appear at the press conference on the morning it was announced.)

The news of the Hagers made up a little bit for my bad news — that the team physician O'Halloran had expected to interview about the project was no longer a spokesman for the College of Medicine. Bernard Aron, at that time still practicing radiology at UC, had been withdrawn, as we have seen, from his public role when it had become known that he himself had been one of the project physicians.

At the Blue Gibbon that Sunday night O'Halloran and his producer Barbara Want had been very nearly flattened out by the long day's journey, and then greatly subdued by the news that Bernard Aron might not meet with them. But we felt that perhaps Aron would keep this one appointment, since it had been made before he had been silenced by the school — and in fact he did consent to be filmed.

On a late Sunday night there were very few others in the restaurant, and under slightly bobbing Chinese paper globes, we had a quiet talk. I had felt all along that O'Halloran was a very quick study, and yet there was a lot more reading and studying to do, it seemed to me, before the team could possibly start filming. I did not see how they could do it in a matter of days. They were happy indeed to hear about the Hagers and would call them up right away, they said. They started a tape going, and we talked about the case from its beginnings up to the present.

By the time we went out to sit in the front foyer of the Blue Gibbon, to wait for the taxi that would take the two of them back downtown, the lights had been turned down and the staff was closing out the cash register. I was finding it interesting to learn how BBC teams went about making those rather famous documentaries and what the reporters' lives on the road were actually like.

O'Halloran is a tall, long-legged fellow, witty and friendly and ironic; he is an Oxford man. He sat quietly for a time, and then he said he was thinking of his baby girl, left behind only that morning, and the funny little playful ways she displayed, especially at mealtimes. He said he was already lonesome for her.

Want and O'Halloran knew my friends in London, Caroline and Tony Benn. The only reason I know the Benns, I told them, is that Caroline grew up in Cincinnati and I had met her through a small magazine my husband and I had edited for a time, the *Cincinnati Review of Politics and the Arts.*

Tony is a Member of Parliament. O'Halloran said he did know Tony Benn — of course! — that everyone knew Tony Benn, and told me what a great sport Tony was, what a good show he was on television, and how everyone wanted to have him on their programs. Benn is a well-known socialist throughout Europe, respected as a brilliant spokesman for the long-time European dream of a democratic society designed for common people, where everyone can lead a decent life, have their basic needs met, and develop their abilities. In Britain this dream, this grand idea, had grown not just out of Marx, but out of the indigenous radical traditions of workers, women, artists, and intellectuals, and had been nurtured by such heroes as the Welsh miner Keir Hardie. My friend Caroline Benn, I told O'Halloran, had just written a fine biography of Hardie that I thought would live on for a very long time.

Waiting for the taxi, the three of us talked a little bit about our views of things in general, and I said that if they cared to know how a person like myself sees the world, I saw it pretty much as the Benns did. "I'd like things to be quite different from what they are," I said. Julian O'Halloran chuckled comfortably at that. "My mom couldn't agree with you more," he said. He said his mother thought Tony Benn had written the book on society, that he was right on everything and always would be.

The next morning the team appeared at my door, a foursome now including the two technical men. They were all rested and ready to go and it was an entirely different scene from what I might have expected the night before. They brought a bursting agenda of things to do and see and find and seemed to set about them all at once. Barbara Want got on the phone in the kitchen and stayed there most of the morning dialing and checking and talking and making notes, and then dialing again at full speed for hours. She was mapping out, it seemed, with a number of individuals, the team plans for not only Cincinnati but the other sites on the tour as well.

The two friendly technical men seemed to be all over the house at once, searching for good filming locations upstairs and down, looking over and under things, trying everything out for good sound and sight, giving the whole house a close clinical examination. While all this was going on, O'Halloran and I camped in the living room amidst a mass of papers and files, all of which he seemed to read simultaneously. He called for things and I went to find them and then he called for something else. He scanned and skimmed and talked to himself while the whole melee progressed, or seemed *not* to progress, and someone said, "Would there be such a thing as a cup of coffee in the house, do you think?" I put on my apron, made coffee, and took some rolls out of the freezer to zap in the microwave—with papers still under my arm half the time, no doubt sometimes zapped in their turn along with the comestibles.

One of the first things O'Halloran had asked to see were the research reports to the DOD signed by Bernard Aron. "Do you think you could turn those up?" he asked, but of course they were easy enough to produce. Aron had signed, along with eight other researchers, the last three reports to the Department of Defense; and later on, when the original hospital records were released to the families at last, we saw Aron's name turning up with some frequency.

O'Halloran exclaimed aloud when he saw Aron's name on the reports. He thought it was amazing, he said, that the school would try to put him over as a neutral spokesman, defending the research of other doctors. He remarked that his own country had its cover-ups too, to be sure. "But even the London Police," he said, "are a bit cleverer than this." O'Halloran had already contacted the school and knew that they were still expecting him and Aron to meet the next day.

The staff meanwhile had fixed upon my dining room as the prime location for filming. O'Halloran and I would sit at the end of my dining room table over a scattered set of patient summaries, including the history of Catherine Hager's father. (Want had already reached the Hagers and made an appointment with them for later in the day.) But the technical men still had the soundtrack to worry about, and they detected, in my dining room, a very grave thing—a slight whirring sound. We traced it, finally, to the fan on my furnace in the basement, and this fan was duly disengaged. But then a secondary whir, which had gone undetected under the buzz of the fan, became discernible to the trained ears of the men. This offensive little noise was tracked to the refrigerator in the kitchen. (One of these men, a most courteous fellow, said, "I need to unplug this cord, but I'm afraid of leaving you with an unconnected appliance." He found his jacket and tied the arm of it around the cord as a reminder. "We won't be leaving without that, will we?" he said. We had about a foot of snow that day.)

So after all this hurry and hustle in the house, the coffee and papers and phonings, the soundings and measurements over the whole place, I was instructed to take off my apron and sit down with a now neatly jacketed and groomed O'Halloran, for my expert professorial commentary on radiation in Cincinnati—with very little breath to tell it with. We must take it from the beginning, O'Halloran said, and so I told the whole tale again—the documents discovered, the radiations stopped, the long lapse of years, then the blowing up of a new storm around the tests, the local press finally getting its hold on things, victims and families found, the invisible army reforming in its ghostly ranks once more.

O'HALLORAN PRODUCED a good film, and it was shown throughout the British Isles a few months later, in March 1994. The Benns in London saw it and were amazed at the whole Cold War story (and not least in seeing on their screen a familiar Cincinnati face). The film was titled "The Sacrifice Zone," a twenty-five minute documentary on the *Panorama* show. O'Halloran himself was the onscreen narrator, looking very composed, sounding low-key and a little bit gruff, in the familiar British way. I had known nothing of television production, and this order out of the prodigious chaos I had seen in Cincinnati seemed altogether remarkable to me.

It was not until I saw the film itself that I realized how it had gone with O'Halloran and Bernard Aron over at the College of Medicine. Aron is a gray-haired, round-faced man, who in 1994 would have been in his sixties, soft-spoken, a little bit unsteady on his feet. On the BBC film, he walks O'Halloran gingerly down a hushed corridor of the medical library past the portraits of the distinguished physicians of the past. "There have been very great men here," he says solemnly, reverentially, almost in a whisper. We watch the two men then sit down and begin to talk about the experiments. Aron repeats his earlier remarks to the local press about the desperate state of the patients when irradiated. It seems clear that he has not expected O'Halloran to know that he himself had been an investigator. When O'Halloran suddenly asks him point-blank if he had been, Aron replies quickly and rather fretfully:

ARON: I was not involved in the reports to the Pentagon. I was in the Department of Radiation Oncology from 1969 and it was the usual thing for all reports to be filed under everybody's name.
O'HALLORAN: Are you saying you had nothing to do with the experiments?
ARON: My involvement as a department member was perhaps in the tail-end of the last few months of the experiments. [A pause.] Basically, in the last few months of the experiments. I was not involved in the vast majority of the experiments.

This gradually ascending avowal by Aron of his own part in the experiments was the last we would hear of him as a spokesman for the project.

During this year and the year that followed, citizens in the wider United States were hearing little at all of this subject. Most people knew almost nothing about what the British and Japanese were learning of the deliberate Cold War exposures of U.S. citizens by their own military, in collusion with American doctors.

BUT DURING THE SAME MONTH O'Halloran was in Cincinnati, the existence of the Clinton committee began to be noticed, at least, by National Public Radio. It would be of interest to know how and why Richard Harris, among the various science reporters, was assigned the story. Harris's reports hardly ever have any edge to them. He specializes in soft honorific stories on the winners of Nobel prizes and so on, alleged breakthroughs in cancer treatments, new forays into space, and matters of that type. He is clearly not one of those who is comfortable criticizing science and scientists, or inclined to doubt that technoscientific progress is always progress. He likes to admire things and to explain them in an animated, classroom sort of way, and he is good at that. All is for the best, he seems to say, in the wonderful world of science.

His brief initial report on the forming of the Advisory Committee was in this style; he told listeners, or at least strongly implied, that it was unlikely any real wrongs had been committed by the scientists involved or that any bona fide injuries would be found. He did not expect the Committee to have much to do.

I happened to hear this report and I found it exasperating. To complain about a story to the national press is usually not worth one's while, but this time I did protest; I left a message at my local public station, and that night was called by Harris. I told him that if he thought no injuries had been sustained by people deliberately exposed to radiation, I would like to tell him about Cincinnati and also send him some documents. He was willing to talk and to hear what I had to say. He knew about the American College of Radiology review of our case and confessed that he would be very surprised if the ACR was found to have acted irresponsibly; he had long respected the integrity, he said, of a leader of this group, the well-known radiologist Henry Kaplan. Well, but Kaplan had directed the on-site review of the Cincinnati tests, I told him, and had submitted a very strange critique, full of what would turn out to be patent untruths and relying entirely, judging from the internal evidence, on information supplied by Eugene Saenger.

We talked a little more, and I gave Harris the outline of our case. I then faxed him the JFA report and in a few days he called back to say he was feeling differently about the matter and would like to include me in a brief forum on the air. For this report, he talked to several "ethicists" as well, who were inclined to take such a case as ours seriously, as far as they understood it, and it was a decent beginning.

But during the next year there followed from Harris other stories on Cold War radiation that picked up again the original pooh-poohing, downplaying tone of his initial report and revealed nothing specific about any of the radiation populations and what people had suffered or were claiming to have suffered. No victims or families of victims were interviewed. Harris focused on the releases of the Advisory Committee itself and their puerile discussions about any and everything *except* the actual documented tragedies of exposure around the country.

When the court ruling against the Cincinnati doctors was made in 1995, Harris was sent information about it and phone numbers and profiles of our families in Cincinnati, but none were ever contacted by this "grassroots radio," as they were by the media in England and Japan.

In 1997, when the fairness hearing on the proposed settlement was held in a federal court in Cincinnati during two long days in February, a senior editor, Gwen Tompkins, of *Weekend Edition*, took notice of our legal action. I believe it was David Egilman who contacted this show or sent them a copy of a Cincinnati report. Tompkins contacted me, and I went over a few days after our hearing to a public station near my home and talked by phone to Scott Simon in Washington for about thirty minutes. He permitted me to tell the full truth about what had happened, let me describe the evidence against the doctors, the findings of the federal court, and the nature of the proposed settlement. The staff did not edit out the more incisive exchanges—everything was there that needed to be. Maude Jacobs's story was told in bald unequivocal terms, for instance. I was grateful for that, and felt a certain sense of relief that another small step had been taken in bringing our case before the public.[6]

The NPR afternoon news show *All Things Considered* continued to be deaf and dumb to the real radiation stories while accounts were being broadcast in large and vivid detail in England and Japan. It seemed that this show was too busy simply forwarding to its listeners the official releases of Washington to catch up, not only on Cincinnati, but on the Navajo miners, the Atomic Vets, Nevada, Hanford, Nashville, and so on.

THE COLLEGE OF MEDICINE had insisted all along, from the time I had first called on Edward Gall years ago, that normal people—journalists, English professors, patients—could not understand medical research. *You will not be able to understand it,* Gall had said to me, in effect and in so many words, over and over again, and this was the major defense, if it is a defense, the school was still mounting in 1994.

Do bear in mind, they kept telling Reeves and Rusconi, for instance, that the criticism of the project had come only from nondoctors. Look at the Suskind Report, they would say (the internal review commissioned in 1971 by the president of the university). Look at the report on us by the American College of Radiology. These reviewers were scientists and they said things were all right here. Only those *other* people, their argument went, in that junior faculty group, and a few sensation-hunting reporters from out of town, have attacked our work on radiation. Do by all means remember that that Stephens woman is not a doctor, though she seems to want people to think she is. Why do you suppose, they had asked Julian O'Halloran, she wears that white jacket of hers on television? I had been seen a number of times in an old white cardigan sweater of mine. (I am still wearing it today—and still not a physician.)

The general public and the surviving families, the school contended, might well have very curious ideas about what had taken place years ago when their relatives were ill; such people were confused and misled, they said, disturbed unnecessarily over things they were not equipped to understand.

But the problem for the researchers was that the press in Cincinnati was *not* confused. That was the deadly truth of the matter, and while it had seemed crucial, even so, in the first weeks of the evolving story to find doctors who would back up the original charges against the school, and Peg Rusconi, for instance, had looked high and low for a physician in Cincinnati who would speak, she had never found one, and after a time enough study had taken place in newsrooms so that medical doctors were no longer necessary.

We were more than aware, all the time, that all too often this kind of reportorial study does not take place and that the companies that own our media, and depend for their profits on their advertisers, customarily protect everything in the world *except* people's health and well-being and their basic need for information as to what is happening to them. We know how many decades it took for the awesome hazards of tobacco to be leaked at long last to the public—many years after journalists and researchers had known of the dangers it posed and had attempted to let people know.[7]

If, in the Cincinnati case, there had not been daily journalists assigned to study the detailed technical records of the tests and able to master them, to learn for themselves, finally, with the initial help they were given, what some of us had learned years ago, what chance would this history have had of being brought to light by any other means? Were medical insiders themselves ever going to tell what they knew to the public at large? We have no reason to believe they would ever have done such a thing.

There are many morals to the Cincinnati story, but one of them is surely this: that we cannot achieve any control over dangerous medical experiments, or of any other kind of systemic abuse, medical or otherwise, *unless we have information.*

It is not the working journalists, of course, who stand in our way.

African Americans Lost and Found   67

Once reporters had been freed to take hold of the Cincinnati story, Peg Rusconi and Nick Miller, for instance, they had cut quickly to the bone of the matter; their coverage was not tabloid-style, entertainment-style journalism—it was accurate and restrained, respectful of the technicalities involved.

Yet the doctors at the College of Medicine counted for the containment of this story on the medical ignorance of the press, of public officials, and of people at large. They banked on the incapacity of those who were not doctors to grasp what had been done, and so they gave out their casual generalities, declining, as Aron had with Julian O'Halloran, to be drawn into any substantive discussion of the case. Yet this may have been a serious error. For too many weeks the newsrooms were left to study on their own, with myself and others to instruct them in the basic facts of the case. If the researchers had put up complex technical smokescreens early on, while the press was still new to the fundamental ideas of the project and hardly knew what total body radiation was or if it could hurt anyone, they would have had a chance of deflecting the whole campaign. But in his early reports in the *Post*, Nick Miller, for instance, had little he could cite of the positions of the College of Medicine:

- Officials from UC and Defense Department did not return telephone calls today for comment on this story.
- The *Post* made repeated attempts to talk with Saenger; he declined to be interviewed.
- The Medical Center issued a statement Thursday calling reports on the study "old news." The statement said consent forms were obtained from patients for experimental cancer treatment. It makes no mention of the Pentagon's involvement.
- "The doctors were attempting to treat incurable cancer using radiation at a time before chemotherapy was available as it is today," UC Medical Center officials said in a recent statement. "The objective of the treatment was to kill cancer cells and at the same time study the effects of radiation on blood and urine. . . ." [But] Medical Center officials have declined to answer specific questions about the program. The project's director, Dr. Eugene Saenger, also has not responded to requests for interviews.[8]

"It's a terribly mismanaged issue over there," Peg Rusconi would finally say that winter about the school. In the early weeks she had made a point from time to time of recalling to herself and me that after all she was a journalist and had no *personal* view of what had happened, was only trying faithfully to present both sides of the issue. But in time her patience with the school had worn away. She saw that one side could not *be* covered, and that—finally—there was no other side. We talked frankly about the meaning of such things as had happened in our hospital, and as the publicity she had evoked streamed out, she was happy to have forged the path she had at Channel 12. "Look what we popped off," she would say.

Rusconi had studied political science and journalism at Syracuse, but it seemed she had not forgotten the laboring roots of her immigrant family. Somehow I felt that she, like many young journalists, wanted to do work that meant something and generally could not, within those one and two-minute flashes reporters are trapped in, on those long hours of newsbite news.[9]

Rusconi was still hoping for scientists to speak to. Couldn't I call the unnamed medical professor we had referred to in the JFA report? she asked. In time I did contact the individual who had first helped us, secretly, back in the seventies. He had read the final draft of our report and assured us we had gotten things right. Only one flaw, he had said: we had not mentioned the lack of autopsies for most subjects. We saw that in a genuine cancer study, those would have been done, and we had written in a line about the missing autopsies. This individual was now retired and living in California, and I was able to reach him there.

Could he speak up now? I asked him. He was *needed*, I said; the newsrooms were trying to tell the truth now, at long last, and they needed a medical scholar to back them up. He was retired; was there any reason he could not speak out now about what he knew?

But he could not, he said. "I know you're not going to understand," he said, "but Martha, I can't do that. I'm going to be ashamed of myself, but still—I just don't feel I can do that. . . ."

That same week I had an exchange with a Cincinnati physician named Huxley Miller. He was known in town as a progressive doctor who would help out with the medical problems of Central American refugees. But he too quickly said no, rather coldly; he could not help, he said. He was not a radiologist, he explained.

BUT THERE ARE many bizarre twists to this story, and as curious as it seems, we would soon learn, in this winter of 1994, that we in the JFA had had doctors all along to validate what we had charged, if only we could have known it.

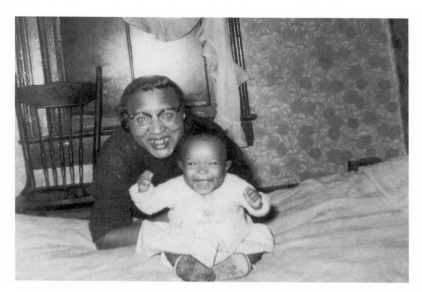

Lula Tarlton and family tot in a happy moment in Cincinnati's East End. Tarlton would develop breast cancer and be irradiated over her whole body in 1960, the earliest female victim of the tests to become known. See the Prologue of this volume. (Courtesy of Barbara Ann Mathis)

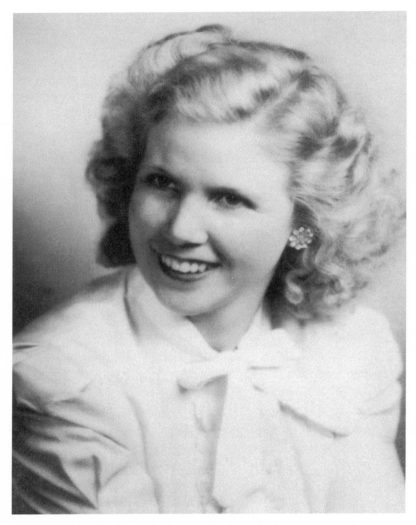

Maude Jacobs as a young woman. At forty-nine she would develop breast cancer, receive in 1964 a large dose of whole body radiation, and die twenty-five
days later, leaving seven children, including three young daughters at home.
(Courtesy of the Jacobs family)

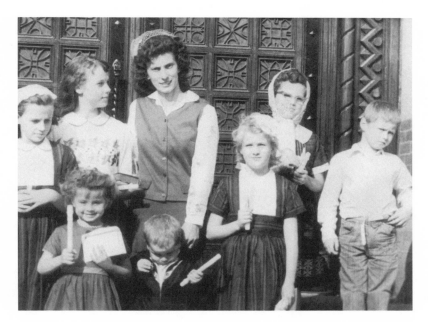

Children and grandchildren of Maude Jacobs near the time of her death. The older woman in back, Lilian Pagano, has brought the children to St. George's church to be baptized. When Jacobs died, three of the daughters shown here were placed in homes by Catholic services. (Courtesy of the Jacobs family)

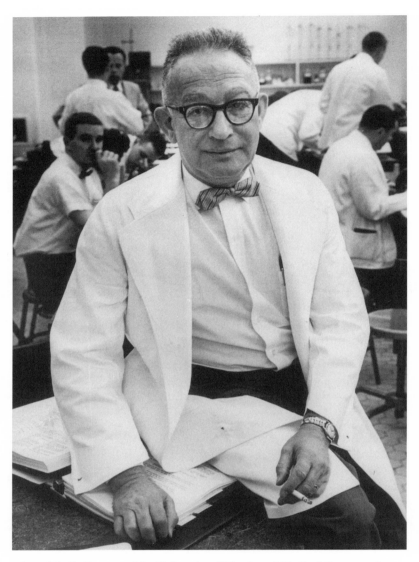

Edward Gall, director of the University of Cincinnati Medical Center and a pathologist, at work. This photograph was taken not long after the radiation project was halted by the president of UC in 1972. Gall performed some of the blood studies on radiation subjects. (Courtesy University of Cincinnati Archives)

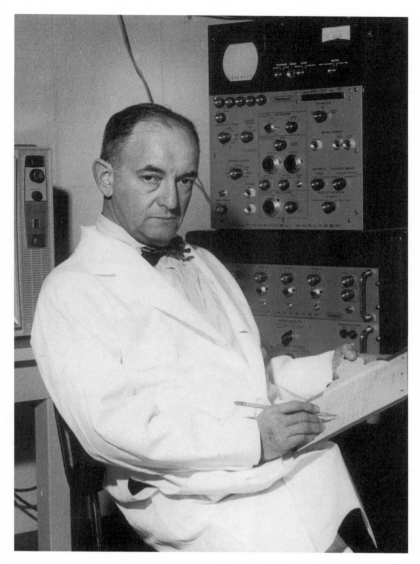

Eugene Saenger at whole body radiation controls in 1961, during the early years of the radiation project. (Courtesy University of Cincinnati Archives)

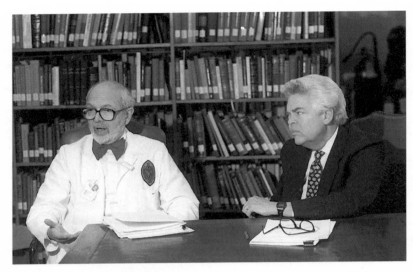

One of the radiation doctors, Bernard Aron, a UC radiologist, meeting in 1994 with Representative David Mann. In this early interview, both men gave assurances that nothing unusual was being uncovered about the project and that further inquiries would be unnecessary. (With the permission of the *Cincinnati Enquirer*)

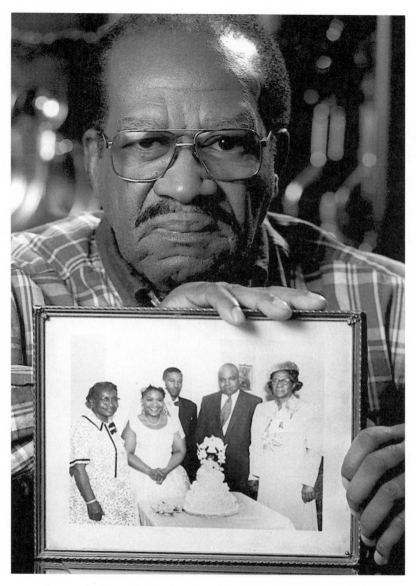

Leon Thomas displaying his wedding picture for reporter Linda Dono Reeves in 1994. The caption over this *Enquirer* photo read, "The very money I paid in taxes they used to kill my mom!" Thomas is shown third from left and his mother, Willie Thomas, on far right. Willie Thomas became radiation subject #068 in 1966, developed severe mental confusion, and died two months later. (With the permission of the *Cincinnati Enquirer*)

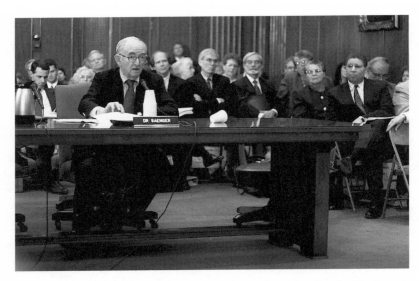

Eugene Saenger testifying in 1994 at a congressional hearing in Cincinnati. (With the permission of the *Cincinnati Enquirer*)

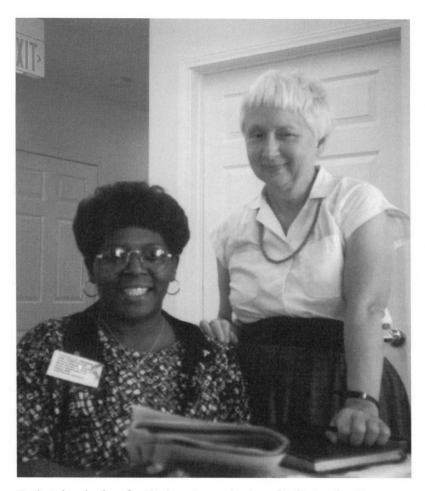

Doris Baker, leader of a Cincinnati organization of radiation families, meeting with Martha Stephens before a press conference in 1995. Baker's great-grandmother, Gertrude Newell, was irradiated over her whole body for colon cancer in 1962.

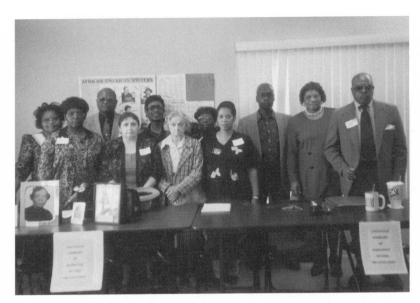

The steering committee of radiation families at a press conference in 1995. At front, from left, are Doris Baker; Barb Tatterson and Bertha Jungnickel, the cousin and mother of young victim David Jungnickel; and Gloria Nelson, who testified at the congressional hearing about her grandmother, Amelia Jackson. In back are six members of the family of James Tidwell, who was exposed over his whole body in 1960 and died thirty-two days afterward; and near the middle of the back row, Ernestine Goodwin, whose mother Estella was irradiated in 1966. (Martha Stephens)

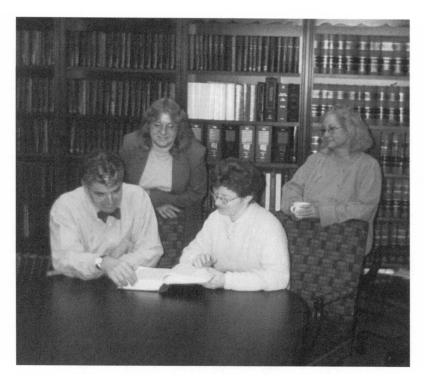

In the library and conference room of the Cincinnati law firm Newman and Meeks. This is the entire staff. Lisa Meeks is seated beside Robert Newman; behind is secretary Beth Wells and, on right, paralegal Jennifer Thomas. (Courtesy of the Office of Newman and Meeks)

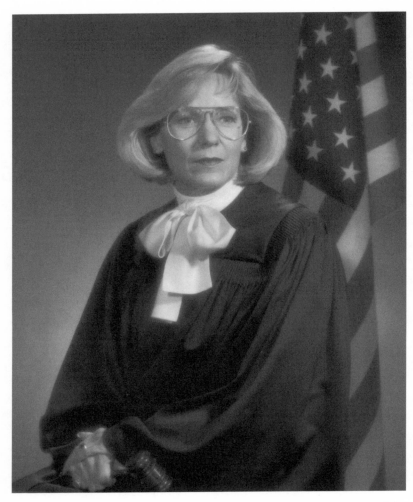

Sandra Beckwith, federal judge in the Southern District of Ohio who heard the radiation case 1994–99. Beckwith's ruling in 1995 denying the motion of the researchers to be dismissed as individual defendants cited at length the Nuremberg Code. (Courtesy of the Office of Sandra Beckwith)

5

The Back Files

In my own mind, this project borders on what happened at
Auschwitz.—VERNON STROUD, Theatre Arts Department,
UC, April 24, 1972

On March 1 an event took place that no one had expected, and it provided new evidence against the doctors that was extremely damaging.
At ten o'clock that day UC held its own press conference and turned
over to all comers copies of a massive set of documents on radiation.

The first two months of the public crusade against the experiments
had played out an ever-evolving and heightening drama, yet there had
been almost nothing but silence from the university. By the time of the
UC press conference, however, the doctors and the medical school had
been beaten, in effect, to a puling pulp by the relentless battery of the
press and of the outraged families, and the university had apparently
come to feel that there was no way out but to distance itself to some
degree from the distinguished radiologists on its medical site. The two
men who met the press at ten o'clock on the morning of March 1 said, in
effect, "We're coming clean now—we're giving up everything we have
on this case."

One thing about the press conference was somewhat mysterious: no
researcher joined publicly in the act of disclosure. Neither of the two
individuals meeting the press that day was a physician or representative

of the College of Medicine. One was Joseph Steger, the long-time president of the university, and the other Stan Chesley, a well-known class-action attorney who had recently completed a term on the UC board. Chesley told the press that day that he was acting as advisor to the president and that, as the *Cincinnati Enquirer* phrased his remarks, "the release of the documents was intended to demonstrate the school's commitment to openness."

This first release, which would be followed by two smaller ones, included about five thousand random and unorganized papers on the radiation project from what appeared to be the administrative files of the school. It is a strange fact of the legal campaign against the researchers that such a release was made; the lawsuit was only two weeks old, and certainly no disclosures had been compelled and might never have been compelled.

The medical school would not have had access to the personal files of the individual researchers, but the main office files of the school contained plenty of correspondence, memoranda, reports, and other materials that add quite significantly to our knowledge of the case. Other papers seemed to have come from the files of UC medical professors not part of the project.

The most interesting documents were, without a doubt, the reports and correspondence exchanged among the faculty members periodically reviewing the experiments and reporting to Edward Gall and Dean Clifford Grulee. It was not until midway through the eleven years of the study that these reviewing committees had begun to meet, when new guidelines from NIH had made such reviews necessary.

Certain physicians then assigned to review the whole body project, and becoming familiar with it for the first time, are on record in these papers as being greatly disturbed by what they found. Some attempted to send a prickly alert to Dr. Gall, as chair of the Faculty Research Committee, and Gall is on record as early as 1966 as expressing grave concerns of his own. "It is not certain," he wrote to Dean Grulee on May 6, "whether the patient is advised that no specific benefit will derive to him and that there are, indeed, risks involved in the procedure proposed."[1]

In the spring of 1967 a battery of sharp, sometimes caustic critiques was aimed at the investigators by a new team of reviewers. A professor of Internal Medicine, George Shields, observed, for instance, on March 13,

in a confidential letter to Gall, that a large number of radiation subjects had died shortly after treatment. "I recommend that this study be
disapproved," he wrote, "because of the high risk of this level of radiation." He felt that though risks and benefits were sometimes hard to
calculate in such studies, nevertheless "a twenty-five percent mortality
rate is too high." He had found the protocol "difficult to evaluate," he
said, the purpose of the study "obscure." He added this:

> If it is the consensus of the investigators and the review commit-
> tee that a 25% mortality risk is not prohibitive, then the experiment
> could be reconsidered from the standpoint of informed consent—
> provided the patient is appraised [sic] of this risk in a quantitative
> fashion. I believe that the conditions of informed consent will have
> been observed if the authors changed "all patients are informed that
> a risk exists, but that all precautions to prevent untoward results will
> be taken" to the equivalent of "all patients are informed that a 1 in 4
> chance of death within a few weeks due to treatment exists, etc."

A detailed report that anticipated the charges that would be made in
1972 by the Junior Faculty Association was written on April 17, 1967, by
Dr. Thomas Gaffney, director of Clinical Pharmacology. It is strange to
know that this letter rested unknown in the back files of the school for
nearly twenty-seven years:

> I cannot recommend approval of the proposed study entitled "The
> Therapeutic Effect of Total Body Radiation. . . .
>
> The applicants have apparently already administered 150–200 rads
> to some 18 patients with a *variety* of malignancies and to their satis-
> faction have not found a beneficial effect. In fact, as I understand it,
> they found considerable morbidity associated with this high dose of
> radiation. Why is it now logical to expand this study?
>
> Even if this study is expanded, its current design will not yield
> meaningful data. . . . It will be difficult if not impossible to observe
> a beneficial effect in such a small sample containing a variety of dis-
> eases all of which share only CANCER in common.
>
> This gross deficiency in design will almost certainly prevent mak-
> ing meaningful observations. When this deficiency in experimen-
> tal method is placed next to their previously observed poor result

and high morbidity with this type of treatment in a "variety of neo-plasms" I think it clear that the study should not be done.

And yet of course the project was not halted; new people were regularly brought in for radiation, made ill in one way or another, often severely, as we have seen, and their injuries studied in various ways. Blood and urine samples went back and forth across the corridors, and the later subjects were given daily batteries of mental tests before being more or less abandoned to their cancers. As in the past, some sufferers would continue to succumb within a month of their "treatments." This would be true up until the final year, 1971, when events finally closed in on the researchers and the radiations ceased.

Other reviewers than Shields and Gaffney wrote serious critiques of the project and were also more or less ignored as they were. The reasons for this do not come clear in the correspondence but often seem largely attributable to *meetings* between the reviewers and Saenger or Edward Silberstein, and to the two doctors' "oral testimonies."

The reviewer who persisted longest in challenging what was being done was a professor of Immunology, Dr. Evelyn Hess, a native of Dublin, Ireland, and graduate of University College there. She had not come to the U.S. until 1958, and had taught first at the University of Texas. At UC in the mid-sixties she was working on new drugs for joint disease and was the subject of good-news media reports on the cures that seemed to be coming along for rheumatoid arthritis. Hess chaired the Faculty Committee on Research during what would turn out to be the final year of the project, 1970–71. The radiation doctors had made several unconvincing attempts to produce a control group against which the beneficial effects of radiation could be measured, and in the protocol for Hess they made new comparisons with a set of cancer patients treated with a chemotherapeutic agent, 5-fluorouracil. Hess wrote the researchers in February 1971 that information about the effects of 5-fluorouracil itself had not been provided and that, as far as she knew, the controls had been given nothing more effective than "mud packs."

As late as July 22, 1971, Hess was still declining to grant final approval to the project. "We are not much farther ahead," she wrote the researchers after reading a revised proposal from Edward Silberstein. "The whole problem concerns the lack of understanding of what is to be done. If evaluation of whole body radiation is the main point, then the proposal should so indicate," she wrote; and indeed, a number of reviewers seem to have had trouble understanding the point of the project and what exactly was being studied. In the records provided, there is generally no indication that the review committees knew of the doctors' study of radiation injury for the Defense Department.

In any case, Hess notes in her letter of July 22 that Silberstein has reported that "preliminary results published by Dr. Saenger have suggested an effect of prolonging life. However, upon reviewing Table 2, we do not find any evidence of prolongation of survival." She then invited the investigators to meet with the committee and "simply outline (perhaps on a blackboard) what you want to do."

Apparently this long-delayed meeting took place, for less than two weeks after the probing communication above and the almost year-long seige of questions and criticism from Hess, she too agreed to the continuation of the experiments. She wrote Clifford Grulee a letter of two sentences, stating that the protocol of Silberstein and Saenger had been reviewed and that her committee "recommends its approval of this project." On the same day, August 3, 1971, Hess wrote a short note to Eugene Saenger saying that Silberstein had met with committee member Harvey Knowles and that "all questions now appear to be answered." That was all. "We would like to thank you for your complete cooperation with the committee," she concluded.

Hess's doubts had apparently been allayed or she or her committee mollified, but we do not know exactly how doubts were allayed or she mollified, or how the doubts of Gaffney had been allayed in 1967.

Did Saenger and Silberstein provide the committees persuasive oral information they were not prepared to put in writing? Did Dean Clifford Grulee come to the team's defense? Did Defense Department officers get in touch with the school each time such a crisis arose and say, "Do please explain to your committees that this study is needed for the defense of the country"? Did Eugene Saenger lean on Gall and Grulee not to interfere with important military research, bringing in a good sizable grant from the DOD each year and enhancing UC's reputation, as he would have argued, among the nation's community of radiologists? We do not know.

Thomas Gaffney had ended his resistance to the project with a final sour note to Edward Gall on May 18, 1967: "The only proviso I would suggest is that the applicants give at least some consideration to the basic rudiments of experimental design which are necessary to the completion of studies of the type contemplated." This, however, was, as far as we know, the only protest he permitted himself.

No doctor spoke out to the public at large.

Gaffney capitulated, and in that same year of 1967 George Shields had already extricated himself from the situation by withdrawing from the committee, "for reasons of close professional and personal contact with the investigators and with some of the laboratory phases of the project." He informed a reporter in 1994 that he had known nothing more of the project after 1967 and had been surprised to learn in 1972 that the radiations had only recently ceased.[2]

As publicity began breaking out in 1971, both Hess and Harvey Knowles, professor of Medicine, would be appointed by Grulee to the internal review requested that fall by President Bennis. Hess would compose that December a historical overview of the project and its faculty reviews, but in this document of six pages there was no mention of the severe criticisms of Gaffney and Shields.

After Thomas Gaffney's complaints in the spring of 1967, at least thirty-five more citizens had been drawn into the experiments, and of these new subjects ten had died within thirty-one days of their radiations.

ON MARCH 1 the reporters went to work on the disclosures. Within a day or two of this release of chaotic papers from UC, Nick Miller at the Post and Steve Bennish at the Enquirer had already located the telltale letters of the faculty reviewers.

Miller has said that he went over to the press conference early that morning and was able to pick up the two cartons of materials at eight o'clock. He then raced back to his desk while a fellow reporter stayed to hear the remarks of Chesley and Steger. Miller had already had a folding banquet table set up by his desk—the staff asssumed there was going to be a party—and he dumped out the whole contents of the cartons onto this surface and began tearing through them.[3]

Along with Miller and Bennish, the Enquirer's Tim Bonfield also turned up some interesting materials, including papers that suggested, for the first time, how the doctors had reacted back in 1972 to the charges of the JFA. "Radiation Docs Felt Victimized" read his report of April 7, and he found evidence that Saenger had wanted to reply to the JFA report but that friends had advised him not to do so.

Bonfield also quoted from the 1975 letter to Silberstein by his physician friend in California, William H. Crosby, in which Crosby comforted Silberstein in his travails by assuring him that he was cast in the role of a saint—Saint Sebastian no less—and had been on the receiving end, not of arrows, but of "one custard pie after another pitched by a pack of sly, self-seeking, savage clowns." (We had not specifically identified any savage clowns among our junior faculty group, but of course such persons might well have gone about in clever professorial disguise, a situation not unheard of in universities. Indeed, some would say that in any academic grove there's more than one circus in town at any given time and fully operative.)

I recall that Linda Reeves apologized to me for my not having been given a chance to reply to these insults; the *Enquirer* had attempted to reach me, she said. I assured her no reply was necessary.

FROM THE UC DISCLOSURES of March 1 we also learned a great deal about a quite different matter from the internal reviews: the panic, that is, in the main office of the school during the fall of 1971, not many months after Hess's final pursuit of Silberstein, when the first twists and tremors of the quake to come were being felt. The public learned that fall that Senator Kennedy had begun to target the UC tests for probes by his committee and that Senator Robert Taft (Republican-Ohio) was upholding fiercely the honor of his proud hometown institution. Very little, though, was being revealed about the even deeper challenges being presented behind the scenes by Senator Gravel. It would have been unclear to anyone reading the Cincinnati press what the doctors were actually being accused of doing and whether whole body radiation posed any serious danger, and Saenger and Silberstein gave cheerful local interviews about the beneficial powers of their total body treatments,[4] and indeed during those early years the College seemed staunch and untroubled in the doctors' defense.

In 1994 I would draw up, for a small-panel meeting in Cincinnati of the Clinton committee, a detailed statement about what we had learned during the preceding eight months of that year's campaign, and I recalled some of the new information that had emerged in the disclosures of March 1:

> Because of what the families have told us about the victims and because we now have their full medical records, as well as a mass of long-secret letters and documents from the medical school, we can fill in a great many details of the picture some of us had tried to sketch for the public years ago.
>
> Behind the rather placid public demeanor of the medical school back in 1971 and '72, we know now that there was intense secret manoeuvering to try to put a decent face on what had happened over the eleven years of the experiments; memos flew thick and fast, phone messages piled up, statements of explanation and defense were drafted and re-drafted, discarded, rescued, and drafted again.
>
> The most intense effort of all was that of keeping investigators of the case away from the victims, an effort involving the entire cadre of doctors, administrators, and public relations people for the whole half-year period of the defense and cover-up beginning in October 1971. On December 20, for instance, a decision was painfully reached in the front office of the school to hire a Washington attorney to shore up the wall between patients and potential interviewers, and ten days later we see a move to keep this hiring itself a secret (Ralph Bursiek's memo to the UC Board of December 30).
>
> Doctors Saenger and Silberstein constantly urged non-compliance with the requests for interviews and claimed ever-mounting evidence that patients were repeatedly refusing to be known.
>
> This winter, of course, readers of the local papers found out *why* that massive fortification between public and patients had had to be built up.

Senator Kennedy's attempts in late 1971 to gain access to the living victims of the tests had excited a great many intense exchanges between the radiation doctors and the College of Medicine administrators. The argument of the doctors was that it would be harmful to patients to have to discuss their illness and treatment with outsiders and to think of themselves as "guinea pigs." Documents of all kinds, and correspondence from colleagues around the country, were produced to support this contention. I count at least forty communications on this crucial theme, beginning with a nine-page memorandum from Saenger about a meeting of himself and Silberstein with Kennedy aide Ellis Mottur and a physician working with the Kennedy office.

In this meeting of December 8, Saenger reports—writing on the same day—that Silberstein had described a lengthy two-day consent process, and outlined the thoughtful, sensitive manner in which the subjects were treated and the many special services he personally provided them. When at the end of this elaborate meeting, Mottur asked if the Senate committee could talk to the subjects directly about their understandings of the treatments they were getting, the meeting seemed to turn somewhat sour. Permission would have to come from Dr. Gall, Silberstein said, but that he himself was concerned "about the anonymity of the patients" and what they would regard as "political footballing."

It was "grossly unfair," he went on, according to Saenger's report to Gall, "to bring patients into this entire matter." Saenger adds that in his mind the meeting made it "reasonably clear" that for Kennedy the project's DOD funding was the real issue. "If they could block the DOD in this research, they could hobble the DOD in all other biomedical research whenever they would choose to do so."

There followed many other communications of Saenger and Silberstein to Gall and others on this topic, and it proved to be capable of endless variations and interpolations. We find here the first letter to the school from the new president Warren Bennis, writing on this subject to Gall on December 20. The next day we find Harry Horwitz of the radiation team writing to Saenger regarding interviews of three children, and we find a doctor who was a major member of the team until his departure to the University of Tennessee in 1968, Ben Friedman, writing to Saenger from Memphis with copious explanations about the careful treatment of patients during the seven years of his participation.[5]

We also have Gall's letter to Kennedy on December 22 officially disallowing any interviews with patients or the release of any patient names, and we have letters from various university legal counselors on what Kennedy might be able to subpoena, what legal help UC might need, and whether this legal advice would need to be made public.

Many of the other disclosure documents are interesting reading in one way or another. A Saenger letter to Gall on January 13, 1971, opens as follows: "There are two occasions in the past decade of this program when I must confess to having been naive." Edward Kennedy is wanting to know why a television crew could interview UC subjects but a Senate committee could not, and Saenger is confessing to Gall, for the first time, to having allowed a crew from National Educational Television to work on a documentary in the radiation laboratory during the past September, and to have had "access to patients." (Saenger's second episode of naivete had been to place his trust, he said, in reporters Thomas O'Toole and Stuart Auerbach of the *Washington Post*.)

As to the NET team, Saenger writes:

In answer to the specific question (1) as to why the t. v. team had access to the patients, but access to the patients (or to their families) was denied when it was requested, in the public interest, by a Senate Sub-Committee, the patients initially were delighted to appear on t. v. because they were appreciative of our work. Subsequently, the unfortunate publicity afforded to this study and the use of such terms as "guinea pig" applied by the press have caused patients to shy away from any type of inquiry demanding personal interviews. After we consulted special legal counsel in regard to permitting patient interviews as requested by Senator Kennedy's staff, I was surprised to learn that I had apparently erred in regard to Ohio law in acceding to the request of NET in September, 1971. I would suspect further that many of us have behaved similarly. . . ."

Still, it is his "personal belief," Saenger goes on to say, "that information obtained by Federal funds should be made available both to the scientific and lay public, and obviously to public officials. We have scrupulously adhered to this policy as shown by our many scientific communications, none of which have been classified or secret." It is, of course, one of the many somber ironies of the radiation case that this latter statement of Saenger's is in fact largely quite accurate.

Among the other treasures of the March 1 papers we find an unsigned memo dated December 3, or an early draft of some such memo, in which the writer is brooding on the difficult matter of whether the appointment of a faculty review committee by President Bennis should be made public. This was the group later referred to as "the Suskind Committee," led by Raymond Suskind, a UC environmental scientist. "The one problem to be avoided at all costs in the further saga of this matter is that of secrecy," says the writer, and somehow this question relates to the troubling intervention of the JFA. "A conversation with Dr. Suskind this morning once again raises the question of secrecy. Dr. Suskind says that a group of young faculty members on the campus see the whole body radiation project as a devise [sic] for stirring up a fuss. There is some question as to just how Dr. Bennis will deal with this matter."

ONE LETTER IN THE disclosures touched for the first time, as far as is known, on a Nazi analog for the Cincinnati tests.

This is a letter to the provost, not from a medical professor but from a faculty member in Arts and Sciences, Vernon Stroud, who was director of Speech Pathology and Audiology in the Theatre Arts Department and was serving on an all-university research review committee recently set up by the new administration. Stroud was writing on April 24, 1972, to the new provost, Robert O'Neil. "I have given considerable thought," Stroud began, "to the discussion which occurred during our recent meeting of the subcommittee on human research," and he continued as follows: "I have formed an opinion toward the whole body radiation study which I am sure is not in agreement with those involved with the research and possibly some of the members of the committee. In no way can I condone such a project regardless of whether it is supported by the Defense Department or the University of Cincinnati."

Stroud went on to complain of a number of problems with the project that he feels were not being clearly addressed by the Suskind Committee. He noted some of the serious contradictions in the Suskind findings regarding the basic *purpose* of the project. He felt information was not being given about "the manner in which the subjects were selected." He objected strongly to the findings of the psychiatrists on the mental and emotional effects of radiation. He asked why more information had not been sought about the way the research had been reported. Stroud appears to have read the Junior Faculty review, which was made available by our group to all faculty, but not the original reports to the DOD.

Stroud closes with remarks that indicate that he was having serious difficulty accepting a decision already publicly sketched by Bennis a few days earlier to the effect that he would act according to the various Suskind recommendations and would close off funding from the DOD but leave the door open for other sponsorship:

> These are just a few of the points I will mention at this time, since it is important to get this to you prior to the President's decision.
>
> In my own mind, this project borders on what happened at Auschwitz. It differs primarily in that the subjects there were much more sophisticated. Further, I feel that continuation of this project, regardless of the source of funding, can be devastating to the University, especially if the composition of the population becomes known to the general public. . . .
>
> I sincerely hope that Warren will take these matters into consideration before making a decision.

In 1994 the Stroud letter with its Auschwitz lines was seized upon quickly by the reporters. A few of us had known of it in the past and were not unhappy to see it entered now into the public record.

About the Nazi analogy, it might be mentioned here that two years later, that is, in the fall of 1996, the *Journal of the American Medical Association* would devote most of its November 27 issue to the fiftieth anniversary of the Nuremberg Code, with papers by a number of scholars. (It was in November of 1946 that the Nuremberg Doctors' Trial had commenced.) The JAMA writers seemed to be disturbed by a constantly recurring thought that we in the United States today might not remember how medicine had gone wrong—so tragically—under national socialism, how much collusion there had been between physicians and nurses and the Third Reich, and how vigilant *we* have to be to be sure we are not following in those sinister footsteps.

Do we too, they asked, have among us populations of citizens we are coming to feel are expendable? Are we in the process of writing off anyone who may be, not only too poor, but simply too ill, too elderly, or too frightened to resist crude experiments—along with cheap medicine, and assisted departure from life—in the name of the larger and larger profits that must be taken by the health and insurance industries?

If—these essays seem to be asking, point-blank—we decide to *neglect* certain people to death, where are we then?[6]

VERNON STROUD'S CORRESPONDENT Robert O'Neil came on as the new provost (or vice president for academic affairs) during this winter of 1972. His first day on campus was the day of the release of the JFA report, January 25. That afternoon he walked over from the administration building to our press conference in the student union. We made note of a tall, rather gangly figure sitting in the back row of the room, but had no idea who this individual was. O'Neil, who would in later years become president of the University of Virginia, was known to have said that the report he had heard at this event was not a very cheerful welcome to the University of Cincinnati.

He had been brought in as provost by Warren Bennis, the new president who had himself only arrived in September. On campus one would sometimes hear reports, in later years, that walking into the radiation turmoil had been extremely agitating for Bennis and caused him at times almost to become ill. Bennis came on as UC's first and only Jewish—and liberal—president; he clearly valued his standing as a modern, progressive leader, and found himself in a serious quandary about the irradiations of low-income citizens taking place in his new medical school. To extract himself from this quandary, he eventually enlisted, as we have seen, the help of Ohio governor John Gilligan, who intervened with Kennedy to release UC from the Senate investigations.

Some time before this meeting of minds that spring—*all us fellow liberals getting together to resolve things, and fashion a reasonable exit for all from this unhappy situation*—Bennis had set up his blue ribbon committee to study the project under Raymond Suskind. But before this committee could report, the review from the junior faculty was issued and was reported in the national news. The general quandary thus deepened, and Edward Gall, as it turned out, had a draft of the Suskind Report on his desk when the JFA charges appeared, and realized that in this new context the Suskind findings were not going to be credible. "Editing would be desirable," he wrote to Bennis the next day, saying that only certain *pages* of Suskind need be actually released.

Two medical students friendly to the JFA had surreptitiously stuffed the JFA paper in the mailboxes of the medical faculty, and many, perhaps most, of that faculty read in this document the true details of the experiments for the first time. In the disclosure letters we see Dr. Gall now brooding and suffering over the vaporish and inconsistent findings of Suskind, the only "objective" reply available to him to counter the JFA. Still, this was all he had, and a week later he issued a *summary* of the Suskind report at a news conference on February 2.

Letters in the March 1 papers show that he was turning back all requests coming in for the JFA review, and then even for the unreliable Suskind Report. He wrote the French Embassy in Washington on March 1 (1972) that he could not send them this entire internal review because it was "voluminous"; it could only be examined in the school library, he said. Senator Kennedy wrote asking for Gall's reply to the JFA charges and *was* sent the Suskind Report, with an assertion from Gall that it would constitute the only reply that would be made to the Junior Faculty Association. Dean Grulee, we note, wrote Gall on January 31 about a call from *Medical World News* asking for the Suskind Report; it was not yet ready, he told them, adding that he had taken the trouble to read his caller the letter from the dissident JFA member Dodd Bogart, "indicating that the other report which has received so much publicity in the East was not an official position of even that small splinter group in our faculty."

The Suskind Report had included no one from outside the university, and a reporter for the student newspaper, Lew Moores, worked hard to track down the activities of the various Suskind members and was able to show that half of this rather large contingent had had connections of some kind with the radiation project itself or with its faculty reviews.[7] One of the Suskind reviewers was Bernard Aron, a member for several years, as we have seen, of the radiation team itself and a signer of the doctors' final three reports to the DOD.

The Suskind papers were an extremely labyrinthine set of comments, obviously from a number of different hands. What would be given by one writer would be taken away by another, and the "summary" at the end of the report was no true summation of what had gone before. Nevertheless, the report succeeded in recommending that the project continue, though in a limited way, concentrating on certain cancers that were said to have shown evidence of being "palliated" by the exposures, but that funding be sought outside the DOD.[8] When Bennis finally made it clear several months later that he was accepting the funding recommendation, Gall, who had opposed that part of the report, knowing it would be a death-blow to the project, nevertheless let Eugene Saenger know immediately that relations with the DOD would have to end.

This brought about a near break between Gall and Saenger, an angry letter, for example, from Saenger on April 24, attaching a budget for new radiations for the year to come, which he said he was expecting the College to fund in place of the DOD. "Attached is the budget for the year beginning April 1, 1972 terminating on March 31 1973 which was to have been covered by the DOD contract until we had an opportunity to seek other support." The opening clause of Saenger's next paragraph tried hard the already much-tried patience of Edward Gall: "Since you have decided to deny renewal of this contract without permitting us sufficient time to make any other arrangements. . . ."

Gall replied coolly a few days later that he found that charge an "interesting interpretation of the circumstance" and advised Saenger that "the proper channel" for his activity was "through Dean Grulee."

The question of funding was of course crucial, and the many anguished vacillations on this point within the main office and possibly within the Suskind Committee as well are clearly illustrated by a series of drafts of an unsigned, unaddressed memo simply marked "Confidential." The first draft, going back to April 11, requests the full implementation of the Suskind Report, including its recommendation on new funding outside the DOD, but also the expansion of the committee to include an attorney, a "social scientist with interest in ethical issues," a "physical scientist" experienced in radiation, and a "distinguished physician not in the College." In the next draft the paragraph on cutting ties with the DOD is scratched out; and in the next, on the same day, that paragraph is restored.

A week later (on April 18) there is another unsigned note to the effect that Bennis is known to be "getting worried" about certain items of the above conclusions and that a funding source other than the DOD "is necessary in this instance." Is this Gall himself drafting and redrafting for the president his position with respect to the DOD? We do not know.

There followed new disputes about who in the College could and could not sign contracts with funding agents. Gall quickly circulated a ruling on April 25 that before an agreement on research funding could become a contract, "it must be signed by senior administrative officials of the university." As late as the following July Saenger was still disputing this ruling, writing that "no manual of administrative procedures has ever been made available to UC medical faculty members concerning these administrative routines," and reminding him that the Hess committee approval of the radiation project on August 9, 1971, had never been rescinded, and that patient studies had ceased only upon Gall's verbal instructions.

On May 1 Gall addressed to Saenger what he apparently expected to be a letter of conciliation. "This has been a long and harrowing experience for many of us," he wrote in closing. "I think you will agree that much foresight and wisdom has gone into the [Suskind] conclusions." He extends his "best personal wishes" and signs himself "Cordially, Ed."

For me, Dr. Gall remains a figure of mystery in this case. It is difficult to understand such a man. He was a courteous and patient individual, likable and respected, it seems. He was very courteous to *me* when I first went to see him for information. He wished to think well of all his colleagues, it would seem, and unlike Grulee declined to insult even our young faculty group. Asked in 1972 whether the JFA was a "responsible" organization, he said that yes he felt sure that it was.

But what can have been his feelings, his real beliefs, about the citizens of his town who became the secret soldiers of these tragic tests, thrown into a medical combat from which many would never return, by their doctors, their government, their medical school, their public hospital, which after all they themselves had helped to build? *Do* scientists actually train themselves, are they trained by society, in that time and this, not to feel as others feel? Not to question, ponder, weigh — reflect on their actions?

It is never quite clear whether or not Gall had ever read for himself over the years, or even in 1971 and 1972, the doctors' full reports to the Department of Defense. There would, of course, have been plenty of research of all kinds to ponder and worry over in a large teaching hospital; free-flowing experimentation is what teaching hospitals have been largely about. At UC there were hardly enough patients to go around; the radiation authors remark on this themselves, as I have noted, in their reports to the DOD. They tell their sponsors that their need to compete for subjects limits the options for their research; this competition no doubt accounts in part for the extremely variable conditions of the patients brought into the tests.

There is a curious fact, an anomalous fact in a way, about the role of Edward Gall: he was himself engaged in some of the patient blood studies, and yet this fact is never broached, in writing at least, by him or by the other doctors during the turmoil of 1971–72. We can see Gall's role rather clearly in the full hospital records. These records, of course, were kept by and belonged to the institution, not to the research team, who composed their own more limited histories for the DOD. In these records, Gall is sometimes consulted about radiations being planned for certain patients. As a pathologist, he performs blood studies for a number of others, and he seems to have been personally involved with at least one subject of the tests.

This individual was Gertrude Newell, who became in 1962 the twelfth individual irradiated. We know Newell's case rather well, partly because her great-granddaughter, Doris Baker, a leader of the family organization, has had much to tell about her grandmother's illness and death. Baker was seventeen when her grandmother was irradiated, and she was closely involved with her during her illness. (Newell, Baker says, was a plump, humorous, unusual woman with a lively personality, and Baker was greatly attracted to her.)

Newell was sixty-nine when she first went to Cincinnati General Hospital with strong symptoms of rectal cancer. A few months afterward, she had a "combined abdomino-perineal resection," and two months later she received two hundred rads of total body radiation. This was a high dose indeed and Newell might have died of it. Almost half of the subjects who received this dose expired within about a month. Ten days after her treatment, Newell's blood counts began to drop, but gradually they recovered, and after sixty days were at normal again. Even during this hazardous period of immune system decline, Newell was started on radiation to the region of her primary tumor—the treatment that would in fact have been applied several months before, we have to assume, had she not been entered into the DOD study. Before the tumor treatment could be completed, Newell moved down home to Tuscaloosa,

Alabama, and did not return to UC until over two years later. Back in Cincinnati, she returned to General Hospital with "constant abdominal pain," and her death came two weeks later.

During these years, Doris Baker met Edward Gall from time to time at the hospital; she recalls vividly her grandmother's decision to go back to Alabama after her whole body treatment and Gall's efforts to keep her in town. This kind of close contact between patient and doctor is of course unusual in any setting, and we can be sure it was extremely unusual at this public hospital, but Gall telephoned Newell repeatedly, Baker says, urging her not to leave the city. We can rather imagine why this might have been the case, with a radiation subject whose records would have been expected to go with her, but we cannot know precisely what Gall's reasoning was.

It is also hard to know whether or not Gertrude Newell could be said to have had incurable cancer when taken in for whole body radiation, or to know the full effect the radiation had on her. She was certainly not one of those acutely ill patients the doctors often publicly described— Dr. Aron, for instance—to reporters in 1994. She was not by any means so ill, that is, that a desperate, last-ditch treatment had to be tried even though it might have ended her life within a matter of weeks. Radiation to her primary tumor, not to the whole body, appears clearly to have been the right therapy for her after her surgery, and yet this treatment was first delayed, then administered when her system was already compromised by total body exposure—a painful administration that may have been the cause of her decision not to complete the later and more appropriate course.

Gall's name appears on other patient records as well. We note that on those of Mike Spanagel, who died thirty-one days after radiation, there is a memo citing B. I. Friedman as "operator" and evaluating Spanagel's bone marrow status after radiation. This memo reads "Attn. Dr. Gall" at the top and then "Intensive Study," a code name for the radiation project.

Gall's specialty was pathology, and as noted above, it was he, at least at times, who studied the blood samples of the irradiated subjects. A man named Louis Romine was irradiated on May 8, 1965, and Gall submitted to the team pathology reports on the condition of Romine's blood on May 20, May 26, and June 3, then once more on June 8, three days after Romine's death on his twenty-eighth day after radiation.

Clearly Gall knew a lot about the course of certain patients after radiation and knew that their bone marrow had suffered terminal damage. It is just possible, perhaps, that he did not fully understand the awesome degree of risk for those given the higher doses, or that the studies being carried out were not focused on cancer but on radiation injury. It is even within the realm of belief that Gall learned, in 1972, more about the true parameters of the project from the report of the JFA, and to some extent of Suskind, than he had ever quite known, or allowed himself to know, in the past.

When Laura Schneider and I went over to the UC archives to try to learn a little more about the personae of this drama, we found Edward Gall—a major figure, after all, in College history—to be the subject of a rather thick file of old clippings and notices and oddities of all kinds. We learned that a Cincinnati astrologic society had once named a minor planet for Dr. Gall.

Gall seemed to have grown up among common people, but in time he was to attain a considerable degree of national standing. He grew up in New York City and went to City College. It was not in the east, however, but at Tulane Medical School that he became a physician, though afterward he was affiliated for a time with medicine at Harvard. He left there in 1941 for Cincinnati, and by 1948 had become head of the UC Department of Pathology.

Gall was a captain in the Army during World War II, and in the sixties a consultant to the surgeon general of that body. In 1964, in the midst of the radiation project for the DOD, Gall made a five-week tour of inspection of all the Army's medical installations in France and Germany.

It can hardly be insisted too strongly that the doctors who carried out the radiation tests, or administered the College where they took place, were not by any means alienated or marginalized physicians. They were graduates of Harvard and other prestigious schools; Saenger was a Harvard undergraduate, and Edward Silberstein a graduate of Harvard Medical School. The team investigators published in received journals and often served their profession in national posts. Their views, feelings, predilections, and habits of mind with regard to their patients and their research subjects must be assumed to be the views and habits of mind of many in their profession, in that time and this.

It is strange to find that during the year of the first public revelations about dangerous irradiations in his College, Edward Gall was serving as president of the American Association for Cancer Education. A few years later, he was presiding over a national group of cancer doctors, the American Federation of Clinical Oncologic Societies.

Leafing through the papers UC holds on Dr. Gall, I came upon a large black-and-white photograph of him in his lab. It is a huge slanting close-up of the doctor in his later years, perched on the corner of a desk against a busy background of young women and men working among slides and microscopes. Gall looks exactly like the man I remember from 1971. Under his disheveled white jacket shows a rather crooked bow tie. The expression he turns to the camera is rather vague and a little surprised or disconcerted. A cigarette is burning out between his fingers as they rested on the desk; he would die in 1979 of lung cancer. In his file were contact shots of his memorial service at the College.

It is impossible to know how Edward Gall rationalized the existence of the DOD tests and his own part in them, or whether he failed, somehow, at least in this early period, to understand the real dimensions of what was taking place.

Not long after the disturbing publicity of 1971–72 and the ignominious end of the military research in the radioisotope lab, a search commenced for a replacement for Gall as director of the UC Medical Center. In 1974 a man named Stanley Troup was brought on from the University of Rochester, an individual with a more ebullient style who was also felt to be more in touch with national standards of ethical research and patient care.[9]

Edward Gall, then, was soon relieved of his position, and even before the year 1972 had come to an end, Clifford Grulee had resigned as Dean of the College of Medicine.

WITH THE LOSS of monetary support for their work in 1972, Saenger and Edward Silberstein set about to try to tell their own story.

In 1994 Tim Bonfield's *Enquirer* article of April 7 ("Radiation Docs Felt Victimized") first alerted us, I believe, to the existence in one of the UC releases of a manuscript the two doctors had coauthored in 1975 and continued down through the years to try to get colleagues around the country to publish. This article was carefully and rather artfully composed as a narrative of persecution—of a serious miscarriage, that is, of medical justice. Certain of the events recounted above are told as they were felt and experienced at the time by the two researchers, and what is rather curious is that the writers provide a wealth of information about attacks on them of all kinds that might otherwise have hardly become known. France landed its own blows ("Les Cobayes de Cincinnati," L'Express, October 1971), and in London and South Africa and elsewhere stories ran that did not mince their rhetoric as most papers did in the U.S. But we also learn that The New England Journal of Medicine had printed a harsh editorial.

We find in the disclosures a letter to Dr. Saenger from a fellow radiologist at the University of Michigan to whom he had sent the manuscript in question, a twenty-four page piece titled "Ethics on Trial: Medical, Congressional, and Journalistic."

"Your letter of May 8, 1975, makes me realize for the first time," writes William Beierwaltes, "what a nightmare you have lived with for such a long time." Even so, Beierwaltes says he cannot recommend the narrative's publication; it would simply stir up new controversy. The press must always be told simply "no comment," he says. "Publishing the paper would increase your workload and not increase your happiness," he writes.

An interesting point about this letter is that Beierwaltes assumes that the malignancies the team had treated over the years were "mostly leukemia" and that the purpose of the radiation was "to impair the vitality of small metasteses," but he advises Saenger to spell this out in his paper. In fact, the patients in the study had, not leukemias, but radioresistant solid tumors. Nor had the radiation been given in the divided doses needed to protect the patient and to block constantly developing new cancer cells. The crux of the matter is that the authors of "Ethics on Trial" provide almost no concrete information about the experiments themselves or what exactly was administered, and discuss no individual patient case or death.

In "Ethics on Trial" we see Saenger and Silberstein still smarting and suffering under the loss of the whole body project and almost incredulous that with the nearly uniform medical support for their work in

Cincinnati and around the country things could have come to so sorry a conclusion. The authors are profoundly contemptuous of the Junior Faculty Association and still astounded that anyone would have listened to such a group:

> . . . on adding up the result of the multiple investigations the only unfavorable comments had come from a handful of local, and non-medical junior faculty members. The UC Faculty Committee on Human Research, the Cincinnati Children's Hospital Medical Center Committee on Research, the American College of Radiology, the American College of Physicians, the American Association of University Professors, an Ad Hoc Committee of our own peers at UC, two separate General Clinical Research Committees of the UC Medical Center and Children's Hospital Medical Center, and the General Accounting Office of the United States Congress (ten groups in all) indicated no violation of medical research.

The authors complain as well about our "surprise press conference," saying that what might have been expected was "the open forum" they "assumed a university offered." They cite only one sentence of the JFA report itself, so that anyone reading their paper would hardly know what kind of attack had been made on them. Yet they include the full statement circulated by our dissident member Dodd Bogart.

In an oblique reply to our charges, the two doctors say that "it is true that some patients with metastatic cancer died in one or more months (or years) after TBI," but that "to infer that our patients were killed by TBI one should have to compare survival of this group to a similar sample of patients with metastatic cancer." The concept of such a comparison had "eluded" the JFA authors, they say, as well as "the press who uncritically publicized this 'report.'"

THE ABUNDANCE AND SIGNIFICANCE of the disclosure materials of March 1, 1994, has perhaps been made more than clear, but the scope of these papers may be gauged, too, by the fact that a member of Robert Newman's staff, paralegal Jennifer Thomas, devoted almost all her working days for over a month to their cataloguing, and that her summaries and indexes alone mounted to nearly a hundred pages.

In the winter of 1972 and for twenty-two years afterward, the existence of these documents—the internal reviews, for instance, where College doctors themselves privately counted up the deaths following radiation—remained unknown to all but those directly involved within the school.

AS TO THE ROLE of Warren Bennis, it must be acknowledged that for a new president of a large university to wage an all-out war on his own medical school would have been a very odd phenomenon. As we have seen, Bennis took the middle road of severing the team's ties with the Defense Department but protecting them from any further investigation. Later he clearly wished it to appear that nothing untoward had happened at UC. Late in 1972 he penned an article for the *Saturday Review of Education*, arguing that media sensationalism had created all the difficulties and casually setting aside the notion that anyone was misused:

> Some terminal cancer patients, with their consent, had been subjected to whole-body radiation as possibly beneficial therapy. Since the Pentagon saw this as a convenient way to gather data that might help protect civilian populations in nuclear warfare, it provided a series of subsidies for the work.[10]

Was this research already in progress when the DOD became involved? Certainly Bennis knew otherwise. The university's own reviewing body, the Suskind Committee, had written that the "systematic investigation of whole body radiation at the University of Cincinnati General Hospital did not begin until the project was funded by the Defense Atomic Support Agency of DOD in 1960."

Patients gave their "consent"? When and where—and to what? It was "civilians" the investigators wanted to study and protect? Jerone Stephens wrote about Bennis's rationalizations in an article in *Politics and Society* in 1973. "Power over poor, sick and helpless people," he said, "is the issue in human experiments. This exploitation will continue until the issue is joined on the basis of power, rather than over smokescreens such as consent forms."

In the summer of 1973 the Kennedy hearings on human experimentation took place, and we learned a great deal about the alliance of U.S. Public Health doctors and Tuskegee Institute. But the bargain between

Kennedy, Gilligan, and Warren Bennis had been struck, and nothing was heard of the radiation injuries and deaths at Cincinnati General Hospital—nor of the other medical crimes of the Cold War era, where American doctors, not Fascists abroad, had conspired with their military to use their own patients in dangerous experiments.

6

Testimonies

It was purely an ambitious and callous act. — Hearing witness
GLORIA NELSON about the radiation of her grandmother,
Amelia Jackson, case study 067

David Egilman in Massachusetts also studied the UC disclosures of
March 1, 1994. At the congressional hearing that followed on April 11,
he entered into the record passages from the letters of Gall, Gaffney,
Shields, and Hess, and made a fierce frontal assault on the whole total
body project. This physician said unequivocally that "cancer therapy
was not the purpose of this research" and repeated his testimony from
the Sharp Committee in January, citing passages from early studies of
whole body radiation that had long since ruled this kind of radiation out
as treatment for solid tumors at the dosage that could be used without
protecting the bone marrow.[1]

Egilman was, however, the only physician who emerged to mount
such an offensive, and the tried-and-true support for the Cincinnati
doctors from the American College of Radiology was again manifest,
this time in the person of Dr. James D. Cox. Even in the face of all that
had been learned about the deaths in Cincinnati, Cox stood loyally by
his fellow radiologists and submitted the following statement:

Radiation therapy is an important part of the armamentarium of
physicians in the care of patients with cancer. Because of its effec-

tiveness in the treatment of local-regional tumors, whole body irradiation has been a subject of research for decades. A bone marrow transplantation is considered a standard part of treatment of many patients with leukemia, lymphoma, and Hodgkin's disease, and is under investigation for myeloma and cancer of the breast. In the era prior to the establishment of bone marrow transplantation to support such treatment, lower (sublethal) doses of total body irradiation were explored for patients with advanced cancer as a possible alternative to no treatment or treatment with cytotoxic chemicals or hormones. The University of Cincinnati studies of total body radiation, conducted between 1960 and 1971, were based on a reasonable hypothesis, were conducted and reported in the scientific literature in keeping with clinical investigations of that period, and seem to have used the accepted standards of informed consent for that period. One might judge them harshly from a perspective 20 years later, but they were reviewed and repeatedly approved by peers of the investigators at the time the studies were conducted.[2]

The Cincinnati hearing was conducted by Representative Jack Brooks's Judiciary Committee and its Subcommittee on Administrative Law and Governmental Relations led by John Bryant, a Democrat from Texas, who conducted the meeting along with David Mann, also a Democrat, and Rob Portman, a Republican. Mann and Portman both represented districts in the Cincinnati area.

This hearing was the largest media event of the crusade, with a gallery full of newspeople. Keith Schneider of the New York Times was present, and the Times printed a detailed article on the day of the hearing and another on the day afterward. These were accurate fine-mesh reports as far as they went, with proper "balanced" quotes from each side, but they left readers pondering whether any serious injury had in fact been sustained by those irradiated.

Three family members were asked to speak to the congressmen, and they gave interesting testimony; but no one from the families of those who died quickly, whom I have referred to as the "short survivors," was invited to appear.

Catherine Hager told the congressmen that while her father, Joseph Mitchell, was being used in U.S. military tests that "shortened or ended his life" (Mitchell lived seventy-four days after radiation), two of his sons were themselves in U.S. military service. One son was in the war zone in Vietnam, and when his father died had to be located by the Red Cross.

An African American woman named Gloria Nelson testified about her grandmother, and when she was questioned about the consent process, told the congressmen that her grandmother could not read or write but that a signed consent form appeared in her records. Nelson also said this:

> The family of Amelia Jackson would like for this committee to know that for the entire 163 days after receiving the radiation, her condition continued to deteriorate. We feel that the 100 rads of partial-body radiation administered to her was cruel and didn't help her condition in any way. It's our belief that she may have lived longer if this experiment had not taken place.
>
> A doctor is someone you trust. His job is to do everything in his power to alleviate your pain and suffering. . . .
>
> Ms. Jackson was used to further Dr. Saenger's professional goals. It was purely an ambitious and callous act.

Joe Larkins, who had driven up to the hearing from Florida, spoke angrily about his father Willard, a Cincinnati craftsman of a certain kind of handmade "picture ring" that could hold a tiny photograph. Larkins had almost escaped radiation; he was among the last five subjects enlisted—all of them treated even while the probing Hess review was taking place. Joe Larkins said plainly that no one in his family, including his mother, had any knowledge that his father was being used in an experiment. "No person," Larkins said, "and I emphasize NO person would willingly consent to a treatment with any degree of fatality involved."

President Steger had just testified to the cooperation and complete openness now being manifested by the university, but Larkins informed the congressmen that after repeated requests his family had yet to be provided their father's hospital records. Over two months had elapsed since Laura Schneider had located this family and they had joined the lawsuit and begun to seek their records. "I beseech you to order the University of Cincinnati to release the patient records," he said; "they are hedging to save their own skin."

Before the hearing, I had been away in Central America, had not known I was being invited to appear until two days before the proceedings, was greatly troubled by the lights, and did not feel I was a very effective witness. But it was good fortune that the three family members seemed to be troubled by very little, had carefully prepared, and spoke with wonderful feeling and confidence.

I expressed regret at the absence of testimony from the families of short survivors, and I discussed the case of Margaret Bacon. Bacon was the African American schoolteacher who, though not at all severely ill when irradiated, had died only six days after her treatment and the accompanying operations on her bone marrow, the shortest survivor of all.

Bacon had only recently been identified, and her family was not yet known to the press. In the crowd that milled in the room afterward, I met Joseph Willis, Bacon's great-nephew. I knew Willis had been living with his aunt at the time of her death, and I wanted him to talk to Linda Reeves of the Enquirer. Reeves was hobbled by recent surgery on her foot, but she propped her cane against a chair and got out her notebook to talk to Willis. Within the mass of radiation newsprint the next day, we saw a good report on Margaret Bacon and her nephew.

I also met that day for the first time one of the most hardworking journalists I ever expect to encounter, Akira Tashiro. Tashiro is the senior staff writer for the Chukogu Shimbun, the daily paper of Hiroshima City, which prints 700,000 papers each morning and another 100,000 in the evening. Tashiro would later come one day to my office at UC, and I learned quite a lot about him. He had already written a great deal about radiation issues around the world and showed me an English translation of a volume recently published by the Chugoku Shimbun. It was titled Exposure: Victims of Radiation Speak Out (The Chugoku Newspaper, 1992.) It featured five pieces on U.S. radiation traumas, including "Hanford's Hidden Past," "Uranium Mining on the Navajo Reservation," and "The Burden of Nuclear Supremacy." The volume also included chapters on radiation disasters and issues around the world: "The Spread of Nuclear Contamination over Sweden," for instance, and such pieces as "Thorium Contamination in Malaysia" and "Namibia's Uranium Mines."

Tashiro would be in the United States for a hundred days, he said, covering all the new findings about our Cold War radiation. Months later he would call me from Hiroshima City still trimming up a series of articles on Cincinnati. His extremely detailed reports on U.S. radiation would run daily in his paper for many months and would constitute the most comprehensive studies yet done on our Cold War tests.

EUGENE SAENGER APPEARED at the Cincinnati hearing and made the only public presentation he would make on the UC experiments. I had never encountered Saenger in person until the morning of the hearing, and I have seen him since only once — in another federal courtroom the following October.

Dr. Saenger is a hometown boy who went to the public college-preparatory school, Walnut Hills, graduated cum laude from Harvard, returned to UC for his medical degree, and became a professor there soon afterward, in 1949. His whole career was then forged at UC, except for a two-year break as an Army major during and after the Korean War, at Fort Sam Houston in Texas (1953–55). He was chief of the radioisotope laboratory at Brooke Army Hospital there; he did not serve in the combat area itself. (He had not volunteered for duty during World War II but stayed on as an intern in Cincinnati and then a resident.) His consultantships in radiology at Oak Ridge, with the Defense Atomic Support Agency, the Atomic Energy Commission, and other military agencies and hospitals, are manifold. He has in fact been closely involved with the U.S. military virtually all his working life. His record of memberships, lectureships, papers, and publications is a highly complex one with a great many honors and distinctions in his field.

In 1987 Saenger retired from UC, and at the time of the hearing in 1994 he was seventy-seven years old. He was seen that day to be a slight man of good bearing and appearance, almost elegant in dress. He spoke somewhat softly and mildly but with confidence and composure. He was assisted with his documents by his son, who seemed attentive to his every need.

Many members of the local progressive community were among

those present in the room that day, people involved over the years in human rights issues of various kinds, and there was clearly great attentiveness to Dr. Saenger's presentation. The five-minute allocation for testimonies had apparently been held not to apply in his case, and he read a detailed version of the ten-page testimony already sent to the panelists. This prepared testimony was made available at the hearing, as is the custom, and was handsomely packaged within a thick volume of related documents, including a massive curriculum vitae of thirty pages.

What was almost surprising about Saenger's presentation was its very positive tone, not quite what one might expect from a man being tested before the bar of medical justice. The opening of his prepared testimony sounded much like an upbeat, good-news report on new treatments for cancer:

> I am Eugene L. Saenger, M.D. of Cincinnati. It is a privilege for me to speak before the distinguished sub-committee of the Judiciary Committee of the U. S. House of Representatives to present a summary of our work on the treatment of far advanced cancer and the effects of wide field radiation therapy, work which I was privileged to direct and the results of which I am proud.

Saenger went on to describe his training, his professorships, consultantships, and awards—the de Hevesy Nuclear Pioneer Award, for instance, of the Society of Nuclear Medicine—and his one hundred and eighty-seven publications, with colleagues, in the scientific literature.

In both his prepared statement and his oral delivery he then outlined "several important points" summarizing the work of the radiation project:

> A. One purpose of the study was the treatment of patients with far advanced cancer for whom the goal was the relief of pain, shrinkage of cancer and improvement in well being.
>
> B. A second purpose was to study the systemic effects of radiation on the patient.
>
> C. Treatment was given only if benefit to the patient was anticipated.
>
> D. Patients were chiefly from the Cincinnati General Hospital.

Selection was based only on the presence of advanced cancer and where no other therapy was considered to be as or more efficacious than then available chemotherapy. Race, IQ, or socioeconomic standing were not selection factors.

E. Treatment was paid for by Cincinnati General Hospital and the National Institutes of Health. No Department of Defense funds were used for treatment or patient care or decisions regarding therapy or patient reimbursement.

F. Patients were told that the treatment might help them and were cautioned that it might not. Some patients chose not to be treated.

G. There was nothing secret about our work. There was nothing secret as to its being conducted. There was nothing secret about the findings obtained.[3]

For those who had followed the developing story of the tests, there was one considerable surprise in Saenger's presentation, and in fact he diverged from his written text to state this point most emphatically: he now felt, he said, "upon reexamination of the records," that the eight deaths he had himself effectually conceded to radiation in the past were not radiation deaths at all but simply cancer deaths. ("Saenger: Tests Didn't Kill" said the *Enquirer* the next day.) Saenger stated that patients were receiving other forms of treatment at the same time, and that their cancers were growing "exponentially." For these reasons, he continued, "it is not possible to identify a single form of treatment or the rapid growth of cancer as being the single contributing cause of death. It most likely would be the rate of growth of the cancer itself."[4] (The full text of Saenger's prepared testimony can be read in the appendix to this volume.)

If this volte-face on the question of loss of life from radiation seemed far-fetched, another aspect of Saenger's testimony proved for some, for a time at least, to be somewhat more disconcerting. Dr. Saenger stated that total body irradiation for cancer treatment had been used in many hospitals around the country with good results both in the past and present, and that at the time he spoke much higher doses were being applied than ever contemplated by the UC team. He listed in an appendix to his prepared statement many citations in the medical literature concerning total body radiation for cancer.

But this claim was made with only passing reference to a number of salient differences between these applications and that of the UC team—to the fact, for instance, that this type of radiation, generally given in divided doses and for nonlocalized tumors, is applied only where the bone marrow can be protected and the patient shielded from deadly infection in a number of ways not employed in the project at UC.

It was gratifying to see that for this hearing David Mann had prepared himself quite admirably. He no longer felt that a person who was not a doctor could not ask questions of those who were, and he was ready with sharp sallies that cut right to the bone of the matter, and if he did not like the answers, he probed and probed again. Why had there been nothing in the DOD reports about treatment for cancer? Why had Saenger himself noted in 1973 that eight patients may have died of radiation, and yet was now refuting his own calculations? Was it not true that the alleged cancer treatments had not begun before the military funding came in, and had not continued after these funds were lost? If this new treatment was beneficial, Mann asked, why wasn't this knowledge shared with other hospitals in town?

Mann also had sharp interrogatories about the Suskind Report, and he noted that Raymond Suskind was in the room. Did Dr. Saenger disagree with the Suskind Committee statement of 1972 that other hospitals had not been treating "localized cancers" with whole body exposures? "Do you agree with that statement?" Mann asked.

DR. SAENGER: Well, there are three references that are cited there. We have cited in the documents that we have prepared for this a great many papers on this subject. And this was written by the committee. It was not written by me.

MR. MANN: Do you disagree with this statement, sir?

DR. SAENGER: All I can say is it is the committee's opinion. I did not write this report.

MR. MANN: Yes, sir. Do you agree or disagree—

DR. SAENGER: I don't have to agree or disagree with it. Their survey of the literature is their survey.

MR. MANN: I am asking you, sir, whether, in your professional judgment or professional opinion, do you—you—I am asking you to develop an opinion. Do you agree or not agree? (p. 280)

John Bryant had blows of his own to land, but Rob Portman, the Republican, appeared to have no serious concerns with the tests; his respectful questions seemed calculated to give Saenger plenty of room for long, unchallenged responses.

Bryant, the Democrat from Texas, grilled the witness repeatedly about the care and treatment of patients. Why were they not routinely given nausea medicines? If they "complained," they *were* given such medicines, Saenger replied. Were they or were they not "psychologically isolated," as the DOD reports had suggested? Saenger felt the radiation patients were better treated than most and "were certainly not isolated or disregarded."

"Why," Bryant asked, "weren't these people told they might die. . . ?" Saenger said he had looked at a great many consent forms and had yet to see one in which "the risk of death was explicitly stated." He said, "I think we explained to the patients that they might benefit and they very well may not benefit from the treatment."

TO BECOME A WITNESS at a congressional hearing, as no doubt many people know, is not necessarily an agreeable or logical experience. This affair was poorly arranged, and the staff never succeeded, for instance, in organizing the written testimonies properly or negotiating with any coherence the printed transcript that followed.

My own experience was probably not very different from that of others, but in order to have the JFA report included in the hearing record, as was originally agreed would be done, I had to seek the help of the panelists. The proofing copy of my testimony was a badly mangled draft and was first sent to the wrong address; by the time it reached me it was already due back at the printer—and so on and so forth. Even the original inquiries from the committee had been confused and condescending. I was called weeks beforehand to see if I would be available but not informed as to whether I would be invited or not. (It was as if a friend should call to say, "We're having a get-together over at our house and we'd like to know whether you'd be available if we decide to invite you.")

During the question-and-answer period following my own testimony, John Bryant gave me very short shrift and grew terse and testy when I said that I felt nothing would prevent the kind of abuse of sick people we had had in Cincinnati except a national health service, where everyone could go to doctors of their choosing and not be trapped in public hospitals or low-budget HMOs, where new captive populations for research might increasingly be found. Bryant said, in effect, that all that was irrelevant and he had hoped not to hear a word about it, nor was he interested in my recommendation that we have common citizens on all boards that decide how hospitals, universities, and medical services are organized. "If we can't do that," I stated, "we are not a democracy, in my opinion."

Such recommendations as these are just common sense, surely, and would meet with most people's approval, yet of course our leaders purport to find them ridiculous.

I was still being asked, this time by Portman, if I were a physician. No, I was not, I replied, I was an English professor, but medicine was not, it seemed to me, a "magic science," a body of knowledge "different from all other bodies of knowledge that only certified people can understand." I added that there was, needless to say, a great deal I had not studied and did not know about cancer and that I was happy to be working with David Egilman.

The room in the federal courthouse in which the hearing took place was far too small for all those who wanted to attend. Many of the families and friends of the victims were excluded, and they and others lined the corridor outside, where a loudspeaker was supposed to keep them abreast, but did not seem to work. Local politicians and dignitaries, with nothing personal at stake, were, on the other hand, ushered courteously inside.

AT THIS HEARING of 1994, no physician but David Egilman spoke on behalf of the subjects, and those of us critical of the tests continued to work, just as Saenger and Silberstein had said we had back in the seventies, within a veritable blockade of expert opinion about the injuries sustained. Of course there were medical doctors on the national committee formed that winter by President Clinton, and for a time we vested considerable hope in them. But sadly, as we shall see below, the two physicians most active on the panel were radiologists known to Eugene Saenger, intent on containing the charges against him.

I viewed that spring on C-Span a four-hour session of this committee, and after that I knew it would be a fierce challenge to extract anything from this official group that would help resolve our case or any other case. Obfuscation and general beating around the bush of every kind is an ever-present fact of life in the academic world from which these specialists came, but for any group to spend no less than four long hours saying exactly nothing was a triumph, I felt, of smothered speech. That these individuals had before them or expected to have before them any actual real-life population injured by radiation—brought upon them by their own government—no one would have guessed from the discussion that day.

If the last refuge from human reality is high-minded philosophy and abstraction, we had plenty of that. First, last, and always, such round-abouters must define their terms, and definitions were definitely the order of the day. What is a human experiment? What is informed consent? These were the questions being wisely pondered and re-pondered on that occasion, as if no one had ever reflected on them before. Human pain, injury, and death did not enter the picture and would seldom enter it in the year and more to come of these deliberations.

The Cincinnati case would become the single case most studied by the Committee, and after the congressional hearing of April 11 the swayings and swingings back and forth during the periods when the group was examining our case became the major focus of the continuing publicity around the tests. Had there been wrongdoing in Cincinnati—and if so, was the U.S. government implicated in any way, along with the researchers? These questions were asked and reasked, but we read in the Cincinnati papers that they were very difficult, very complex questions, and could not be resolved without massive research into the state of medical affairs during the years the experiments were taking place.

All summer we read about this stalwart search of the Committee for answers to our case and others, but answers always eluded them. The answer was, we began to see, that there was no answer. The tasks the Committee needed to do to resolve these questions, it had not been charged to do, as it turned out, or was not equipped to do. It could not possibly examine hospital records, for instance, or the cases of any individuals said to be injured. And yet the charge to the Committee was apparently not so very narrow as that. Speaking of President Clinton, the Committee said in its preface to the Final Report, "He urged us to be fair, thorough, and unafraid to shine the light of truth on this hidden and poorly understood aspect of our nation's past."[5]

When the Committee first began meeting in late April 1994, I had assumed, once more, that my own work around these tests would now be taken up by individuals much more knowledgeable than I was about medicine and human research, and that I would become an interested observer. But that was a strange delusion. I eventually came to feel that doctors on the Committee were constantly issuing opinions that played fast and loose with the facts of the case as I knew them to be, and with what I was learning from the hospital records and the conditions of the victims before radiation, and so it was inevitable that I would in time come to enter into a good many dialogues with Gary Stern, the staff member of the Committee who was coordinating the study of our case, and to attempt to reply through him to the Committee radiologists, as they set about to protect the researchers instead of their victims.

IN OCTOBER the Advisory Committee on Human Radiation Experiments 1944–74 sent three of its experts and a group of Committee staff to Cincinnati for an all-day public meeting on our case and other cases in our vicinity. Any citizen who had a radiation story to tell was granted five minutes of testimony, and even for this slender slot people came from far and wide to tell their stories.

Many of us in Cincinnati heard for the first time, for instance, the story of the Atomic Veterans. We heard of the tragic exposures and accidents at the nuclear plant two hours away in Portsmouth, West Virginia. We heard of the body-snatching of deceased workers from the nearby Fernald plant—for the sake of the secret testing of certain body parts for the study of radiation injury.

On this twenty-first day of October, 1994, the Committee sent us a retired bank vice president from Omaha, Lois L. Norris, and two physicians: Reed Tuckson, president of Charles Drew University of Medicine and Science in Los Angeles, and Mary Ann Stevenson, assistant professor of Radiation Oncology at Harvard. But these individuals added nothing that day to our understanding of the medical facts of our case or any other case; we never knew what they personally thought or where they stood, and their infrequent and somewhat faltering questions did not reassure us that they had even read our materials. It seemed obvious that they had not studied; they had not bothered to prepare themselves. In good hearing form, they simply sat on their risers in our local hotel meeting hall; they listened (we presume); they called our names and watched us take our seats before the TV lights. The leader of the panel assured us of their "concern" and that each one of our testimonies would be most carefully attended to.

We never knew anything at all of the feelings, views, and reactions these panelists had to the long grievous train of wounded statements they heard that day.

Eleven Cincinnati family members spoke, and they gave sharp and compelling testimony. It had become known that Eugene Saenger was suffering from bladder cancer, and Joe Larkins, who had also spoken at the April hearing and whose father Willard had lived eighty days after being irradiated in 1971, told the panel he would like to know whether Dr. Saenger had been himself treated with whole body radiation. We had bladder cancer patients among our victims, and I thought it was a fair question to ask.

In my own statement I asked the panelists not to be part of the continuing cover-up. *Tell the country the truth about us,* I said. I reminded them that 42 percent of the patients who received the higher doses of radiation had died within a matter of weeks, and said I felt the doctors should have experimented on each other or on themselves—a practice not unheard of in human research after all—or if they truly felt these treatments were beneficial, on the cancer victims within their own families.

I spoke again of Maude Jacobs, the mother with kids at home who got herself to the hospital on her own for her treatment and died twenty-five days later, in pain, and suffering the mental derangement the doctors were studying for the military. I could not say a great deal in the time allotted, but because the Jacobs family were present that day, I was remembering every detail of their ordeal.

When her mother had been admitted to the hospital the day after her radiation, Lilian Pagano, Jacobs's oldest child, had packed her bag and her coffeepot and moved into her mother's hospital room, and I knew that she remembered her suffering all too well. "I feel like I'm on fire, Lil," she had told me her mother had said—and that she had had all kinds of strange hallucinations. She imagined that one of her babies of years ago was in the hospital room. "Don't drop the baby, Lil," she had cried out one day. "Put him on the bed!" Somehow, when the priest came, her mother's senses would seem to return. "Are you ready, Maude, to meet the lord?" he asked her, and her reply seemed beautiful and good: "Yes I am, Father." [6]

I was remembering all this as the Jacobs's turn to testify came up and three of Jacobs's children moved forward to confront the panel. But when they would start to speak, hardly any voice would come from them, and finally they simply sat weeping helplessly. There was a very long silence in the room, and other heads were bowed as well.

Of course none of the eleven researchers made an appearance that day or had anything to communicate, though we later learned that on the day before the meeting Eugene Saenger had given a private interview to members of the Committee staff; according to Gary Stern, one condition Saenger had set for this meeting was that he not be questioned about any individual subject.

The only satisfaction for the people who came to speak their griefs that day in Cincinnati was the presence of cameras, which might show on the evening news a minute or two of what was said. Peg Rusconi stood up front beside her cameraman all day, and filed a detailed report which she edited to her own liking. Linda Reeves sat on the front row with her notebook for the entire proceedings, which went on into the very late afternoon, and she had a full notebook and a great deal to write about when she returned late that day to her newsroom, but it happened that an *Enquirer* night editor killed most of the story as she was just sitting down to compose it. It had been a hard painful day; this was too much, Reeves said, and she wept with frustration. "I really lost it," she said.

As to physicians, we had had, on this occasion, no doctor to speak up for those irradiated. One local physician, Judy Daniels, Medical Director of the Cincinnati Health Department, had agreed to speak. Daniels was serving on the local panel set up by City Council, had read the DOD documents, and had spoken out quite clearly about the unconvincing defenses of the researchers.

But on the day of the hearing, this doctor did not appear, and the reporters said she was answering no calls that day. Daniels told me later on that city attorneys had called her in on the afternoon before the hearing and made it more than clear that she must not participate. The city, as past owner of the hospital, had become a defendant in the lawsuit, and Daniels was given no choice but to withdraw. She was told that it would be her "personal responsibility" if, because of her testimony, things went wrong. It was contended that the university might choose not to cooperate in the city's defense, in spite of agreements made when the contract between the two entities had been signed back in 1962, when the management of the hospital had been given over to the control of the university.

"I am not proud of this," Daniels has said, "but under the circumstances I did not feel I could go against them."[7]

IN OCTOBER 1995, a year after its Cincinnati small panel meeting, the Advisory Committee on Human Radiation Experiments (ACHRE) made its report to President Clinton on the deliberate exposures of people by their government during the three decades following World War II. The report fills a volume of 925 pages.

Over the year and a half of its endeavors, the Committee had heard voluminous testimony about the Cincinnati case. Twice members of the organization of surviving families had traveled from Cincinnati to Washington to speak before the Committee. (They paid their own way, or accepted donations from those of us back home, and shared their hotel rooms. They were not of course on anyone's per diem.)

David Egilman spoke to the Committee several times, as did one of the Cincinnati attorneys, David Thompson, and a publicist for a California firm representing a set of families, Geoffrey Sea. It happened that an individual living in Washington, D. C. and working in a hospital there, Gwendon Plair, had learned that his mother Beatrice had been one of those irradiated in 1964, and Plair made a number of appearances before the Committee and attempted to act as liaison between the Committee and the families back home.

Two members of the ACHRE staff, attorneys Gary Stern and Jonathan Engel, interviewed Eugene Saenger and myself during their stay in Cincinnati in October, and Saenger had also consented earlier that fall to be interviewed by a Committee staff physician, Ronald Neumann. Though all activities and records of the Committee were supposed to be public, the first Saenger interview remained unknown for some time, and neither of his interview transcripts were made available for many months after the events, in spite of repeated requests for them.

Stern and Engel spent several hours with me in my office at UC taping my "oral history," as these sessions were being termed. I felt we were at that time definitely at a low point with regard to the kind of explorations the Committee was willing to make. What we were reading in the papers was, as suggested, less than encouraging; we read of extended Committee debates as to whether the UC investigators could have known in 1960 that total body radiation was harmful in the doses they expected to apply and not considered useful, anyway, for radioresistant cancers.

The simple commonsense reply to this was that if the doctors had not known of these dangers in 1960, they did know by 1961 and 1962, when patients were already being lost, and yet they had proceeded with the radiations for another ten years. The doctors and their supporters had never been able to show that other hospitals were administering whole body radiation as routine cancer treatment for breast cancer and other solid tumors, but the Committee said it could not be sure this had never taken place, and so their search for such hospitals had to continue.

We must not charge doctors simply with not knowing in the past what we know today, this argument went. Well and good — but in our case, this presented itself as a remarkably unproductive argument, and more than anything else simply a last-ditch struggle of the radiologists on the Committee to degrade once again the climate of debate. I had long since begun to feel very tired of all this, simply bored by the incredible repetitiveness of the decades-long united front of medical people to explain away the obvious causes and circumstances of the Cincinnati deaths, beginning with the 1972 review by the American College of Radiology, the archetype of the various cover-ups, and a gushing fountain, it seemed to me, of falsehoods and fabrications.[8]

I said all this in very plain terms to the staff interviewers that October. I felt there was no longer any reason not to, and apparently such arguments as I was making had some effect on my interlocutors that day, and all in all, those of us who continued to press and press again the feet of the Committee to the fire of the plain truths of the Cincinnati case did keep the radiologists in the group from succeeding in pulling another thick coverlet over what had taken place.

As their report developed, the Committee staff sent me for my comments the draft chapters on Cincinnati as they came along, and I sent back my critiques. In time I also asked for and received the individual position papers of Dr. Eli Glatstein, a physician in Radiation Oncology at the University of Texas in Dallas, and Dr. Henry Royal, a specialist in Nuclear Medicine at Washington University School of Medicine in St. Louis. It seemed to me that these two physicians were attempting to water down, if not wash completely away, the staff findings they did not like.

Glatstein felt strongly that it was not so much work for the military that had led to the Cincinnati tests, but the availability in the late fifties of "new technology" for radiation treatment. He wrote on March 30, 1995, in his comment on the draft final report of the Committee, that "inasmuch as Dr. Saenger himself was not part of the physician group that made decisions about which patients to treat, we have no evidence that these physicians did not think that they were offering their patients an effective form of treatment." He thought it likely that the doctors believed "there was some slim hope" that their subjects would benefit. Patients can tolerate the doses applied, he said, though they need "intensive support" throughout the procedure that was not being provided in the 1960s. "I am not trying to justify what they have done," he wrote to the Committee, "but I do not think we are giving them the benefit of any doubts, and I believe there are many doubts." The draft report was "a bit unfair to the people from Cincinnati," Glatstein wrote. "Dr. Saenger did not give those patients cancer," he said. "That does not excuse him from at the very least what must be construed as poor judgment, and possibly malpractice." [9]

Henry Royal saw in the tests a great many complexities that made it difficult to condemn what had taken place. Experimental treatment in the interest of the patient does sometimes result in death, he reminded the Committee, and we must look at the "net benefit" and "net harm," an equation he said was hard to calculate for the Cincinnati tests. On the issue of the purposes of research, he wrote, "The universal problem is the conflict between what is best for the patients and what is most desirable for science. That problem has not gone away and will not go away." [10]

The radiation oncologist from Harvard who had heard testimony in Cincinnati, Mary Ann Stevenson, was somewhat more inclined than her associates to regret what had taken place. "Given what we know now," she wrote the Committee, "the UC tbi study probably should not have continued for over a decade, with no clear benefit for patients and no appreciable results for biomedical research." [11]

When the ACHRE report was issued, I was asked to serve as the spokesperson for the Cincinnati families, and in many ways a show was made of valuing my input and participation; indeed the JFA report remained a primary guide for the writing up of our case, and many of the passages I had originally gleaned from the doctors' DOD reports—if not the critical ones on death-by-radiation—reappeared in draft after draft just as I had formed them. Yet I knew that all any of us could hope to do was to moderate the effort being made to protect the researchers from any final judgment, and it must be said that in the end such truth as emerged was varnished to a rather high shine.

Some clear history was composed, by staff writers, of the somewhat complex events within the military that had led to the original sponsoring of our tests and others, but again, the specific outcomes for victims remained largely hidden from view.

It was not clearly recommended that the surviving families in Cincinnati be offered even an apology, much less the financial compensation many thought the Committee might ask Congress to provide—and so it was in most of the other cases as well. Still, taking it all in all, the final Committee report was not nearly so problematic for our cause as it had sometimes promised to be. It was possible for us to acclaim it in the papers as "a victory for the families," and it probably wrote an end to the willingness of the doctors' backers and insurers to take their case to trial. Glatstein and Royal were overruled on a number of points even as they prevailed on others, and in spite of the curious contradictions of the report's finale, anyone reading closely the factual record it provides will be able to piece together rather tightly the events that had taken place in our hospital.

George Annas has noted that Joseph Heller, in his funny and satiric novel *Good as Gold*, describes just such a presidential committee. The character Gold is writing up the commission's final report, and he receives these instructions from the group:

Make it short . . . and make it long. Make it clear and make it fuzzy. Make it short by coming right to each point. Then make it long by qualifying those points so that nobody can tell the qualifications from the points or ever figure out what we're talking about.[12]

In certain individual passages the ACHRE report was highly critical of the UC tests—censorious and condemning, one could say—but in other sections there was more than a touch of just the kind of circumlocution Heller describes.

At the time of this report in 1995, no public funds had been vouchsafed, or even proposed, for radiation victims or their surviving families, yet by the end of fiscal year 1995, $6,188,988 had been contributed by the taxpayers to fund the Committee itself, large hourly fees and per diems, of course, for the specialists involved, and smart salaries as well for the very large staff.[13]

For myself, I have been able to say that I have never received any pay for my own work on this case; no one hired me to look into the matter, sit on panels, consult on lawsuits, write or speak. But after all, I was being paid a salary by the citizens of Ohio for my endeavors in their university. I felt that it was only reasonable that I try to protect their interests there in whatever ways I could, and I assume that they expected me to do exactly that. Indeed I often said in 1994 and '95, when people asked me why I had involved myself in this case, that I was just trying to earn my pay at my university. I have often explained, or tried to explain, that I believe that social change can take place, and that we need only look about us to see that a great many nonexperts and ordinary people, active around issues of justice and fair play in their own communities, are finding ways to move things along, even in the very dark times in which we are living.

During that fall of the October meeting of the Clinton Committee, I was reading with a class a book I especially liked to read with students, Kurt Vonnegut's Slaughterhouse Five, which describes the bombing of Dresden by U.S. forces during World War II. Vonnegut draws an awesome picture of American violence in Dresden, and in fact the only good life that can be imagined in the book is in the fantasy land constantly daydreamed by Billy Pilgrim after the war, where "everything is beautiful and nothing hurts." Still, Vonnegut's narrator contends that there are three things in life we cannot change — the past, the present, and the future. It may certainly seem this way at times, yet Vonnegut himself has shown by his own rebellious acts that he does not believe that change for the better cannot be brought about and is not worth struggling for.

WHEN THE ACHRE REPORT appeared in 1995, one item I read at once was a statement in the back of the volume by Jay Katz, the only Committee member represented by an individual statement. This article of eight pages was by way of dissent, I think it could be said, from the findings of the Committee on an issue that was for Katz of primary importance: the question of whether or not human research in the nineties and beyond was still something to be feared. Clearly, Katz does not think our troubles are behind us.

The Advisory Committee commissioned a study of the proposals for human research sent to a large number of hospital review boards, and of these proposals, Katz says he found fully 50 percent "ethically unacceptable" and another 24 percent "of concern." Katz wrote that what had been learned, in part, from the hospital radiation tests of the Cold War, along with other post–World War II medical experiments, was that sick people — simply patients, that is — were the most vulnerable population of all. Sick people are the most easily deceived, he said. The more ill the patient, the more easily drawn into dubious or dangerous experiments, and whether patients are helped or hurt, their "remaining quality of life" is seldom even a consideration, he wrote.

Katz is an emeritus professor of law and medicine at Yale. He was a contributor to the Nuremberg issue of the *Journal of the American Medical Association* in 1996 and is the author of a well-known volume of studies on the legal issues of human research, *Experimentation with Human Beings* (1972).[14]

An editorial in the JAMA issue on Nuremberg also asked some radical questions about the frightening forces coming down today on people who are ill. In this statement, coauthored by Michael Grodin and George Annas, we read this: "The fact that we are not Nazis does not mean we are immune from seduction by social, political, or economic organizations that seek to corrupt medicine for their own ends."[15] George Annas is the lead author of the definitive study of modern-day medical law, *American Health Law* (1990), a volume dedicated to "all those who struggle for justice in health care."

One may well ask what new cover-ups of what *new* medical crimes are in the making now, even as we study the deadly assaults of the past.

AS TO THE NAZI ANALOGY, we find it, from time to time, within government dialogues on human experiments during the Cold War.[16]

When David Egilman first read the JFA Report in the late eighties, during his years in Cincinnati with NIOSH, he came out to my house one evening to see the DOD papers and to take away copies of patient profiles. In turn he showed my husband and me a certain very curious letter addressed to a doctor in the Atomic Energy Commission. This letter had become known among various people studying the Defense Department and was sometimes referred to as "the Buchenwald touch letter." It was written in 1950 by a well-known radiologist, Joseph Hamilton, to the director of the AEC medical division, Dr. Shields Warren.[17]

Ever since the U.S. nuclear attacks on Japan, the U.S. military had worried greatly over what would happen if *we* became the target of a nuclear bomb. Atomic scientists in the United States had frightened themselves, along with the rest of the world, with the savage power they had helped unleash on Hiroshima and Nagasaki. Hamilton was estimating for Warren the amount of radiation it might take to incapacitate "military and civilian personnel" during a war. He said that 150 roentgens "would be pretty much of an incapacitating dose" but that this dose would be "unlikely to lead to an appreciable number of fatalities," except for individuals whose health was already compromised.

Roentgens are a measure of the radiation dose emitted by a machine; a *rad* represents the estimated radiation actually absorbed by the tissues of the body and is the measure used most often by the Cincinnati doctors. According to Eugene Saenger and others, it takes more than one roentgen to effect a rad, and thus we note that over thirty Cincinnati subjects received a dose of radiation larger than Hamilton's 150 roentgens.[18]

More information, Hamilton said, was needed about the dangers at this level, and he discussed the pros and cons of irradiating chimpanzees. "If this is to be done in humans," he said, "I feel that those concerned in the Atomic Energy Commission would be subject to considerable criticism, as admittedly this would have a little of the Buchenwald touch."

Hamilton assumed that in such human research "volunteers" would be used and he felt they should be "on a freer basis than inmates of a prison." But he added that he did not have "any very constructive ideas as to where one would turn for such volunteers should this plan be put into execution." Thinking of the long-term side effects of radiation, he said that there was "much to recommend the use of adult males past the age of fifty in good physical status."

We know now, of course, where in the country these "volunteers" were eventually found, that ten years after this discussion took place, close to a hundred cancer patients would begin to be recruited in a hospital in Cincinnati, and that about a quarter of these subjects would die within a few weeks of being irradiated. In 1963 the Cincinnati doctors would write of their studies that they were designed "to obtain new information about the metabolic effects of total body and partial body irradiation" and that this information was "necessary to provide knowledge of combat effectiveness of troops." [19]

During the October hearing of 1994, eleven of the Cincinnati families remembered their dead mothers and fathers and other relations, and struck angrily back at their assailants.

A man named Herbert Varin, who had been twenty-two when his mother was irradiated in 1967, told the panelists that he was his mother's only child and close to her in her illness and death, along with an aunt, and that neither he nor his aunt had any idea that with any of his mother's treatments an experiment was being performed.

When Varin finished his testimony, he thought of something he wanted to add. He said that his mother had always remembered John F. Kennedy's appeal for people to ask not what their country could do for them, but what they could do for their country. But did that mean, he wondered, that people were being asked to give up their bodies to military tests? "I don't believe that saying meant—that people should be total-body irradiated," Varin said. [20]

Back in Washington that November, the ACHRE panelists and other Committee members had a long round-table talk about the Cincinnati tests. Gary Stern had come away from this meeting, and from our talk at the university, with clearly disturbed ideas about what had happened in Cincinnati. In Washington Stern put the case against the researchers to the Committee quite firmly and repeated my own charge that regardless of what the doctors knew or did not know about the dangers when they began, they had continued the radiations long after people had begun to be lost and injured.

But Ronald Neumann, along with Glatstein, Royal, and others, went on equivocating and clouding over once again the plain facts of the case, saying that all they were looking into as a committee, anyway, was whether people had given their *consent* to the exposures. Neumann, in his introductory statement to the group on November 14, said, "it's extraordinarily difficult to prove and we've not tried to prove individual harm with any of the subjects in these experiments because the fundamental question comes down to again informed consent. . . ." He reminds the Committee that "in spite of their apparent good health," the patients used "all did have advanced metastatic carcinoma of one type or another whose outlook long term certainly wasn't good." Even analyzing the researchers' attempts at bone marrow replacement would be "fraught with difficulty," he maintained, if the Committee were to attempt to do it "on a medical or scientific basis." [21]

Most Committee members appeared to agree that the "science" could not be studied and that the issue was simply whether or not "ethical informed consent" had been attained, and even that was said to be a difficult matter to decide. Ruth Macklin tried rather hard, without much success, to probe the issue of whether or not victims were truly sick and dying when exposed. Without such knowledge, she was asking, how could risks be assessed, or the question settled as to whether individuals had given their consent to these risks? [22]

From time to time Committee member Jay Katz struck quite a different note from the others. He said that "in a sense poor Dr. Saenger was really a triple agent here. I've talked about the problems of physician investigators being double agents, both committed to science and to the patient, and here he's also committed to the defense establishment, and I was struck, perhaps even more than you were, by his use of relatively healthy cancer patients." [23] But many Committee members did not share these concerns of Dr. Katz.

When Gary Stern wrote up for the Committee the story of the hospital radiations during the Cold War and their origins in the debates within the Defense Department, he included, in certain drafts, Joseph Hamilton's letter of 1950, with its line about the "Buchenwald touch." At times this letter disappeared from the running drafts, but when the final version of the Committee's report appeared, the haunting image of Buchenwald, and a passage from Hamilton's letter, had been restored.

IN 1995 FEDERAL JUDGE Sandra Beckwith, denying the Cincinnati researchers' claims of immunity from prosecution as public doctors just carrying out their normal functions, would write that "the Nuremberg Code is part of the law of humanity." "It is inconceivable to the Court," she wrote, "that the . . . Defendants, when allegedly planning to perform radiation experiments on unwitting subjects, were not moved to pause or rethink their procedures in light of the forceful dictates of the Nuremberg Tribunal. . . ." [24]

As for Joseph Hamilton's formula for using "adult males past the age of fifty in good physical status," one is moved to reflect on whether Hamilton and his correspondent Shields Warren had considered that they themselves fitted this profile. Eugene Saenger fitted this profile. Edward Gall and Clifford Grulee were also good fits, as was the supervising physician for the radiations up until 1967, Ben I. Friedman. As deeply concerned as these men were about the defense and well-being of the country, none, as far as we know, ever offered up his own body for whole body exposure.

7

Author's Intermezzo

And what shoulder, & what art, could twist the sinews of thy heart?—WILLIAM BLAKE, "The Tyger"

The two hearings in Cincinnati in 1994 were vivid events: certain personae of this drama had been seen on a public stage for the first time. No concessions had been wrung from Eugene Saenger, of course, but the president of the university, in his own testimony before the congressional committee, had kept a careful distance between himself and the doctors, and in fact, the disclosures of March 1 had already marked a retreat in UC's long battle to cover over in thick wrappings of evasions, irrelevancies, and downright untruths the real facts about the radiations in the whole body room down the narrow winding tunnels underneath the hospital—the catacombs, one could almost say, of the radiological laboratories of General Hospital.

This labyrinth of strange metallic-looking tunnels, with long sheaths of exposed pipes overhead, had been constructed years ago when contagious diseases were a serious problem and some patients needed to be isolated. The hospital of that day had been built to include separate annexes, or "pavilions," for certain patient populations; and these pavilions, as they are still called today, were connected to each other and to the main building by the tunnels underground. It was these old tunneled corridors I had walked down years ago to see Edward Silberstein in his little nook of an office down there; but in the later incarnation of the radiation publicity in the nineties, I did not visit those precincts again.

During that bitter winter of 1994, the temperatures in our valley sank on some nights to twenty below, and looking out the window of my back door, I could see rows of great sharp icicles bristling down from our stoop like giant stalactites. So strange they were that I went out on the porch one day to take their pictures.

The days were often full of radiation tasks of the kind I have been describing, but in the late nights at home I began editing, little by little, in a rather chill room upstairs, a long novel about life in the balmy south where I grew up. It was a story based closely on the lives of my mother and father, working-class people of Waycross, Georgia.

This book on Cincinnati radiation has had to be, in part, a personal narrative, since I was myself involved in the long course of events described, and perhaps a sketch of my own life and affairs during the campaign of 1994 and '95 will help to explain why I concerned myself with this affair as I did.

As to the novel I was writing about my parents' lives, I should say that my mother had grown up in the white slums of Jacksonville, and that my father's father, on the other hand, had run a prosperous general store on the outskirts of Waycross but eventually lost all he had in the Depression. I tend to chart the beginnings of my own radical consciousness, such as it is, to what I learned as a child through my grandparents of the Great American Depression, and also to what I would hear in our small Protestant church, every Sunday morning and every Sunday night, of the teachings of Christ and the deep and beautiful songs of the Broadman Hymnal. Over the years, and though I did not remain a true believer in the Christian miracles, I gradually came to accept, as a perfectly serviceable gospel for the world today, the communal and collectivist ideas within the moral teachings of the church, even if not very often the worldly *practices* of the church.

The title of the book I was writing, *Children of the World*, had been taken from a little song familiar in all the Protestant churches of the south: *Jesus loves the little children, all the children of the world; red and yellow, black and white, they are precious in his sight; Jesus loves the little children of the world.* In the novel this song is sung on Sunday nights by the children, standing up together, shyly, in front of the small sanctuary; and for the mother of the tale, who would wish to believe the promise of the song but cannot, hearing it in the small broken voices of the children is a sorrowful and paradoxical experience.

But in short, if it has appeared, from what I have been relating, that my life in 1994 and '95 was given over entirely to work on military radiation, the actual case was somewhat different from that.

A few weeks before the appearance of the first newspeople and the opportunity they gave me to tell, at long last, the story of the UC tests, as far as I understood them, this book about south Georgia, long in the writing, had been contracted for by a university press, and I had begun to consider the final form in which it would appear. I expected to be quite occupied with this manuscript in the months to come and to put other things more or less aside. I felt it was good fortune indeed that in the winter I would have only one course, an easy-going class in the beautiful writings of Conrad, Lawrence, Mansfield, Mann, Chekhov, and that company, the modern masters, in short, of the story-telling trade I was trying to follow.

In a desultory way, I was also thinking ahead from time to time to a trip to Central America during the March vacation.

Radiation struck, so to speak, on the first day of the quarter, as I have related, but late-night work went forward on my manuscript, and calls and letters went back and forth to the editors at Southern Methodist University Press. Was my title really the right one? Should there be so much music in the book—hymns galore, and Bing Crosby too, and could we get permission for the Crosby songs? Was there too much Georgia speech? Would everyone catch on to that? What would we put on the jacket and who would provide the blurbs for the back cover? SMU Press has become practiced in the art of fiction publishing and is publishing little else but fiction, much of it set in the south. Though my first novel had been brought out by Macmillan and condensed in *Redbook*, this was a new age where serious fiction was concerned, and SMU seemed a good place to be.

BUT AT SCHOOL, and in late afternoons at home, Laura Schneider and I went to work in the detection field and began looking for the relatives of the people irradiated. Laura had found the name of Irene Shuff right away and the current address and phone number of her sister.

But where we had names of victims but no relations, we had to contact the funeral homes we could identify. Some of these did not want to be bothered to search their back files, but others were willing to help.

One late afternoon we set up at a desk in the main English office and made, rather tensely, certain important calls. We felt they were calls that simply had to work if Laura's labors down at the Cincinnati Court Index were to count for anything. When we knew we were getting somewhere, we would whisper intently, cupping our hands over the phone, and then exclaim aloud at times with satisfaction. Later we wondered what in the world the office staff had thought of us that day.

Laura had told me a small tale about her day down at the Index that I felt Herman Melville and Charles Dickens would have wanted to hear. The Court Index press was in an office down on Ninth Street, a strange archaic little place that few people seemed to know about. When Laura arrived one day at the main counter upstairs, a young man with dreadlocks was there requesting a form for changing his name. He wanted to change his name to "God," and the odd thing was that the clerk accepting this information seemed to have no reaction to it at all. Perhaps this is simply the famous low affect of Cincinnati; Laura gathered that so many bizarre things happened up there that no one even noticed any more.

When Laura asked for the court bulletins for the years back in the sixties, she was shown to a back closet and a hidden-away stack of huge dusty books that had not been opened in some years. Just lifting them out and onto a table was hard dirty work, but then, after hours of looking and leafing, the initials of our invisible people began to assume the shapes of actual names. We had the dates of death, but Laura did not know, of course, the dates when the Index might have printed its brief notices of these deaths, and since its printing patterns were quite as eccentric as everything else about the place, several weeks of bulletins usually had to be scanned to find each of the matching names we sought.

At home, Linda Reeves began to bring the morning paper, or stopped in with it at night and stayed, sometimes, to study with me the new data about the case.

In time families were reached. The lawsuit was filed. The university released its files, as its long, carefully stitched cover-up came apart in its hands, and the disclosures of March 1 made me ponder many events of the past and reflect on the characters of the whole affair once more.

In late March, while the print reporters were still piling through the disclosures and bringing up new bits that sometimes surprised me very much, and my own cartons of these papers, brought to my house late one night by my friend David Logan, once of the JFA, had been stowed away in my dinette for later study, I went away for two weeks to Costa Rica.

MY HUSBAND, Jerone Stephens, is a political scientist and was spending a sabbatical year in Central America, studying the various elections there, riding the smoky decrepit buses of those mostly forsaken lands, in and out of the mountain towns of Nicaragua, Salvador, Honduras, and Guatemala, putting up in small hostels, resting well enough, he said, on thin mats on narrow wooden cots, eating his rice and beans, and trying to gauge the mind and mood of the people, their feelings about their governments, the degree of interest they had, when they had any at all, in such changes as elections might bring.

By late winter he was working his way down southern Nicaragua and planning time off from these endeavors in the comparative civility of Costa Rica, that long slender arm of a country which divides the two great seas of the Atlantic and the Pacific.

Jerone had been making visits to Central America since 1984, when he had become an official observer for the Nicaraguan elections, and since that adventure of his, the two of us, and our son Daniel as well, had made many trips back and forth, together and apart, to Nicaragua and other lands of this beleaguered world. For two years Dan had worked for Witness for Peace in Nicaragua. I myself had spent a month, just before the 1990 elections, living with a family in Managua, through a Nican program to help deluded North Americans like myself experience the severe realities of Nicaraguan life. *Live as we live*, the Nicans seemed to say to us, *for at least a time; feel what we feel; learn what we think, what we need, the collective life we're trying to build; then go home — help stop the war against us . . . speak, write, witness.*

The idea of the witness was indeed the powerful idea that had sprung up among North Americans and their Nicaraguan friends after the Nican revolution of 1979.

We can do very little about the human pain we see around us every day. Few of us today—perhaps tomorrow will be different—feel we can do very much to challenge the forces in control. And yet at least to *witness*, to be able to say, "I saw this — and will tell what I saw," counts, we felt, for something. In the early eighties people from churches and colleges in the U.S. had gone to the Nicaraguan border with Honduras; they had stood beside the people in the villages that were under attack by the Contras, the counterrevolutionary forces armed by the United States. These border-walking Americans did not bring arms; they brought simply themselves, their presence, their bodies, their *witness*. They walked the violent border of the two countries and were subject to the same attacks as their Latin friends. They saw what was not meant to be seen, told what was not supposed to be told. These were the beginnings of Witness for Peace.

A great many North Americans eventually followed in this path, in small ways and large, in the decade to come; and in later years the idea spread to struggle for solidarity in many countries. Delegations flew around the world, came home and told what they had seen; told what could not be read in the *New York Times*; wrote to Congress, gave their talks, showed their slides, got out their newsletters, spread the word.

If Nicaragua itself was, finally, not invaded, the revolution not crushed until much later on, through the long war of attrition that finally wore the people down, the presence there of credible North Americans to *know*, to witness to what was really being done, counted, it would seem, for more than anything else to keep our planes at bay.

My own family had friends who were giving years of their lives to keeping this witness and working beside the Nicaraguan people, and we too wanted to be, in a small way, among the witnesses for peace and justice; for myself as a writer, it was a concept that had a deep appeal. In recent years many of my writings for small papers and magazines, and for our solidarity newsletter in Cincinnati, have been of my personal experiences with the struggling people of Managua and Cuernavaca, Guatemala and Cuba. In 1990 I brought back photographs and notes from Managua and wrote an illustrated narrative for *World Magazine* about life in a neighborhood of the middle sector of the city, a somber piece called "Family Life in Managua on the Eve of the Elections." These were the elections that were to end the Nicaraguan dream of a society that would care for all its people.

As to the witness idea, I began to feel that through my novels themselves I had been trying all along to bear a witness of a kind to the life of common people in my own small town in the southern United States. Then, in such political work as I had been able to do in Ohio, often with my husband, then also with my son, and in time in collaboration with my two daughters as well, students at UC, and of course with many friends, I was attempting, as they were, to bear witness to the growing exploitation of the people of Cincinnati and Ohio and within our own university. In many small writings for papers of various kinds I told of the economic struggles of our students; of our clerical workers to form a union; of the campus campaign against the war in the Gulf.

Once in a while I thought, whenever I thought about those years at all, of the seven-page report I had written decades ago on events in our medical school, where I had *witnessed*, in a sense, if one wanted to think of it that way, to strange and secret deeds on my own campus.

IN COSTA RICA, my husband and I spent four days in the coastal park on the Pacific, Manuel Antonio—very hot under the naked sun in that season, but not intolerable at the big shaded tables in the open-air concessions (where the fruity drinks, the *batidos*, are cold and fluffy, at least, if blended up mostly from concentrate). As everywhere in the tropics, there is the vague smell of sewage and of ripe fruit and rotting fish. The Pacific there is a violent sea. "When it is angry," people told us, "never go out even a little ways, or you'll certainly be drowned." The sea did not drown us—quite, for we did not tempt it very far. We walked on the beach and took our ease at the tables under the sheds of the beach bars and concessions; we drank batidos and read, and spoke of many things in the contemplative way people do speak when away from home. We reflected on life in the tragic and beautiful countries where my husband had been sojourning, and we spoke too of life in Cincinnati, Ohio, and especially about the events around the medical research we both had studied years ago.

After the JFA report in 1972 and the events that followed that winter and spring, the president's decision to end the tests, for instance, and the failure on my part to find attorneys who might represent the victims, assuming they could be found, I had considered the matter closed, and my husband had taken to his own university in Bowling Green, Ohio, the papers I had acquired and had begun work of his own on the political issues around these tests and human research in general. He wrote for a 1973 issue of *Politics and Society* a paper called "Political, Social, and Scientific Aspects of Medical Research on Humans," with the Cincinnati tests as a primary focus. A related study of his appeared in a volume called *What Government Does* in the *Yearbook in Politics and Public Policy*. He presented papers at various conferences, including the annual meeting of the American Political Science Association. In the summer of 1973 he attended the hearings on human experiments led by Senator Edward Kennedy. He studied drug trials and visited officials of the Food and Drug Administration. He read massively in journals and transcripts and books of all kinds on medicine and research; he read the records of the Nuremberg doctors' trials.

But during his travels in Central America in 1994 he had known little, except for what I had been able to relate during two brief staticky phone calls, of the new events taking place. I brought him a set of clippings on the Cincinnati tests gathered up by David Logan, and he read them with great interest and surprise.

As for myself, Jerone thought it was amazing that I had found myself in the center of a new maelstrom of publicity and had succeeded in working as I had with the local reporters.[1] He admired the work of Nick Miller at the *Cincinnati Post* and Tim Bonfield at the *Enquirer*; and he felt that at the *Enquirer* Linda Reeves's interviews with families were crucial to public understanding of the case and the failure of consent. It was just as we had thought, he said: "These patients knew nothing of what was happening to them."

Jerone recalled for me the modern-day history of the *Enquirer* and of the leading figures of Cincinnati's ruling caste who were enmeshed with it—Carl Lindner, for instance, the multimillionnaire of Chiquita Brands fame and the American Financial Corporation, who had bought the paper in the early seventies and later sold it to Gannett, and Lindner's long-time associates, attorneys William and Charles Keating. William had been brought in by Lindner as the *Enquirer's* publisher and remained on for a time as an executive with Gannett. His brother Charles

—founder in Cincinnati of Citizens for a Decent Literature—is the Charles Keating of Savings and Loan fame, convicted in federal court in 1991 on seventy-three charges of fraud, conspiracy, and racketeering, in connection with the collapse of American Continental Corporation and its Lincoln Savings and Loan, as the *Enquirer* itself was to report when Keating left prison in 1996 to await a new trial.[2]

During the early radiation campaign of the seventies, *William* Keating had been the First District congressman. By the time of the new campaign of 1994, he was no longer an elected official but was president and publisher of the *Enquirer*, and also serving, as it happened, on the UC board of trustees, an appointee of Republican Governor George Voinovich. In his new role at UC, Keating presided in late 1996 over the "privatization" of University Hospital, once Cincinnati General—over the transfer, that is, of the hospital and all its facilities and assets to private entities for one dollar a year. (Shortly afterward, a lawsuit was filed on behalf of Hamilton County taxpayers to attempt to return the hospital to public control, but it did not succeed.)

As for the leadership in 1994 at the *Enquirer*, I could report that Linda Reeves had given me this sketch: in 1992 the *Enquirer* had been selling fewer papers in Cincinnati than *USA Today*, and publisher Harry Whipple had moved editor George Blake to a newly created job upstairs and hired to replace him Lawrence Beaupre, from the Gannett papers in upstate New York. The Charles Keating debacle and conviction had at that time never been reported in the *Enquirer*, but when Beaupre came to town, he said, according to Reeves, "There's no news in this paper," and coverage of Keating's travails—and certain other neglected events—commenced in a prominent way.

But the conservative positions of the paper in most respects changed but little. As with most newspapers today, there was in 1994 no reporter for labor, and seldom any news from the point of view of common people seeking to resist the assault on their incomes and way of life. One could read very little from the vantage point of the low-income people in Cincinnati's downtown neighborhood Over-the-Rhine, for instance, who have been locked in recent years in a bitter struggle over their housing and neighborhood supports with business developers and the Chamber of Commerce. Critics of the *Enquirer* feel that the interests of the business community remain the focal point for virtually all news.

(Robert Dole, it goes almost without saying, was the *Enquirer's* candidate of choice in 1996; Clinton's positions were said to be full of "shallow trash talk" about Medicare and other nonissues, as the *Enquirer* sees such things.)

My husband and I spoke of the rather amusing way the paper had been backed into the radiation story by the *Post* and the floods of print they had then expended on it. We reflected on the feelings of the doctors as they read about themselves day after day in the press—an awesome sentence indeed, it seemed to me, about as severe a punishment as one could devise, but Jerone said he did not necessarily see it that way: "They probably don't feel any more remorse than they ever did, but regard themselves as martyrs for the defense of the country." Of course it is a fact that in the forties, fifties, and sixties the whole atomic world was intently focused on the finding of precise answers to the continuing riddle of radiation injury, and that the Cincinnati doctors had been drawn into that. (Scientists are still wanting to know today just how much radiation it takes to make people ill, in the shorter term, and how the amount absorbed might be measured.) [3]

THE REMAINDER OF OUR stay was in San Jose, in the fine climate of the highlands. We walked around the town and visited parks and markets and street affairs. I went to an Easter Mass. We talked to people here and there, at the Quaker house, for instance, where the local newsletter we picked up told of the many battered women of the city and the severe treatment of prisoners, and detailed the tragic decline during the eighties of living standards in Central America.

In a back foyer of the small hostel where we stayed, I sat some afternoons on an ancient divan and read the poems of John Milton for my spring class. My vision has been impaired for many years, due to dystrophy of the cornea and dysfunction of the tear glands, but in the dry season of the tropics, where moisture hardly ever condenses into rain but is suspended heavily in the air, and where, in the highlands at least, windows are open and artificial climates unnecessary, I found I could read my enlarged sheets of poetry with considerably less effort than at home. I traveled, too, with a low-speed tape recorder from the Library for the Blind and good books from their library. I wanted to understand, as far as possible, the unexpected press campaign on radiation still forging ahead, I assumed, in Cincinnati, and I was rereading my tape copies of Ben Bagdikian's *Media Monopoly* and Michael Parenti's *Inventing Reality*, both of them deep-cutting critiques of the U.S. media.⁴ On a later trip to Central America I would take with me Robert Lifton's book on the Nazi doctors and their strategems for composing their minds as to the awesome deeds they were committing.⁵

The local Quaker materials we were reading spoke of the "U.S. terror" the countries of Central America were suffering, constantly undergirded by the propaganda machine of the U.S. media. For these people, we North Americans are exporting our "violent culture," and doing so "through the most technologically advanced news apparatus that humanity has ever known." In the small sitting room of our hostel it was CNN, indeed, that seemed always to be playing on the telly.

On the other hand, it was good to find that in San Jose combative newspapers could still be found, a whole batch of them with different postures and constituencies—a print media not yet swallowed up by Murdoch and Gannett and company (though perhaps the next time we go, it will be). As in much of Latin America, there still exist, as well, journalists of conscience. A television reporter was fired while we were there for "conspiring," as the charges went, with other journalists to describe certain financial affairs of the well-known political leader Jose Figueres, and the very strange thing, for North Americans, was that when this reporter left, her editor—also a woman—said *If she goes, I go,* and in fact they both went.

For after all, people must have information. Without it how can we act to defend ourselves or try to change the world we live in? It is this basic right, this *need,* to know what is really happening to us and to those around us that is a primary theme of the present study and which led to its undertaking.

IN MY OWN MIND, the public information campaign about the tragedies of radiation within our school was a valuable part of the crusade to redress the balance of the past; such a campaign could play a small part in helping people understand the continuing need in our own decade, the ever more pressing need in fact, for a measure of public authority over medicine—and all the other systems that control our lives. The public and press campaign was essential for the initiation of the lawsuit and the search for surviving families. Though the suit began as the offspring of the early publicity around the case, it then helped create, and was also in a sense enveloped by, a public "outcry" that reached to some degree into every part of the city.

It reached the court. Sandra Beckwith opened her crucial ruling of January 11, 1995, with a reference to "this well-publicized case." She too could hardly have failed to have known of the UC experiments before they came before her court.

By the time the first families had appeared to initiate a legal action, attorneys had read about the tests in the papers, had already become acquainted with the parameters of the case, and were prepared to take on the front expenses of an action that might otherwise have looked, after the lapse of over twenty years, dim and doubtful.

As for the Cincinnati corps of press, if we ask again *why* this story could be told in 1994 and could not be in 1971 and '72, it can only be said that some of the reasons are obvious and some are not. But it must be readily apparent that to bugle out over the town a scandal of this kind from the past is not nearly as difficult as to disturb the quivering muck of the living moment, where much more may be at stake with a paper's owners and advertisers. We must reflect on the full-page ads of the great insurance companies, the spreading wastelands of print of the health conglomerates and the HMOs. The pharmaceuticals. To rake *their* muck, if I may repeat the metaphor once more, would be a different thing indeed, and you have to take care not even to scratch against it. To attack a public hospital for its crimes of the past is something else entirely.

In spite of the massive Cincinnati reportage on UC radiation, there was also a tight lid on the ways the discourse could be extended. I for one tried again and again to insert remarks on national health insurance, which the country was still trying to debate in early 1994, before the media shut down any bona fide discussion and simply gave way to the millions of dollars the health industry was spending to block a national discussion. In Cincinnati and elsewhere, in Gannett territory in general, the health industry would not go for such a debate, of course, and their advertising dollars are as eloquent as anyone's in town.

No one could say in the papers or on TV that had national insurance of the Medicare type existed in the sixties for all citizens, young and old, as it did in the other developed countries of the world, people would not have been trapped in charity hospitals and had to take the risk of being experimented on, dying painfully, and being miserably doctored; they could have gone to doctors of their choosing—and in other words, people like Maude Jacobs and Margaret Bacon, Evelyn Jackson and Mike Spanagel, James Tidwell and Louis Romine might not have lost their lives in the way they did.

No, one could not say such things as that. "Oh that's not relevant— that's another issue," reporters would say. No one could publicly rec- ommend that ordinary citizens actually *using* the hospital be included on its board of directors, or even on the local panel of experts reviewing the UC case.

One could, then, certainly not complain about the make-up of the board of trustees of our university, from which, after all, our medical school takes its authority for all its actions. I, for instance, could cer- tainly not discuss in the press the great need to have common users on this board, plain parents and students and staff, not just wealthy lawyers and businessmen with nothing personal at stake, sending their own children off to expensive schools out of town, and certainly not using our public hospital.

REFLECTIONS LIKE THESE come easier, somehow, when we are far from home and looking back as if through space, and almost like strangers, toward the far little dime of a world we have left behind.

My husband and I reflected on the strange juxtaposition of our own lives with those of the radiation families. In the sixties we were not living in the same town as Lula Tarlton, James Tidwell, Maude Jacobs, and company, and had never heard the name of Cincinnati General Hos- pital.

We were Georgians. I had lived in a small south Georgia town all my life and had an image of Cincinnati as a smoky industrial metropolis that would not be a pleasant place to live, where no one should *have* to live. But in 1967 I would go to live there. Without ever visiting this town, I would accept, by mail, a job at the local university, which had hired my husband to teach political science and been willing to employ his wife as well, when most schools would not employ women professors at all.

When we arrived in Cincinnati that fall I was rather amazed to see its tumbling green hills and narrow decorated German houses, its formidable old halls and churches, schools and banks, of a great variety of architectural types and degrees of artistry. Some of these structures, like the turn-of-the-century city hall downtown, with its sharp little gothic towers spurting from every pore, were almost comically ornate, but others were quite beautiful—one of the original structures at UC, for instance, a small, domed neoclassical edifice with high vaulting marble steps and a handsome situation on the wooded upper drive of the campus. Back in the nineteenth century it had been the first library of this city-owned school, which in 1977 would become part of the state system of colleges. The great tilting lawn leading down from the main drive to the city street far below was a vista of beauty that would become a major landscape of my life.

Back in 1964, when Maude Jacobs had gone into the hospital for what she thought was a treatment for cancer, and died of it twenty-five days later, we had been living in Bloomington, Indiana, on a sprawling estate of rather rough-shingled two-floor buildings called Hoosier Courts, which had once been army barracks. We remembered an odd little march for peace which took place on that estate—we women in the Courts had rolled our infants around the grounds with Mothers for Peace signs jutting out of our strollers. (We did not produce any spectacular effect.) In the years to come, like many other families, we would take children on marches of all kinds, and as to radiation, would form part of a huge crowd that marched from Cincinnati to a proposed nuclear plant in Moscow, Ohio, a town just up the road. That movement had splendid leadership among the Quakers and various religious, socialist, and environmental groups and succeeded in permanently blocking the operation of the plant as a nuclear facility. It would later be converted to electricity.

During the year Jerone and I began teaching at UC, unknown to anyone outside the College of Medicine, seven more individuals, as we shall see in the chapters that follow, underwent treatment they thought was for cancer, and three died within a month. It would not be until four years later, in 1971, that is, that I would learn about these three individuals and the eighteen others who had died, by that time, shortly after their exposures.

WHEN I GOT HOME to Cincinnati from San Jose, the April hearing was about to take place, and I found in the mail the request for my presence.

That spring and summer I also embarked on a number of exchanges with the Clinton commission by phone and mail and fax, as I have explained, and in the fall the small panel meeting of the Advisory Committee took place in Cincinnati. A British radio team led by John Slater had come for this meeting, and they spent several days in Cincinnati getting their story. Slater became, with his series of programs on U.S. radiation, "Atomica America," aired in England by the BBC in the fall of 1994, an important historian of this aspect of U.S. history. In a number of lengthy visits to radiation sites around the country, he had recorded the views and reminiscences of over thirty victims, journalists, and public officials who had known what was happening when most of the country did not. The rushes for these interviews come to about thirty hours, according to producer Peter Hoare, and are being kept in a special archive available to historians of the future.[6]

The family organization was also planning its events and various testimonies, and I spent time on the phone with the canny leader of this group, Doris Baker. I was getting to know some of the newer families as well, and working, also, with interested students at my university. Young people in journalism and history were writing research papers on the case, and a senior at Northern Kentucky took a long bus trip to my home one night to study the records for his honors thesis. Student reporters came in and out of my office at school along with the regular media, and in a way working with the various interested young people was the part of the campaign I found most to my liking. As a teacher, I liked, of course, to help young people along if I could to understand what our society is all about, and certainly they often helped me. A law student, Michael Beatty, editing a publication on campus called *The Independent*, devoted a whole issue to the UC radiation story and other Cold War sites, and he came upon some materials about Cold War exposures that few of us had known about.

AS TO THE DEEDS of the doctors in the radiation tests—who would claim to understand how such acts could be performed?

Can it really be that there is a deep grain of wrongfulness in some human creatures? Are some of us simply deceived as to our own natures and the pain we bring upon others — so that there is no more to say about us than that? That there are bad men and women and will always be bad men and women, and they must be caught up with — and that's that?

Like many others, I see the matter a little differently, as I shall presently explain. But I do not mean to say that I did not rejoice when these offenders were pinned and pinned again to a public whipping post in the mass publicity of the winter of 1994.

On certain days of the week I would sit down at a lunch counter in a sprawling student eatery near the university, order a late lunch, and look at the poems I was going to be reading with my class that afternoon. I glanced at the newspapers that were lying about (that I declined to pay money for), and the headlines of those papers would often be very gratifying to see. My lunch slipped down my digestive apparatus very smoothly on days like that. What was the headline I enjoyed the most? "Scientists Whereabouts Sought," perhaps — a huge black header on the day the lawsuit was filed and all the researchers' known whereabouts named on the record for the first time. Many of the defendants in the suit had retired or moved away to other schools or practices, but four were still at work in the same medical complex, including Dr. Edward Silberstein.

I remember being very content with a Channel 12 lead-in on the Newsmaker show I have spoken of: "Old General Hospital's on the hotseat tonight!" And I have mentioned another gratifying header in the Enquirer: "Radiation Docs Felt Victimized" — by the JFA. It was impossible not to be more than a little bemused by what the doctors had said about our old JFA in their correspondence of years ago. How tenderly they had despised and feared us, yet how little to be feared — in most respects — we were.

For a time interesting new aspects of the case came to light in the papers almost every day as reporters went through the mass disclosures of March 1, the same tumbled mess of papers that would later give Albuquerque reporter Eileen Welsome carpal tunnel syndrome, almost, just to page through them. (When I spoke to Welsome on the telephone one day, she said she could hardly hold up the receiver — her hands were in splints from turning so many sheets of paper.) What benefits, the colleagues of the doctors had been asking, in those documents of years ago, were the patients expected to gain in exchange for the enormous risks?

One must feel, of course, the mysterious horror of what had taken place. When I think, once more, of the woman named Maude Jacobs, caring for children at home when called in for her treatment, living afterward only twenty-five days, miserably ill and her wits mostly gone; of Louise Richmond, a survivor of thirty-one days, crying out and gripping her bedpost in mortal agony for lack of that full range of vaunted "medical services" the doctors say they freely gave; of Greg Shuff and Elise Feldstrup and Herbert Varin, Greg and Gwendon Plair, and the many other young people suddenly asked to cope, without help, without information, with a strange new crisis in the life of an ill parent—when I think of those things I almost *do* believe in human depravity without explanation. The lethal assault that Jacobs and others suffered, I ask myself—was it any less horrible, finally, than a crazed attack with a baseball bat on someone in a parking lot, a fatal gunshot through the brain on a street or a porch on what we think of as the bad side of town?

The poet William Blake put this question to us in certain lines of immortal verse. Where does the animal of evil come from? he asked. How are we even to imagine its origin in the universe? Who is it who fashions the terrible tiger of sin and wrong and death? *Tyger! tyger! burning bright | In the forests of the night, | What immortal hand or eye | Can frame thy fearful symmetry? | . . . And what shoulder, & what art | Could twist the sinews of thy heart?* Blake was a deep-dyed Christian, and yet he was asking in this verse whether the same god who sent humankind his "little lamb" to save them could have sent the tiger of death and evil as well.

When the legal hearings took place and we saw, at the defendants' bar so to speak, the two long rows of the attorneys of the investigators, one could not but feel content that justice was being served at last. When the doctors effectively ended their long battle to defend themselves and entered into negotiations to settle the claims against them, that was, it must be said, a satisfaction. When an agreement then was reached, all people of good will must surely have rejoiced.

Deliberate medical violence is rarely a simple thing to expose, and in the case of an invisible killer like radiation the offender's tracks are not difficult to cover. Radiation is an agent that generally requires time to do its work, and it was this fact as much as anything else that made possible the assaults in Cincinnati and around the country. And radiation, after all, is invisible. John Slater said it well in "Atomica America" for the BBC: "Radiation is something against which none of your senses protect you. You can't see it, feel it, smell it, hear it or taste it. But its rays invade your body. . . ."

IF WE CANNOT quite believe in human degradation as such, many of us do believe, after all, in the evil we together may make of society. Perhaps we should hold ourselves and all people accountable for not having worked hard enough for a democratic way of life where the lives of all people could be valued, where we are not separated from each other by a massive class divide we may be helpless to reach across.

We must assume that these practitioners had great difficulty regarding their low-income patients as normal people whose lives were as valuable as their own. This was exactly the point of the young African American woman who spoke up in the lecture hall at UC and told the assembled crowd that scientists would not have done even to their pets what was inflicted on her aunt.

When I had been writing about these tests years ago and been vouchsafed the privilege I've described, of speaking to Edward Silberstein down in the basement corridors of the radiology department at UC, I remember that he struck me as an agreeable, unassuming young man, friendly, a rather gently spoken man. He had said he felt he had a special sensitivity to those dying of cancer because his own mother was ill with that disease. When I got home that day, I remember my husband saying to me this: "Well, did you ask him if he had considered entering his mother into this study?"

I had not asked him and perhaps I should have.

Yet according to local reports, Silberstein would, a few years later, involve himself rather intensely on the side, this time, of *victims* of radiation, the Cincinnati-area workers and residents exposed to contaminants at the Fernald uranium-processing plant on the northern perimeter of the city.

Eugene Saenger, for his part, has been described to me by a woman who once worked for him as a man of charm and cultivation, of completely unthreatening demeanor. In the College of Medicine he was a physician with beautiful works of art on his walls; he and his wife were dedicated symphony-goers. There would seem to be nothing about Saenger that is rough or cruel or mean; he is a mild-mannered man, it seems.[7] It became rather clear, as we studied the new materials of the nineties, that he had not personally selected the subjects nor superintended their exposures.

But by the time of the closure of the lawsuit in 1997, a lot of ground had been swept out from under these investigators, irreversibly, and they had no place to retreat to but the one last-ditch island of defense enunciated by Saenger at the congressional hearing—the contention, that is, that there had been reason to think in 1960 that such a "treatment" for cancer as they were beginning to administer might actually help someone.

As the families of the victims began to emerge in 1994, the battle over consent had been quickly lost, and the researchers ceased to argue, as they had when identities were still a secret, that the subjects had understood the risks and opted for the treatment anyway. No families have said that they or the victims understood the awesome risk involved or had any notion that the point of the treatment was anything other than their own improved health.

Linda Reeves of the *Enquirer* effectually settled the consent question on her own with her interviews, there on the record for all to see. These interviews are especially valuable for this reason, I believe: Reeves would usually speak to the families on the very day they learned that a member of their family had been part of the study, before there could be any considerations of lawsuit or compensation. She caught their first fury, their first instinctual outpourings of anger and grief, their first and most uncalculated recollections of that past time. That much was certainly true as well of the families I first spoke to myself. Even when they had been at the side of the victim every day, they rarely knew there was any research involved at all—and certainly not that it posed any deadly risk.

Reeves took, faithfully, a photographer with her when she went out to interview the families, and I see, in my mind's eye, most clearly a huge front-page color photo of a man named Leon Thomas, bursting with rage, towering, glowering over a picture of his mom at his wedding, with these words in large letters over his head: *The very money I paid in taxes they used to kill my mom.* I hear Catherine Hager's words about her father Joseph: "Dad, do you think this treatment will do you any good?" and his simple reply that he had been told by the doctors it would. As to consent, I recall Gloria Nelson, at the congressional hearing, saying of her grandmother that she could not read nor write, and that yet there was in her records a signed consent form.

ON TELEVISION and in the papers, in churches and courthouse corridors, in the halls of the university itself, I could speak in the winter of 1994 of the sore wound of my own that could perhaps begin to heal as the tragic truths of this affair began spilling forth for all to see and puzzle over. It was good to be able to grace with their actual names the once invisible people of these experiments, that secret army of unknown soldiers fighting in a war they did not even know about, who would now have names and human histories.

From among the families of the victims, with their typically modest educations, their typically modest worldly goods, some bold and canny individuals came forward, nevertheless, to work for the common cause. Their stories too must be recounted here.

But first, knowing what we know today, and weaving it into one tapestry with what was known in the past—what exactly did the doctors do, why did they begin, what were they looking for, and what exactly were their relations with their sponsors, the Department of Defense?

Are we quite sure they were not, first and foremost, simply trying to tame a dread disease?

II

The Medical Story

8

The Mother Without a Name: The Earliest Exposures

I want everyone in this courtroom to know that my mother had a name. — LILIAN PAGANO of her mother, Maude Jacobs, "M. J.," case study 045

The story of the radiations that could be read in the documents turned over to me by Edward Gall in 1971 was a large and startling one in itself, but when the new disclosures came along in 1994 and '95, and the testimonies of the surviving families, I could patch together, little by little, an even more graphic picture of what had taken place.

The earliest individual irradiated whose family had been identified was James Tidwell, a bricklayer by day and by night a singer in a small African American church in the West End of town.

In late 1994, after the congressional hearing and then the local meeting of the Advisory Committee, the legal action was going forward, and the family of James Tidwell had become part of the suit. On a certain October day a hearing was held in a Cincinnati federal courtroom on motions to have the charges against the doctors dismissed, and for the first time the defendants came out in considerable force to sit in public view among their attorneys. It seemed to be a sign of their sense that silence and composed indifference to plain people's anger and grief would no longer serve their purposes.

Eugene Saenger sat up in the front row beside attorney Joseph Parker, who led the case for the defendants, and when the session began, a strange rite took place. Parker introduced Dr. Saenger to the judge in a formal, honorific way, noting some of his many accomplishments.

Sitting down near the front of the room as well were members of the Tidwell family, including three of James Tidwell's sons, and it was later said that attorney Robert Newman might have introduced the Tidwells in the same way. He might have said, "Your Honor, I'd like to make you acquainted at this time, if I may, with the family of Mr. James Tidwell. Mr. Tidwell was a gospel singer of Cincinnati and a craftsman of note, and in 1960 he had the distinction of having his bone marrow destroyed by Dr. Saenger and his colleagues at UC. Mr. Tidwell was given one hundred rads of total body radiation by this research team and lived only thirty-two days afterward. He is the earliest victim of these experiments whose family we know. Thank you, Your Honor."

In 1994 two of the Tidwell brothers were in their sixties. They came out to the various actions and events in dress suits and seemed as solemn and silent as undertakers, while a younger, more talkative brother did the communicating.

There were eleven different attorneys for the defendants that day in court and four teams for the plaintiffs, so the lawyers alone made up a roomful of combatants any day of the week.

The argument of the defendants was that they should all be dismissed from the case because they enjoyed qualified immunity as "publicly employed physicians and health care professionals" simply engaged in their "discretionary functions." Attorney Parker asserted, too, that the patients were not coerced into accepting treatment, but were "voluntary consumers of medical services," free to suspend treatment and leave the hospital at any time. He insisted they were patients accepting treatment, not subjects being experimented on.[1]

JAMES TIDWELL, the gospel singer in a small Baptist church and father of nine, was irradiated in 1960 during the first year of the Cincinnati project. Tidwell was the third individual to be used of the ninety cancer patients who would eventually become part of the study. There were ten subjects during this first year, eight of them African Americans. The first two patients were, like Tidwell, males in their sixties, fitting the profile Joseph Hamilton had sketched in 1950 for the "human volunteers" that might eventually be found. These two men each received fifty rads; compared to what would follow, the doctors were proceeding with a certain degree of caution, with doses on the lower side of their spectrum.[2]

Even so, the five subjects who were given, during this first year, one *hundred* rads in a single ministration were being subjected to serious risk, as people who were, after all, already ill. Two of these hundred-rad subjects died not many weeks after their radiation and with their blood counts seriously affected. Tidwell was one of these, and the other was the African American domestic worker with breast cancer, Lula Tarlton.

James Tidwell had first come to General Hospital for treatment back in 1957 and had had part of his colon removed. For three years he had seemed to do well enough, but in October 1960 he returned, complaining of weakness in his legs and "repeated seizures."[3]

Tidwell, of course, had no way of knowing that during his respite from treatment, a new research project had begun in the hospital that would change drastically the way certain cancer patients would be treated. After a fair amount of dickering back and forth between Eugene Saenger of the College of Medicine radiology department and the Defense Atomic Support Agency of the Department of Defense, a contract had been signed, a new machine had been bought that delivered a relatively new kind of radioisotope, and a special lead-clad chamber built for it down in the hospital basement.

Tidwell was admitted to the hospital on October 6, 1960, and though the doctors wrote that his seizures were "well controlled with dilantin and phenobarbital," he was subjected two weeks later to radiation over his whole body, a single continuous dose of a hundred rads, and ten days after that to a series of radiations to the head, since it was thought that his cancer had spread to his brain. In another three weeks Tidwell was dead, thirty-two days after his exposure.

No consent form for radiation was signed by Tidwell, nor do the doctors claim in their reports that in these early years they felt any necessity to tell the patients anything about what was being done. They were not defining the radiation as experimental, even as cancer therapy, but simply as the most appropriate "treatment."

"The patient is told that he is to receive treatment to help his sickness" reads the first report to the DOD in 1961. Tidwell's autopsy shows that he had contracted pneumonia, and if we consult, not just the original patient summaries submitted by the doctors to the DOD, but the full hospital records released to Tidwell's family in 1994, we find a complete record of his blood counts up to his final four days and note that a white blood count of 8100 two days before radiation had begun to drop a week or so afterward and was recorded as 1120 four days before his death. No further counts were recorded.

The autopsy is not absolutely clear on certain points. Although it does report that his cancer had spread to his lungs and brain, nevertheless this man had come into the hospital only a month earlier under his own steam and had not seemed acutely ill. There seems to have been no possible reason to have added to his difficulties with a type of radiation that could not only be painful but could "precipitate his demise"—a phrase the doctors employ when describing the deaths of patients with the "hemotologic depression" that Tidwell's records show, the presence, that is, of falling blood counts.[4]

The researchers were selecting for their subjects at this time, and more or less at random as far as we can tell, patients with varying degrees of illness and a variety of cancers.

Of these earliest subjects of the first year of the project, living and dying at Cincinnati General Hospital so many years ago, the only other one whose family we know was the woman named Lula Tarlton. Tarlton was sixty-six when she too became an unwitting target of this research. As with James Tidwell, Laura Schneider had found the full name of "L. T." in the death notices of the Cincinnati Court Index, in those dusty old tomes in the strange little office downtown. Tarlton's name was then given to Linda Reeves of the Cincinnati Enquirer, and it was at the time that her name first appeared in the paper that her niece Barbara Ann Mathis saw it and began to weep. No one in the family had known, she said, that her Aunt Lula had been experimented on.

Tarlton became extremely ill after her radiation, according to Mathis; and indeed the doctors report that Tarlton vomited for five days after her "treatment," became more and more ill, and died forty-nine days afterward.[5]

For a long time we had not known any family of Tarlton's, though we had her name and had included her profile on the sheet of unidentified victims we circulated at the mass meeting at UC. We knew where

Tarlton was buried and that there had been a service for her in the Second Baptist Church in Cincinnati's East End. On a certain day later on, I saw Barbara Ann Mathis's name alongside Lula Tarlton's on a record of families sent me by paralegal Jennifer Thomas in the office of Robert Newman, and I was able to speak to Mathis at length about the final illness of her aunt.

Tarlton was the first woman to have been seriously injured by radiation. As with the victims to come, both women and men, she was not, as we have seen, "indigent" or on welfare, certainly not in any way the unproductive, unneeded, disposable person the investigators apparently took her and all her race and class of people to be—she was catching a bus to work when she first realized she was ill.

A CERTAIN FEATURE of the publicity around this case has continued to be disturbing: the depiction of the project, that is, as a one-man enterprise, a weird anomaly in medicine, a one-very-bad-apple phenomenon that need not cause us any great distress about our medical research in general.

Readers who examine the first Cincinnati report to the military for 1960–61 are bound to be struck, I think, by the fact that not one but five departments within the UC College of Medicine were participating; during that first year there were twelve investigators, all but two of them medical doctors. The project was said to be a "cooperative study" of the departments of Radiology, Internal Medicine, Pediatrics, Psychiatry, and Preventive Medicine.[6]

Drs. Harold Perry and Harry Horwitz, both assistant professors of Radiology, were directing the therapy and were also "concerned with clinical care of the patient." Perry would remain at this post for the first six years of the project, until he left the college in June 1966, and Horwitz, originally described as Perry's "assistant," would participate throughout the full eleven-year course of the tests. James G. Kereiakes, Ph.D., a radiation physicist, was said to be directing all "physical" aspects of the study, such as the calculation of doses, and would also stay with the project to the end.

According to the team's reports and publications, the correspondence released by the university, and the full hospital records, a doctor who was not a radiologist but an assistant clinical professor of Medicine, B. I. Friedman, played a large part in the research and in the care of patients until his own departure from the college in July 1968. He was replaced by Edward Silberstein and Bernard Aron.[7] In the first report we read that the "selection of patients" and "their workup," along with the supervision of laboratory studies, fell to Friedman and his associate in Medicine, instructor "T. Wright." Three Pediatrics professors were involved, one professor in Preventive Medicine, and two psychiatrists.

The stated aim of the team was to study biological indicators of radiation injury and "the emotional and psychometric response of the patient." Several pages of detail follow about exactly how the early radiations had been conducted and the data studied. No concomitant cancer project is mentioned. A question that naturally presents itself is this: in the cancer study later said to have inspired the project, who were the investigators? Were they the same researchers profiled in this first DOD report as those carrying out the studies of radiation injury? Was the project in reality the "dual-nature research" — on both cancer and radiation injury — it was said to be in 1995 by the national Advisory Committee?[8]

If there existed a parallel study of whole body radiation for cancer, we do not know who the investigators were or how the project was designed, except as it was described in various ad hoc ways in the correspondence with the internal reviewers of the College of Medicine beginning in 1967.

As to the selection of subjects for the project, we read that the doctors are choosing only patients who have "proven metastatic or far advanced cancer" but are in "relatively good nutritional status." They will not have lost weight. We will read in the second report that documented spread of cancer would no longer be required as long as a patient is found to be "incurable."

In 1961 we find another datum about the selection of subjects that is strange to see in what was later claimed to be a cancer study. Certain women would not be used — women with active menstrual cycles.[9] We may well ask what this has to do with the treatment of cancer. The problem is that for the study of radiation injury, and the search for a radiation indicator, such women are not good subjects. Changes in their body chemicals during menstruation might confound the tests for radiation indicators.

In the doctors' second report, we read a long introduction about the project that gives clear notice that the report is being widely circulated to the military, with thirty-eight copies sent out to various bases, schools, and agencies of the Army; twenty-three to the Navy; and twenty to the Air Force.

We do not know of any mailings to cancer agencies.

IN THE EARLIEST GROUP of subjects is one individual whose case we will see reflected in a number of others in years to come: a thirty-nine-year-old woman with cancer of the tongue became the last person to be irradiated during the first year. Like Tidwell and Tarlton, she too received one hundred rads of total body radiation, became quite ill in the days that followed, with nausea and vomiting, weakness and loss of appetite, and then suffered the dangerous decline in white blood cells that was to take away other lives.

But within forty days this patient, Mary Pasley, had begun to recover, and a few months later the "small mass" on her tongue—a recurrence of an earlier mass that had been removed in 1951—was surgically excised.[10] Records show that Pasley then went on to live six more years, but we did not know the date of her death, nor apparently did the researchers, as far as can be ascertained, until the winter of 1997, when the hospital records for all patients were released.

Three others of this group who survived the immediate aftereffects of the radiation lived a long time afterward. The second patient lived over two years, the fifth 438 days, and the seventh 324 days. Looking forward into the second year, the first two subjects there survived for 298 and 885 days. We could go on through the years with this kind of calculation. When patients did survive the radiation, in other words, they often had a fair span of life remaining to them.

What is happening, then? Are the subjects as sick, as close to death, as the doctors have insisted in their public statements? Over and over again, we have been told that the researchers were trying to offer hope to people with far-advanced cancer for whom there was no other treatment left and who had only a short time to live.

The patient Mary Pasley with tongue cancer did certainly have other therapy available to her—she needed surgery to remove a mass on her tongue—and only got it after whole body radiation had been administered, after she had been monitored for the immediate side effects to see how sick she would become, and after the batteries of tests on her blood and urine had been performed for the Department of Defense.

I remember an occasion when Robert Newman and I spoke about the radiation project to a large hall of undergraduates at UC. A new family member had quite recently joined the suit and had come to sit on the proscenium with us just to lend her presence that day. Before the talks got underway I went over to meet her—a pleasant well-dressed African American woman of middle years—and found that she had something really quite astonishing to say: that her aunt, study number 057, had lived nearly twelve years after her radiation.

We had not known this patient's name nor her date of death. I learned that day that her name was Clara Johnson. She had gotten the lower dose of one hundred rads, which, though it had proved highly damaging for James Tidwell and Lula Tarlton, most patients did survive. If she had gotten fifty rads more, this woman, who was not at all seriously ill, would have had little better than one chance in two of living for more than a month.

Since 1994 Eugene Saenger has given, I believe, only one interview to newspapers; in that exchange in the *Cincinnati Enquirer* he said this about the radiation deaths ascribed to him: "Well, if I'm responsible for those who died early, why am I not also responsible for those who lived long?" [11] This is certainly a fair question to ask, and we must continue to explore the issue of whether help for patients was indeed sometimes occurring and was in *fact* the underlying purpose of the radiations.

IF WE LOOK over the records of the second year of the project, we see that in spite of the severe outcomes for Tidwell and Tarlton, the doctors are now doubling the dose of radiation applied.

Five of the ten new individuals brought into the study during 1962 and early 1963 would receive a whopping dose of two hundred rads—larger than the radiation dose Joseph Hamilton had privately told the Atomic Energy Commission back in 1950 would be, in his view, an "incapacitating dose" for healthy young soldiers, and bound to lead to fatalities in people whose health was not good. [12]

Of ten patients treated in this second year, three were lost within thirty-seven days. John Edgar Webster was lost, the country musician and school caretaker whose family would help initiate the lawsuit thirty-two years later. Evelyn Jackson was lost, the African American woman of forty-eight, our "E. J.," who had lived only ten days after her treatment, and who became a focus of Nick Miller's dramatic story in the Cincinnati Post that broke the print coverage of the case in early 1994. John Henry Wells was also lost, an African American man with lung cancer who lived only thirty-four days and whose family we do not know.

John Edgar Webster had had a resection of a bowel mass in January 1962, and he returned to General Hospital a few months later with cancer in his bowel and his lungs and needing help for pain. What he received was a large dose of whole body radiation that made him more ill and destroyed his still-normal white blood cells. According to the doctors' own records, his white blood count "dropped from an average of ten thousand prior to therapy to a low of six hundred, twenty-nine days post TBR." Webster's hospital records make everything clear; abundant notations describe the radiation trauma from which this patient never recovered. Harold Perry reported in his "final notes" on the case in January 1963 that there was "severe hypoplasia of the bone marrow." A hospital lab report is equally damaging. "Follow-up studies of this patient showed essentially no change until the time of total body irradiation, and then the patient on May 4 developed a rather marked but progressive leukopenia . . . ," a reference to Webster's failing white blood cells. Yet another indicator of damage to the blood was the drop in his platelet count, which went down precipitously, we read, after radiation, "and did not recover before his death." [13]

This is a matter of deep tragedy, of course. I have sometimes thought that it was precisely because this record of deaths was so amazing that we could not get even people of good will to believe it for many years. "Surely, surely" —we would hear—"these doctors were just trying to help people." It was hard for anyone who was not studying the medical record itself to credit the fact that such things as were being charged could happen in the high ranks of the profession of medicine—in Cincinnati or elsewhere.

THIS SECOND YEAR of the project was a somber one indeed, but on the other hand, from among the families of these ten victims of 1962–63, two enterprising women emerged to lead an aggressive campaign for public acknowledgment of what had taken place. They had of course known nothing about a dangerous experiment which had touched their own families until they began to read of the radiations during the winter of 1994.

This is a part of the story that will always be good to remember. I would not wish to think that ordinary people who are not among the experts or the authorities, or among the wealthy trustees of universities, could not see through to what is happening to them and find the will to stand up forthrightly to those in control and become their accusers.

Doris Baker is a woman of color and Barb Tatterson is white, but the two of them worked together almost like sisters to solve the problems of keeping the families posted and together, and to help them enter on the historical record the stories of their travails.

Baker was mentioned earlier in this book as the great-granddaughter of Gertrude Newell, who had had colon cancer and been involved with Dr. Gall, and who turns up in our records among the subjects of 1962–63. Newell was irradiated the same week as John Edgar Webster, in April 1962, and only a few weeks before "E. J." As we have seen, she received a high dose and might have died shortly afterward, as Webster and Jackson and Wells did, but her system fought back from the damage to her blood and she lived on for two years.

Doris Baker has only a meager education, but when she learned that her grandmother had been a victim of the tests, she rapidly began to reach out to other families as they emerged and to bring them together into a proactive organization. She became good friends with other members who also wanted to take this insult to their families by the horns, and she did all the things organizing people naturally do, like an efficient general secretary. Baker and I worked together at times, and I began to see her as a person who could rarely be distracted by much of anything and who was not troubled by any reverence for official people or professors of medicine—or English. Baker put her own mind to things, and in fact, it seemed to me, often saw what the experts in government and law and medicine did not.

One of her recruits, so to speak, was Barb Tatterson, who was an advocate for the family of her cousin, David Jungnickel, a victim of the same second period of the tests as Baker's grandmother.

David was the youngest of the eighty-five "adults" who would be swept into the study. He had been diagnosed at fifteen with Ewing's sarcoma, a form of bone cancer, and at seventeen he fell into the hands of the doctors at General Hospital and was irradiated over his whole body. At age nineteen David died. The total body exposure of 1963 was a very painful event for him, according to the doctors' own notations, and then the frequent high doses of radiation to the tumors around his body left him with burns and sores. Indeed David's four last years of life seem to have been a nightmare of pain, excruciating treatments, and day-to-day neglect in hospitals, both before and after his whole body exposure.

Even with the best of humane and tender care, to die of bone cancer can be a miserable way to depart this earth. And if you also live in a society that will not provide the help you need and does not care about your suffering, this is a wretched destiny indeed. And that was David's fate.

Barb Tatterson was a schoolgirl herself at the time of David's illness, but she was often a visitor with her aunt to General Hospital, and then at what can only be called a public holding place, or asylum for the terminally ill, Drake Hospital. Over and over again, Tatterson noted in her testimonies David's desperate, weeping need for medicine for his pain, both at General and then at Drake. His mother's first task whenever she came in to see him was to go at once to find a nurse who could administer medicine for his pain.

Late one spring afternoon in May 1994 Barb Tatterson came out to my house after work. We had not met before, and we talked things over as we walked about in the yard and I put some summer flowers in the ground. I began to learn about David's story, and later that night I read the statements Tatterson had submitted to various panels of experts. The writings she brought were the most graphic and strongly reasoned statements I had seen. She was not asked to testify at the 1994 hearing in Cincinnati led by Representative John Bryant, but her written submission was eloquent:

> I remember visiting David at the old General Hospital. Families would all get to visit on the porch that ran the length of the back of General Hospital during warm weather. All patients that were able would be brought down to visit with their loved ones and friends.

Some would come in wheelchairs and others on beds, so all the children could visit and more than two people at a time.

As time went on it became harder and harder to visit David. I don't remember when the burns and sores appeared . . . but they did. I do remember that he vomited quite frequently and lost a great deal of weight and when he ate, ate very little . . . and vomited it back up shortly afterwards. He begged for pain medicine and most often we found him in tears because he had not received it. My aunt would have to go and get a nurse. . . .

It became obvious after a short period of time that David would not be able to return home. He was then transferred to Drake Hospital.

The first time I went to see him at Drake I felt it was the worst place I had ever been in. It was dreary, dark and scary. You could have had a spook house there and would not have needed any decorations for Halloween. Some rooms had as many as six patients in them, all crying for something and no one helping them. David would be crying to be taken off the bedpan (which he might have been on for several hours), or because of his need, again, for pain medication. When we arrived, other patients would ask my aunt to do things for them, and she did. One patient even asked her to clean his dentures, and of course she did.

David's only relief came when his mother appeared on the scene—to take him off the bedpan and then go and chase a nurse for his medicine. They were careless with him and broke his leg, then did nothing about it. They didn't even try to set it or secure it so that it would be less painful when he was being moved.

I remember David crying to go home . . . and then crying to just let him die. I remember the day before he died, and asking my teacher at school if we could say a prayer for him to die peacefully. The next day they came to the classroom and asked us to go home . . . I knew that David had died.

I found peace within myself knowing that now he would not have any more pain and no one could do anything to hurt him again.[14]

Tatterson says that for herself and her family, "It is still very hard for us to understand how trusted doctors, nurses and other medical professionals, and especially the U.S. government, could be involved in injuring or killing so many of their own people. I see more and more of these 'killing fields' appearing before the public for the first time. Most people do not understand unless they are somehow involved, but thank God some people have found it within themselves to speak up."

One of the worst things about the role of the military, Tatterson says, is that the "crimes against humanity" that took place at Cincinnati General Hospital "did not happen during any war." Senator Kennedy, she writes, was wrong for backing down when Senator Taft told him "that Cincinnati was his territory and he was not to interfere in anything in his territory."

David Jungnickel did not die shortly after his radiation, as some patients did, but he suffered and was ill, and his persistent "anemia" after this exposure, particularly in combination with the effects of his tumor radiations, cannot have lengthened his life.

The doctors themselves write that "severe nausea and vomiting began three hours after exposure. These symptoms persisted for forty-eight hours. Anorexia lasted for seventy-two hours. The patient's complaint of chest pain prior to therapy improved, as did the radiological findings, but recurred in four weeks." Four weeks following therapy, they write, anemia developed, and a fall in white blood cells. "Weakness, anorexia, and depression were prominent." [15]

Is this the increased well-being, the "palliation," the doctors say they were trying to bring about with whole body exposures? The major benefit this therapy was supposed to provide?

DURING THE RADIATION PUBLICITY, I received a number of calls from people who wanted to tell me about their experiences at Cincinnati General Hospital. Some of these callers were interesting, and I listened for a long time and wrote down my notes and impressions.

One such caller was a woman named Ann Weise. Her mother had died in a cancer ward of the hospital in 1961, and though we quickly found that she was not one of those who had been irradiated, Weise's almost total recall about what the hospital had been like for cancer patients at that time was valuable. The terminal ward Weise described was located in one of the "pavilions," or outlying underground buildings connected by tunnels to the main facility.

Weise and her parents had lived in Cincinnati only a couple of years when her mother became ill. They had been farmers in Texas, but the farm, Weise said, "had blown away in a dust storm," and they had migrated to Cincinnati. Weise's father found a job at Cincinnati Milacron, but they did not have much money, and when Weise's mother had become ill, at only forty-one, they did not know exactly where to turn. Her father was a veteran but there was no VA hospital in town that could help, and so her mother ended up at General Hospital. She had become mentally confused and was placed in a psychiatric ward.

Weise's mother was a very intelligent woman, Weise says, and had once wanted to study medicine herself. In the psychiatric ward, she was having a lot of pain, and nothing was being done about it. This was excruciating for Weise and her father, and finally it was recognized that her mother's problems were not simply psychiatric.

On a certain day surgery was performed on Weise's mother rather suddenly, without even a warning to the family, and a large brain tumor was found. After that it was said that nothing more could be done. It was then that her mother was sent to one of the old pavilions. "It was just terrible," Weise says. "My mother died there like an animal." [16]

In the long room where her mother lay, there were forty sufferers, mostly poor black people, Weise says. All down one wall were the beds of the men, and along the other the beds of the women—with so little aisle between them that you could hardly make your way down it. "This was all so hideous," Weise says, "that I will carry it with me the rest of my life." She can still smell the smells, even see the tiles on the floor, she says.

There were very few nurses, and those few were rotated in and out of the ward because the work was so painful. Families often stayed half the night, and everybody tried to help everybody else. In the evenings a cleaning lady named Rose would come, and she would prop her tools by the bed of Weise's mother, sit down in an ancient metal chair, and read aloud from the Bible. Weise thought this was remarkable and that if her mother could hear Rose read, it would have had to be a comfort to her.

Her mother lived only two months after her surgery, and she died there in the ward. Weise does not remember that the doctors ever communicated more than once or twice and says they were rarely seen on the floor. She and her father gave permission for an autopsy, but they never saw the results.

Nothing made very much sense, she says, and she remembers her father, at home, crying hopelessly in the night.

ANN WEISE'S MOTHER was in a large terminal ward, but at times, beds elsewhere in the hospital were found for the whole body patients during the weeks immediately following their radiations.

Various tests were carried out each day to see what the patients were suffering, how much their minds were affected, and whether or not a change in their body fluids would evince any tell-tale sign of radiation. Such an indicator could be used as a test for radiation injury—for troops, for instance, whose degree of exposure might not be known. The search for this marker in the blood and urine was a primary goal of the project; in fact, Eugene Saenger told Advisory Committee interviewers in the fall of 1994 that if the team had found this marker early in the study they might have discontinued the radiations. "We kept being on the edge of finding what we were looking for, so we kept on treating the patients." [17] No indicator of this kind had been found by other researchers, and it was not to be found by the team in Cincinnati.

In the first report to the DOD we read that the Department of Psychiatry had made available a bed for the whole body subjects on the Psychosomatic Ward. Here the patient could be given a "careful psychiatric evaluation and more individual attention." That environment, it is written, "is far more attractive and there are no other patients receiving radiation therapy with whom the patient can exchange experiences. Thus the emotional and psychometric response of the patient can be better evaluated in this milieu."

A year later Maude Jacobs would be given her own large dose of radiation and would lose her mind—and her life, but she would be able to die in a private room. Others were not so fortunate even as that. David Jungnickel, as we have seen, outlived his brief follow-up and was abandoned to wards for the hopeless at General and at Drake. In 1967 Mike Spanagel would be sent home just after radiation, with a nurse coming out to take samples of his body fluids, but in the four weeks before he died, his wife became his attendant and the injector of his medicines for pain; a few months after Spanagel's death, Katie Crews's Aunt Louise would die in pain and neglect, as we have seen, in one of the large wards of the hospital where help was seldom available.

OVER A SIX-MONTH period in 1963 six patients were irradiated in the third phase of the experiments. Perhaps the doctors had read a cautionary tale in the high doses they had applied almost across the board the year before, with such very negative consequences for John Edgar Webster, "E. J.," and John Henry Wells. They trimmed the radiation back down to a level between the lower and higher doses administered to the first twenty subjects. Even so, a sixty-four-year-old African American man, William Rucker, died on his fifty-fourth day.

It was during this third period of the tests that internist B. I. Friedman, along with James Kereiakes, the radiation physicist, and radiologist Harold Perry, began to cosign the government reports with Eugene Saenger.

Perry was the radiologist who eventually left UC in 1966; at the hearing on the proposed settlement of the lawsuit in 1997, he was one of three team doctors defending the study in video presentations to the court.[18] Few people had known before seeing and hearing Dr. Perry onscreen that he was an African American doctor. As a person of color himself, Perry expressed outrage that the study would have been thought to have been "racist," just as Bernard Aron would express, on the same occasion, what he said was his amazement and distress that a Jewish individual would have been thought to have engaged in dangerous experiments on captive subjects. Yet no new information that might help exonerate the doctors was brought forth by either physician, and there continued to be an embargo on discussion of any individual case, even that of Maude Jacobs, the mother of forty-nine with breast cancer, whose daughter was a witness in the same court, testifying at length to the details of her mother's treatment under the doctors' care.

DURING 1964 SEVEN new sufferers from cancer would be taken down to the hospital basement for treatment in the whole body room at the end of the corridor, and three of these individuals would die within a few weeks. One of these was Maude Jacobs.

Jacobs had seven children, all living today. After her death, her three youngest children were sent to Catholic orphanages and then to adopting families. Jacobs had cancer, of course, and might not have lived a long time, but she was living a relatively normal life as parent and homemaker when she was called in for her treatment and put on her hat and called a taxi to take her to the hospital. Afterward, she would spend only one night more with the children at home, and would die in the hospital in the care of her oldest child, Lilian Pagano.

Jacobs's youngest child, Kim Szwedo, has given an account of what it was like to lose her mother, so suddenly, as a child of eight. Szwedo said that back in 1964 a mother of a friend of hers had recently gone to the hospital to have a baby, and that when her mother was taken to the hospital too, she had thought a baby would be coming home.

The family lived in a house quite near Cincinnati General Hospital and the campus of UC. Szwedo has said that she sometimes played on the campus and walked through the buildings. She was frightened, though, by the preserved fetuses displayed in the biology wing, and had the childish fancy that she herself might be captured and preserved that way. On the day her mother died, she ran away from the house to a wooded park across the road and crawled into a large open culvert to hide from all that was taking place. When it became dark, she was afraid to leave this hiding place and spent the whole night there, she says.[19]

At the 1997 hearing on the settlement, Judge Sandra Beckwith listened to Lilian Pagano's long narrative about her mother with what seemed to be intense interest and asked a number of respectful questions. Pagano and two other families had become dissenters from the proposed settlement of four-and-a-quarter-million dollars. Their feeling was that this sum did not represent a severe enough penalty for the doctors and their institutions, and that the memorial plaque to be raised in honor of the victims was far from satisfactory. At the close of her testimony, Pagano spoke derisively of this plaque, which as originally proposed would furnish no information about the experiments themselves or even record the full names of the victims, but only their initials. "I want everyone in this courtroom to know," Pagano said, "that my mother had a name. Her name was not 'M. J.' *Her name*—was Maude Jacobs."

While I knew that most people in the packed courtroom that day did wish the settlement to be approved and the case finally closed, and considered the agreement a victory for truth and some measure of justice, I also understood the feelings of the Jacobs family and was glad that their story could be told in court.

9

The Final Years

I've talked to this pleasant, elderly Negro widow, reviewed her chart and discussed whole body radiation with her. She understands . . . that it will not cure. She has agreed to this treatment.
—DR. EDWARD SILBERSTEIN about Margaret Bacon, case number 090, May 3, 1969

Maude Jacobs received a hundred and fifty rads over her whole body on November 7, 1964, and did not bring home from the hospital a new baby, as her daughter Kim had half expected she would.

When Jacobs was exposed to this dose that would destroy her bone marrow and lead to her rapid demise, twelve other patients had already died within weeks of being irradiated, and yet no conclusions had been drawn, it seems, as to the efficacy of this treatment for cancer. The tragedy that befell Jacobs and her family would befall many others as well before the experiments would be brought to a halt.

We may certainly ponder the fates of two male patients who were exposed in the same year Jacobs was and who died very quickly afterward, one only nine days after his exposure and the other on day fifteen. These men belong to a small set of victims who died within a matter of days after radiation and constitute their own special kind of tragedy.

We have to assume, and the medical records seem to bear this out, that these shortest of the short survivors were very ill and could not withstand even briefly the shock of wide field radiation to their broken bodies. It was the pitiable story of one of these individuals, the woman named Evelyn Jackson, that first came to public notice in Nick Miller's story in the *Post*. Jackson, as we have seen, lived only ten days and died in 1962 in a ravaged state after an exposure of two hundred rads.

But in the middle years of the UC project, the contradictions around the choosing of individuals to expose seem especially dramatic. During the same period that the two men mentioned above died so quickly, doctors also irradiated the woman named Clara Johnson, who lived on for twelve years and could not have been considered by any stretch of the imagination "terminal," "end-stage," or even severely ill. Thus we have a picture of doctors casting about rather freely for subjects and taking on people in various conditions and with various kinds of cancers.[1]

In the downtown offices of attorneys White, Getgey, and Meyer, who represent certain surviving families, one may examine, with the requisite permissions, the full hospital records of those irradiated, including Jacob Heim, the survivor of fifteen days. Heim was a white man of forty-five. His records include an autopsy report not mentioned in the patient summary for the DOD. This autopsy states that at death Heim evinced a "marked toxic depression of bone marrow" and died not just of "extensive carcinoma of the stomach" but in the short term with "terminal aspiration pneumonia." He vomited both before and after his exposure, and—possibly because of the dry throat sometimes associated with radiation and the weakened reflexes induced—choked on his own vomit and drew it into his lungs.[2]

When the radiation doctors had first found Jacob Heim on the Tumor Ward, he had weighed only ninety-seven pounds. In all respects he seems to have been a very sick man. We do not know how he was entered into the study, just that he was attended on one occasion by a "Dr. Montgomery," status unknown.

Jacob Heim had been a severe alcoholic for some years, with liver disease diagnosed at the hospital back in 1960. For some time his cancer appears to have been masked by his state of advanced alcoholism, so severe that during a period when he had lost his job, he began to take no food but to exist solely on alcohol and to develop severe malnutrition as well as "chronic brain syndrome." He had become a "sociopath," said a detailed letter of 1963 from a medical worker at the local Social Security office, but had in fact been helped to a degree by a recent stay in the hospital; his nutrition had been improved and his acute state of confusion relieved.

But by 1964 Heim had become a patient on the cancer ward.

Work with such desperate cases as Heim's is, of course, not easy for doctors, but it was as if the physicians who had examined him when making their rounds on the ward had concluded that here was a man who in his present state was of no good to others or himself, but that society might still make some constructive use of him. Why not give him a dose of radiation for the Intensive Study, which needed subjects and could not afford to be extremely particular about them, and see if any useful research results could be obtained? Very little radiation data was obtained, of course, for Heim died vomiting and choking only two weeks after his exposure.

In 1994 Eugene Saenger would tell fellow radiologist Ronald Neumann, a staff doctor on the Advisory Committee, that patients had been "grateful" for what the doctors were trying to do for them, and that many had experienced positive results, the "palliation," that is, the doctors were seeking for them.[3]

Heim, as we learned in 1997 from his sister, Helen Delph, had been a private in the Air Force during World War II and a mechanic for B-29s. He had always liked to work on cars and machines, she says, had proved to be a skilled mechanic, and had eventually become an Air Force instructor in this work.

Helen Delph and her brother Jacob were born in the German neighborhood in downtown Cincinnati called Over-the-Rhine. Their father was a molder in a foundry, and their mother cleaned offices in the Traction Building at Fifth and Walnut. The family had always been employed, she notes. They had not been users of General Hospital, and she regrets that Heim had ended up there through the painful times that had befallen him.

The individual who died on day nine we now know was Sil Watkins, a sixty-three-year-old African American who also suffered from "far-advanced" stomach cancer. Even prior to therapy, the doctors wrote to the DOD, Watkins "appeared to be deteriorating" and his white blood count was already abnormal. After radiation of fifty rads, he "continued a downhill course" and died soon thereafter.

If we wonder how doctors could inflict what they did on people who were in relatively decent health, as the majority of the patients were according to the researchers' own reports, it seems in a way even more puzzling that they could seize upon individuals in the last stage of illness and subject them to a wracking ordeal that might slit the fragile cords of their remaining life streams. Sil Watkins had not been treated for his cancer; when he came to his public hospital for help, he received nothing but total body radiation—and an end to his travail.

In 1994 Eugene Saenger was questioned closely by three members of the Advisory Committee about how subjects were selected, but his answers were not extremely helpful. "When the cobalt machine was in," Saenger said, "and Dr. Perry was here, who was a qualified user, if we decided that the patient should be treated for carcinoma of the cervix or of the lung or whatever, in the hospital, that patient was in. And if you as a resident made that decision, in my absence or Perry's absence, that patient was admitted." [4] There were no formalities, Saenger said, no particular lines of authority for screening subjects. He made the further explanation that the team were simply "seeing patients, either in the tumor clinic or on the tumor ward" and consulting with other doctors "who thought it might be worthwhile offering whole body radiation." But the struggle against other researchers for subjects was a problem that limited what could be done, he said, and helped explain why team publications on cancer did not appear during the project.

> Competing with this study was another group of people who said, *We sure would like to see what nitrogen mustard would do.* Sometimes we would get the patient, sometimes they would get the patient. We had tumor conferences on a semi-formal basis, not every patient went through every step, but between the tumor clinic and the tumor conference in the tumor ward . . . [sentence not completed]. There were rounds that were made, the rounds with the attending physicians and the residents . . . [and] patients were seen and they were discussed at some length. [5]

What kind of "palliation" were the doctors hoping to provide for such sufferers? What in fact did they mean by this term? The Advisory Committee interviewers plumbed Saenger rather hard on this subject, and he defined the goals of the treatment at one point as "shrinkage of tumor" and "relief of pain," but he could not say how these effects had been assessed. When Ronald Neumann, a staff radiologist, asked him point-blank how he measured palliation over time, Saenger said, "We measured it primarily by survival." Neumann—though he continued to defend the UC team against any charge other than "bad science"—later told the full Committee that palliation was quite distinct from lengthening of life, and that he regretted that Saenger had not provided more information than he had about the medical purposes of the radiation.[6] In any case, the hope of extending life would be an ironic explanation for the fates of people like James Tidwell, Watkins and Heim, Evelyn Jackson, Maude Jacobs, and the many other sufferers who died soon after exposure.

In 1971 Edward Silberstein, the young radiologist who had joined the team only a few years earlier, not long out of Harvard, could blithely report to an audience at the medical school that the whole or half body radiation administered was "to allow patients to be as free of pain and to function as normally as possible for as long as possible."[7] Again, a paradoxical explanation for what happened to Heim and Watkins and the others mentioned above.

On the same occasion, Silberstein stated that, regarding consent, the patients had had the "purposes, effects and risks" explained to them "fully and clearly." But neither Heim nor Jackson nor Maude Jacobs, for instance, were presented with any consent form, and the doctors' reports to the DOD for the first five years of the project, we may recall, reveal that patients were being told simply that "they are being treated for their disease."[8] The written consent forms introduced in 1965 underwent various modulations, and a few at the end of the project included language about the "research nature" of the study, but none ever stated the real risks of the exposures. A risk cited in 1970, for instance, is "the chance of infection or mild bleeding to be treated with marrow transplants, drugs, or transfusions as needed."[9]

IN LATE 1966 THE DOCTORS sent in a major report to the Department of Defense. This was a summarizing paper for the first six years of the project, and it contained abundant analyses of the team's findings on radiation injury as it related to men in combat.

This report had the same title as the previous three communications, "Metabolic Changes in Humans Following Total Body Radiation," and it attached profiles for eighteen new subjects, including Maude Jacobs, Jacob Heim, Sil Watkins, and four others who died within a month. Some of these deaths are among the most clearly documented radiation deaths of the project.

A clear record of rapid and irreversible collapse of the bone marrow can be read, for instance, in the patient profile for a sixty-six-year-old man named Louis Romine. Romine had been diagnosed with tuberculosis in 1960, but in April 1965 he had been admitted to General Hospital "with a six-month history of pain in the right shoulder, anorexia, and weight loss." A biopsy of the lymph nodes in his neck had shown metastatic squamous cell carcinoma:

> Before treatment the patient's hemogram was normal except for a slightly elevated WBC [white blood count] (over 12,500). On May 4, 1965, a total of 217 ml. bone marrow was aspirated for storage without difficulty.
>
> He tolerated three sham irradiations well [that is, rehearsal-type "radiations" to help the doctors discount his psychologic reactions to the large and intimidating Cobalt 60 machine]. On May 8, 1965, total body radiation was administered. The patient received 200 rad midline absorbed tissue dose (316 r midline air dose). After treatment the patient vomited through the evening with nausea and anorexia persisting for three days.
>
> His hemogram remained stationary until six days post TBR. At this time his WBC dropped to 7,250 and remained there through day twelve. He was placed on INH [Isoniazid, a treatment for tuberculosis] three days after irradiation. His condition did not change after TBR.
>
> On the eighteenth day (May 25, 1965) after TBR, the WBC dropped from 5500 to 3250. On May 27, 1965, autologous bone marrow was infused without difficulty.
>
> The platelet count and WBC continued to drop steadily until they reached a low (WBC 350; platelets 8,730) at twenty-six days post TBR. WBC and platelet count remained at the same low level until he expired June 5, 1965, 28 days post TBR.

The paragraphs above are from Romine's patient profile in the DOD report in question. If we study the full hospital records of this patient, we find, as noted in chapter 5, that he was one of the patients whose blood was analyzed for the team by Edward Gall, the director of the Medical Center and a pathologist. The counts above are those provided by Gall on May 20 and three succeeding dates. This was information the team needed in order to correlate the blood findings with various other manifestations of injury from radiation.

(What Gall may not have felt he knew were the offsetting benefits that might be accruing to some patients. Still, two years later, as we have seen, when Thomas Gaffney and others in the school raised this very question—what benefits for such severe risks?—and received no intelligible answer, the director did not pursue the matter.)

In this report of 1966 the researchers comment rather extensively in their general narrative on the injuries to the blood that sufferers like Romine had sustained. It is clear that they knew all along that such injuries would occur. "Hematological changes after TBR have followed those patterns well documented in the literature," they write, and a few pages later they count up the deaths: ten of their first fifty patients have now died within thirty-seven days of radiation (thirteen, if we extend this period to day fifty-two).

The short survivors the doctors identify have suffered, they write, the "manifest illness stage of the acute radiation syndrome," that stage of illness that generally comes on about a month after exposure and is marked by damage to the blood. It is reported that even among those who survived this acute stage, "lassitude and loss of appetite" persisted for 'three to four months.'"[10]

It was in this fourth period that the doctors began exposing some patients over only half their bodies. Jacob Heim was the first partial body subject; he received one hundred rads to his lower body. To irradiate people in this way made it possible for the team to study the differences in full and partial body injuries and to report to the military that their findings "demonstrate the importance of shielding in decreasing the deleterious effect of radiation."[11] In general, though not always, partial subjects did better, and the team told their sponsors that soldiers partly shielded in a radiation zone would fare better at certain doses than those without such protection. Thus their study will now provide "a valuable baseline for the evaluation of a great variety of large area and volume exposures in the human being." [12]

Indeed, in the same passage we read that the researchers can now predict, from the data thus far accumulated, that "combat effectiveness would be maintained relatively well up to 150 rads TBR" and "partially shielded exposures" even better. At or above 150 rads, they assert, half of those exposed would be ill.

The retrospective nature of this fourth report of 1966 shows the researchers acknowledging more fully than in the past the price being paid, over six years of radiations, by their "volunteers." Still, they do not conclude that the study should not continue. No physician review committees then or later pointed out, specifically, that the Phase I standard for continuing new medical trials had not been met by this team and that the research could not properly go forward to Phases II and III. In Phase I work, investigators must demonstrate that a new drug or procedure is not "toxic" — only then can they proceed to Phases II and III to try to show that the new treatment is not only safe but efficacious, and that it compares favorably with a group of untreated or differently treated controls.

The doctors did not decide that because the cobalt radiation had proved highly "toxic" for many subjects, according to their own summaries, they must cease and desist until this toxicity could be overcome. Still, they report that while they proceed they will start attempting to protect the immune systems of future subjects.[13] They have in fact already drawn marrow from the bodies of thirteen subjects before radiation, but have only twice tried to reinfuse the unradiated marrow afterward. This technique was in itself experimental in the sixties, and over the remaining years of the project the team would succeed only five times, according to its own record, in protecting the immune systems of those irradiated.[14]

In sum, only five of the ninety individuals irradiated would be protected from the acute radiation poisoning that represented the major risk.

THE REPORT OF 1966 is the first to attach a list of team publications. Four brief abstracts of the ongoing research have now been printed in *Radiation Research*, and a brief notice on "proteins in the serum of total-body irradiated humans" in the *Journal of Immunology*. The magazine *Science* has used a three-page article on the search for a dose marker in the urine. The only known cancer report that would appear, a piece of only a few paragraphs written by Friedman and Saenger along with a medical student, had been published in 1964 in *The Lancet*, on the subject of certain chromosomes in their "relation to cancer and whole-body radiation."

Considering what was already known about radiation injury, a certain question might well have been asked of the editors of these publications, and of others who brought out the team's findings in years to come: "Did you ask the researchers to explain in their articles *why* they were irradiating people and what the outcomes were for them?"

Apparently no one did ask, and shortly after this period, full-fledged articles would begin to appear in important journals: at least five highly technical accounts of the team's search for dosimeters, and a lengthy article in 1969 in the *Archives of General Psychiatry* on the effect of radiation on "cognitive and emotional processes." This latter report was authored by Saenger and four psychiatric researchers, two of whom did not sign any of the DOD reports but would later become defendants in the lawsuit.

DURING THE YEAR that followed the submission of this major report of 1966, five more patients were irradiated. One of them, Willie Thomas, an African American social worker, died on her fifty-ninth day, and another on day sixty-eight in circumstances we cannot fully delineate. A tragic event for Thomas was that she seemed to lose her mind after radiation.[15] It was one of her children, her son Leon, who would be shown in 1994 in a huge front-page photo in the *Enquirer*, visibly enraged at the doctors as he held up a picture of his mom at his wedding of years ago.

It was at the end of this 1966–67 year in the College of Medicine that the Gaffney committee, an early group of physicians reviewing the project within the school, became disturbed about what was happening in their college. In the end, of course, they gave their consent for the project to continue. The approval granted meant that over the remaining five years of the project—until it was finally closed down, with the help, not of doctors or official review committees, but of journalists and nonmedical faculty—thirty-seven more individuals would be afflicted and ten more victims would die within a month of exposure.

Indeed in the school year that directly followed the Gaffney committee's inquiries, three subjects died early. Three weeks after her treatment, Irene Shuff, the mother of the first named plaintiff of the suit, choked to death in the night at a hospital for the terminally ill. Katie Crews's aunt, Louise Richmond, whose final days of pain and neglect were described by Crews and her daughter at the mass meeting at UC, died on day thirty-one. Grey ("Mike") Spanagel, a salesman for a local television station, was irradiated over his full body for his throat cancer and died at home thirty-one days later of pneumonia and the failure of his immune system.

Before his radiation, the doctors had operated on Spanagel to remove bone marrow and then attempted to reinfuse it after his exposure, but the process did not succeed. His hospital records show that his blood count was normal when he was irradiated but by day nineteen after exposure it had greatly declined, and a week before he died was a tiny fraction of what it had been—a count of 6500 fell to 400 in the last measure taken.

I had been interested in the case of "G. S."—case number 077—for some years before his identity was known, and in the summer of 1994 I telephoned his wife Madge to see if she would care to talk about her husband's death. She wanted to discuss things, and I went over to see her up on the seventh floor of a large apartment building. It seemed to be a reasonably comfortable, if not a spacious, place to live, but Spanagel said she had taken the apartment because it was subsidized housing. She had had to crowd her furnishings from larger rooms into this adumbrated space. After her husband's death, she had in time sold the commodious home they had lived in and moved into an apartment. But she found she could not afford the new place either, and a few years before we met had moved into the subsidized Cambridge Arms.

Spanagel said that when she was a young woman she had wanted to go to UC to study for a profession and that in fact she had been chosen for a scholarship, but that as it turned out, she had had to go to work. Her father had died when she was quite young, leaving five children under the age of nine, and the family needed her help. She was Spanagel's second wife and had one child by him.

Madge Spanagel was seventy-four when we met, and though she looked younger than that, she could not move about very well and had not been able to appear at our meetings and hearings. She said her legs were often swollen because of a five-way bypass she had undergone ten years ago, when veins had been removed from her legs.

Her husband Mike had been sixty-three when he died back in 1967. Though it seems certain that he had had incurable cancer, and had had a tracheostomy earlier that year, Madge Spanagel said he had not expected so rapid a demise and had told her, "I'm going to beat this." The doctors had informed him that at first he would get worse after the radiation, but then he would get better. "But that was not the way it happened," said his wife.

Her bitterest memory was that during the August before her husband's radiation in November, the two of them had gone on the train to visit a daughter in York, Pennsylvania; they had "got along fine, enjoyed going out to dinner, and stayed in a lovely motel." He was definitely not at death's door, she said, when he was irradiated a few months later, and had continued up until September to do occasional work for station WCKY.

When this work had ended because of his difficulty speaking, Spanagel had begun writing a book on selling. He loved to write and wrote a lot of letters, she said; he had often corresponded with an editor at the *Enquirer*, Dale Stephens. Mike Spanagel's mother had been an Emerson said to be related to Ralph Waldo Emerson; Spanagel's full name was Grey Emerson Spanagel. For some years he had been in the movie-booking business with Midstates Theaters.[16]

Spanagel had not had time to prepare financially for his death, Madge Spanagel told me, and as a result a large part of his estate went to two grown children named in an early will. Victoria, the fourteen-year-old daughter of Mike and Madge, was not included, and matters became very difficult.

Madge Spanagel said that she herself had known nothing of what was happening to her husband at the hospital. The day he had his radiation treatment, she had waited in a room nearby. No one offered to discuss the treatment with her, she said.

Afterward, her husband was not the same. She says Spanagel had not been in pain before his radiation, and indeed his hospital records bear her out in this, but that afterward he needed morphine continuously and that she became his nurse and gave him injections. He was at home his final month after radiation. Nurses came out, she said, but only to take away specimens of his body fluids. Once a visit was paid by Dr. Harry Horwitz, but he had had no information or reassurance to offer. Spanagel says Horwitz pulled back the sheet over her prostrate husband, looked over his body, and then strode out of the house. "He didn't say diddle-dee-do," she said.

Spanagel had private insurance and had been seeing doctors in downtown Cincinnati; at first they thought he was simply suffering from sinus trouble. When they discovered his cancer, they sent him to UC for radiation, and he had four thousand rads of Cobalt-60 teletherapy to the site of his tumor. He then had the surgery to place a tube in his windpipe, and we find in his files an October letter from team radiologist Harry Horwitz to a private doctor, Charles Blase, suggesting chemotherapy, that is, "a short course of Methotrexate."

Yet two weeks later Spanagel was admitted "for a full body radiation" at Holmes Hospital, a special facility for private patients in the backyard, so to speak, of Cincinnati General. His bone marrow was aspirated at General on October 31, and though he afterward developed a temperature, on November 7 he was irradiated. The next day he was discharged.[17]

Madge Spanagel did not live to see the conclusion of the lawsuit in 1999. When the suit was filed in 1994, she had been one of the few living spouses of the Cincinnati victims and one of those who seemed to have had a particularly strong practical claim for financial compensation.[18]

IN THE SPRING OF 1969, the record reveals a sad and somber sequence of early deaths. Margaret Bacon died on the sixth day after her radiation, another patient on day seven, and others on day sixteen, day twenty, and day fifty-two. All these patients were women.

The records of Mike Spanagel released to his wife show that his exposure had been supervised by Harry Horwitz and the team internist and chief colleague of Eugene Saenger during the first eight years of the project, Benjamin I. Friedman. But before the 1969 deaths occurred, Friedman had been replaced by Edward Silberstein.

When the legal action commenced in 1994 and Friedman and Silberstein became defendants along with the other investigators, Silberstein was still practicing radiology in the same hospital and still a member of the College of Medicine faculty. (Friedman had been gone for over twenty-five years, and in 1994 the *Cincinnati Enquirer* reported that he had retired in 1993 from the Nuclear Medicine department of Morton Plant Hospital in Clearwater, Florida.)

It was Silberstein who had overseen the final three years of the project, and who negotiated during 1970 and '71 the long-deferred approval of the project by the Faculty Research Committee led by Evelyn Hess. He became the major defender of the tests in 1971, during that "grievous time," as Saenger later put it to the Advisory Committee, when the project was coming unraveled and "Kennedy took it up as an issue — and that woman in the English Department"—and suddenly "all these people were jumping all over us." [19]

At that time Silberstein seemed to speak for the whole course of the project, and most people did not know that he himself had not become a participant until 1968. But in spite of certain changes that had by that time taken place, the effort, for instance, to protect the patients' bone marrow, rapid deaths after radiation had not come to an end.

I recall an afternoon at home on Bristol Lane when Laura Schneider, poring over the DOD documents at my thickly papered dining room table, asked me if I had ever looked at a series of deaths that occurred during the spring of 1969.

We found that during that spring this record of events took place:

On February 25, 1969, Marie Johnson was irradiated.
On March 17 Donna White was irradiated (and is still living).
On March 18 Marie Johnson died.
On April 9 Katie Dennis was irradiated.
On April 16 Katie Dennis died.
On April 28 Edna Anders was irradiated.
On May 14 Edna Anders died.
On June 4 Margaret Bacon was irradiated.
On June 10 Margaret Bacon died.

Silberstein, as the spokesman for the team in the seventies, had been the one doctor I had been able to interview for my report. About the lack of publications by the team on cancer, he had said, in a letter to me on November 14, 1971, "I hope I made it clear to you on Monday that we have not yet published the results of therapy because of the variable duration of patients' clinical course with cancer following treatment and the need to have an adequate sample of patients before one makes any statement about the efficacy of one's therapy. Since I am limited to treating seven or eight patients a year, I cannot, as a responsible scientist, issue claims about what we can do therapeutically for patients over a short period of time."

This statement came at the end of eleven years of radiations.

We should pause to remember one individual from that spring of 1969, Katie Dennis, the African American woman who lived only seven days. Dennis's records are similar to those of Jacob Heim and Sil Watkins, but we have the advantage of being able to read a running daily log about her written by the nurses on her floor. It is a somber document.

I had not seen Dennis's full hospital papers until I began preparing the present chapter and went downtown with Laura Schneider to look at certain records that had only recently become available to us. Afterward, as we drove home, I sat thinking about what we had learned. We parked on the neighborhood street I live on, and I remember looking out on the shady walks and lawns of that green-spangled afternoon. We could gaze up into a luminous blue June sky and see, laid against it, a network of lacy green bows from the great oaks that overarch our street.

I thought about the life and death of the woman named Katie Dennis and the assaults of nature—that nature which could also seem so kind on a summer day—and the assaults of humankind upon itself. We spoke in a desultory way about Dennis's case, and Laura took up the papers we had copied from her file and read from them in a low, murmurous voice. We spoke about how hard it was to understand how such things could have been brought to pass. "I still do not understand these events," I remember saying.

Dennis was fifty-three when she died. She had lost a husband and was staying home with four daughters under sixteen. She liked to sew, her records say. She was a patient on a cancer floor when selected for the Intensive Study. She had lung cancer and about four months earlier had been treated with nitrogen mustard and a tumor dose of Cobalt-60. We read, each day, in the nurses' log that she is "weak" . . . "much weaker"

. . . her appetite "poor" . . . sleeping at times "most of the afternoon" . . . at other times complaining of a "dull pain in her ribs and back."

Two days before her radiation she "appears lethargic" and "is afraid to sit up in the chair." The nurses have commenced the urine collections for the radiation team, but there is little in her body to void. She passes a "quiet evening."

On radiation day we read that "after receiving shock treatment for her psychologic reaction" to the frightening Cobalt-60 machine, "the patient finally received 150 rads of total body cobalt radiation." The nurses record that day that she is in pain and bleeding from the rectum; the next day she vomits "thick dark brown material" and cannot even be given medicines. In the days that follow, she has severe pain in her leg, is soon vomiting again. She cannot turn herself in bed. In due time she is complaining "all night" of pain in her legs, abdomen, and chest, and one evening a nurse regrets that though she needs help, it is "too early" for more medication. On another night the patient "moans frequently" but "attempts to rest when pain is not so severe."

At 11:30 A.M. on day seven after radiation, she is "very weak, unable to expectorate." She has a temperature of 102 and constant pain. At times her eyes "roll back in her head." A nurse is gratified that when her name is called, she responds, but later on this day—Dennis dies.

There is no autopsy. A record of her white blood cells shows that by the time of her death a deep decline had set in.

It is hard to know what is meant by the doctors when they report to the DOD that as to radiation, Study Number 088 "had tolerated the procedure well." She nevertheless "continued steadily down-hill," they write, "and expired . . . seven days post TBR." [20]

Dennis is the shortest survivor of all, except for another African American woman who was irradiated the same spring, Margaret Bacon, the school teacher of eighty who died on day six. Indeed, according to the final hospital summary written by Dr. Frederick Strife, Bacon went into "shock" and suffered "an acute myocardial infarction" shortly after the day's procedures, which included not only full body radiation of 150 rads but operations to remove and then reinfuse her bone marrow.

But how had Margaret Bacon been chosen for the "special study"? Ten days after her admission to the hospital, and evaluation for serious weight loss and other symptoms, a physician had written that the patient had been "seen by Dr. Horwitz. Due to the [illegible] nature of the disease the patient is a good candidate for total body radiation. We will contact Dr. Silberstein in this regard."

A few days later, we find this notation by Silberstein: "I've talked to this pleasant, elderly Negro widow, reviewed her chart and discussed whole body radiation with her. She understands what it can do and that it will not cure. She has agreed to this treatment."[21]

We learn that Bacon had tried to make it clear that she did not want an operation, and she apparently did not know either the risks of the radiation itself or that two operations for storing and reinfusing her marrow would be part of the treatment Silberstein was recommending. She signed a consent form stating that the risks of the therapy had been explained to her and that she understood "the special study and research nature of this treatment."

In Bacon's final hospital summary on June 6, Dr. Strife wrote that "a tumor consult was requested and the feeling was that this patient was in clinical condition as she could undergo total body irradiation which would be palliative treatment." Strife describes the myocardial infarct on the day of radiation and then writes that "one day prior to death it was noted that the patient had left sided facial weakness and it was felt had experienced a cerebral vascular accident."[22]

Of the three other women who died early that spring, we read in the DOD profiles for 1969 that Marie Johnson lived twenty days, with a blood count that "remained stable" until day seven but then dropped precipitously as she went steadily "downhill." Edna Anders, a white woman of seventy-one with breast cancer, died on day sixteen, and Genevieve Stone, who was recruited from Drake Hospital for incurables, on day fifty-two. Though Stone's life after radiation was short, the doctors reported that she did not evince serious decline in her white blood cell count and "appeared protected from the otherwise severe radiation effect."[23]

Evidence from Stone's case and others makes it clear that doctors at Drake, and a number of other physicians not practicing at General Hospital, were cooperating with the whole body project. We do not know why they did so or what information they had about the purposes of the project or the role of the Department of Defense.

During the same school year of 1968–69 the team began the practice of irradiating some patients twice. There would be four such individuals, generally receiving an exposure over the whole body and then one where they were, in effect, partly "shielded." The doctors had been interested for some time in finding out to what degree accumulated wide field exposures of this kind would affect military personnel. Three of the four individuals studied in this way were among the patients receiving successful marrow transplants, and evinced, as far as we can tell, a reasonable tolerance of all these effects; these patients would be required, nevertheless, to spend more days in hospital and under treatment than those only exposed once in the standard way.

All in all, the year 1969 had been a dark and costly one in every respect.

The following year the doses were mostly quite reduced, and yet one patient among the ten new subjects irradiated received a very large dose of 250 rads, the only individual to be given so high a dose. In spite of an attempt to protect his bone marrow, he died thirty-one days later.

This patient was an African American individual named Philip Daniels. Daniels was forty-seven years old and worked at the hospital; he is described in the hospital records as a "janitor" or "in housekeeping." The year before he had been operated on for pancreatic cancer and then followed in Surgery Clinic. Though in the meantime he had lost weight, he was eating well, was "alert and active" and "in no acute distress." All of this we read in a narrative composed by a Dr. Bossert on the day Daniels was seen for the first time in the Tumor Clinic. Bossert writes that Daniels was taking medicines for his condition and had had "an excellent response." [24] No plans were cited for more treatment at this time, even though we read, with some foreboding, that "the patient has been presented to Dr. Aron."

Daniels was asked to return to the Tumor Clinic in three weeks, but this did not come about, since in the meantime he had been admitted to the hospital "for whole body irradiation and marrow transplantation as part of a whole body irradiation study."

We do not know whether, after his radiation, Daniels was able to take up his job again, but three weeks later he returned to the hospital very weak and in "increasing pain." A week later he died there, his blood counts severely reduced. A marrow transplant had been attempted but is notated in a later record as one that did not "take." An autopsy report shows the name "Dr. Gall" at the top.

The year after Daniels's death, I studied the profile about "P. D." in the doctors' papers as I composed the report on the project for the Junior Faculty Association, and I also cited their description of the patients of this late period:

> Several of the subjects were tumor-free and essentially normal (following radiation-induced tumor regression) receiving prophylactic whole-body radiation. The rest had metastatic carcinomas which were inoperable and not amenable to conventional chemotherapy. Nevertheless, these patients were all clinically stable, many of them working daily. (Report #8, 1970, p. 2)

A month after Daniels's death an African American man named Willie Williams received two hundred rads to the lower body and died on day twenty-two, with blood counts that had begun to drop a week after his radiation. Twenty-three years later, and after the doctors had agreed to settle the claims against them, Williams's daughter, Willa Nell Woodson, would contest the terms of the agreement and help bring about a ruling by Judge Beckwith that improvements would have to be made in the settlement terms before it could be sanctioned by the court.

THE LAST YEAR of the project brought in ten new subjects, including Rose Strohm, whose daughter Elise had been located by Laura Schneider and myself early on as we looked for families to help develop a lawsuit, and whose immediate response had been to cry out, "How could they do this to Mom? How could they?" and to insist that the exposures were not just "evil" but "beyond evil." [25]

Rose Strohm had to suffer not only a large full body exposure of two hundred rads but, like many of the later patients, the difficult bone marrow removal and reinfusion. In her case, these procedures did not proceed smoothly, partly because of an error in estimating the status of her blood before radiation. After her exposure, Strohm lived eighty-nine days.

Another of the original four plaintiffs of the suit came from this late set of victims—Joe Larkins, that is, whose father Willard had been study number 109. As I have reported, Larkins, who was fifty-two in 1994, testified with angry mockery of the doctors before the congressional hearing led by John Bryant and then before the Advisory Committee panel as it met in Cincinnati. No one, Larkins said, would have given permission for such a dangerous procedure to be used on himself had the risk been known. Willard Larkins received a large dose to his lower body and afterward was very ill. He lived eighty days longer, and we do not know exactly what the effects of the radiation were.

When I first contacted the Larkinses to let them know what had happened and to be sure they were in fact the family of "W. L.," it became clear that a somewhat unusual situation existed among the children. An issue of this kind can arise in class actions just as it does in the execution of estates. I first talked to a "Joe Larkins" considerably younger than the "Joe Larkins" of fifty-two who would become an activist in the suit. "Little Joe," though, was not a wrong lead from an uninvolved family. He spoke of Willard Larkins as his "father" and had been raised by Larkins and his wife, but it turned out that he was a grandson, not a son.

"Little Joe" had grown up believing Willard Larkins to be his father, and as the last child at home he was closer to Larkins during his last years than the other children were. But he was actually the child of a Larkins daughter, and he has said that he was not told until he was a grown man that he was not his father's natural son. Since he was never officially adopted, and his birth parent is still living, this has meant that he is not in the direct line of inheritance and has received no compensation from the suit.

Little Joe, in 1994, was a long-haul truck driver with the Liquid Carbolic Company. He was divorced and a little lonely. "I come home after a long haul on the road," he has said, "and well . . . I play with the cats, and that's about all there is to my life . . . ." [26]

Larkins was ten when his father became ill with colon cancer, and he remembers the tunnels of the hospital pavilions where the clinics were and playing little scooting games down there while his mother attended his father. He remembers well the whole travail of his father's cancer. He can picture the cancer ward with its long rows of beds on either side.

He wants it clearly understood that his father was a hard worker all his life and never on welfare. For many years his job was with an old Cincinnati firm called the Picture Ring Company, where he crafted orders for special finger rings that could hold a tiny picture.

Yet Larkins was a rough-and-ready man, according to his son Joe, and

when the boy had asked him what the little contraptions were that de-
pended from his body, he had said, "Boy—now you look at this. When
I have to pee, it goes in this little bag see? And when I shit, it goes in this
bag. And boy . . . you listen to me—*life's a bitch*. But what can you do . .
hunh? Sometimes you win, and sometimes—you lose, boy."

Willard Larkins had been Joe's protector in a way. When others tried
to constrain him, his father would say, "Let that boy go." But after his
death, his mother put her foot down. "You're not going to run like you
were! You're going to go to church—and you're going to do this and
you're going to do that. . . ." Or that is the way Joe Larkins remembers it.

Early one morning at home Joe had realized there were priests in the
house. "My father was passing away," he says. His father died holding
his hand.

ANOTHER SUBJECT WHO DIED, as Willard Larkins did, during the
last official year of the project was a woman from Mount Vernon, Kentucky, named Mary Singleton.

It was curious the way her family was found. Laura Schneider, working down at the Court Index at the time when we were looking for surviving families, noticed that one of the individuals whose initials and
date of death matched our records had lived in Mount Vernon, a small
Kentucky town not far from her own town of Lexington. Laura figured
that people in a small town would remember practically everyone, and
indeed as soon as she got in touch with a Mount Vernon funeral home
they were able to tell her about Mary Hampton Singleton.

Her son Sam was still living in Mount Vernon, and Laura spoke to him
on the phone, and then she went over to see him and his wife Vistal. It
had been arranged among them that the *Lexington Herald-Leader* would be
contacted, and the reporter who covered Mount Vernon came that afternoon to the Hamptons's small neat house—the front room plentifully
decorated with little crocheted doilies and other mountain crafts—and
brought a photographer. Gail Gibson of the *Lexington Herald-Leader* went
on to compose a careful and abundant story; in fact, the Hamptons's
story was told in more detail than any other family account. Three days
later the *Herald-Leader* ran a plainspoken editorial. "Nobody's likely to
build a monument to Mary Hampton, but maybe someone should. It
would help remind everyone of just what government of the people, by

the people, and for the people did to some of the people three decades ago. . . . The government wasn't interested in curing Mary Hampton. It wanted information on how radiation would affect soldiers on the battlefield." [27]

In 1994 Mary Hampton Singleton was the subject of a rivalry between the Post and the Enquirer as to the details of her case and whether she was actually suffering from cancer at the time she was irradiated. I had told the Post about the Hamptons, and a weekend reporter there interviewed them by phone. Nick Miller was not on duty, and the paper ran a story that announced boldly that Singleton was not ill when irradiated. The facts had not been checked against the Singleton profile in the DOD reports.

In the days that followed, the Enquirer made a check into their own copies of the records and found that Singleton's profile stated that she had had widespread disease when she was irradiated. Singleton's family might well not have known this or ever seen the tests the doctors were citing.[28]

In 1970 Mary Singleton was living in Cincinnati and had gone to the hospital in the late fall of that year seeking help with various complaints that, as it turned out, stemmed from the colon cancer she had had surgery for five years earlier and had thought was cured. The primary treatment she received, though, when she returned, was a very large dose of radiation over her lower body. A few weeks after this radiation injury had been inflicted, she had needed gastric surgery for her cancer. She did not make it through this further ordeal and died the day after the operation.

Singleton did not trust doctors and wanted only a minimum of treatment, her family have said. She was extremely unhappy in hospitals, didn't want to spend Thanksgiving at Cincinnati General, wanted to be able to eat a little holiday dinner back home in Mount Vernon, smoke her cigarettes and visit her kith and kin, be with her grandchildren.

AFTER EXPOSURE, Singleton, like Larkins and the others of the latter half of the project, was subjected to a long series of testing sessions to see how much her injuries from radiation had affected her mind.

A paper specifically about the mental effects would be included in the report to the military in 1971, while the tests were still being conducted. It was circulated, we assume, as other reports had been, to a large number of U.S. military departments and divisions. In 1969 the psychiatric researchers involved had also published a detailed article in the *Archives of General Psychiatry* on the mental testing of sixteen patients. Two College of Medicine professors who signed this article but who had not been authors of the government reports would become defendants in the lawsuit, Louis A. Gottschalk, a psychiatrist, and a psychologist, Theodore H. Wohl. By the time of the 1971 report, submitted not long before the first public inquiries, the team was able to report that forty-three patients had been studied for the effects of the radiation on their "cognitive-intellectual functioning."

When it came to mental capacity, it seemed important to the team to study the minds of whites, not blacks, and so six of the seven new subjects were white:

> In terms of the characteristics of the overall sample, the addition of the new patients will serve to improve the ratio of whites to Negroes, to increase slightly the average educational attainment, and to decrease the average age. The trend noted in the 1969–70 report toward recruiting patients in comparatively better physical condition has continued. (Report #9, 1971, p. 72)

For these mental studies, thirteen testing occasions were required of each patient, beginning during the week prior to radiation and continuing for six weeks afterwards.

Even aside from the assault on life itself that the radiations represented, we have to consider that the subjects were given a heavy roster of duties to perform for the sake of the team's reports and publications and having nothing to do with their personal therapy. Mike Spanagel's records, for instance, show that had he been able to do so, he was expected to return to the hospital *seventeen times* over the weeks following his exposure, to provide samples of his blood and urine in aid of the search for a radiation indicator. He would also have been one of the patients tested as to the degree of nausea he suffered as well as to his mental impairment.

For the mental tests, the patients were first "interviewed," as the doctors put it, just after irradiation. The nausea and vomiting induced by the exposures proved to be a serious hindrance to these initial sessions:

The problem of handling nausea as a factor . . . continues to be a provocative and challenging one. To the extent that nausea is an intervening variable at crucial times in the psychological testing schedule, it causes considerable ambiguity in interpreting test results and . . . assessing the effects of varying dosages of irradiation on cognitive functioning.

Since the winter of 1967, all subjects have been interviewed very shortly after their release from the cobalt 60 teletherapy unit where they underwent irradiation. . . . Of the 25 patients for whom we have records, 15 exhibited some nausea. . . . Of the seven patients studied this year (1970–71) only one did not exhibit nausea and three (subjects 107, 109 and 111) had ratings for severe or marked nausea. (p. 71)

It was Rose Strohm who suffered the "severe or marked nausea" attributed to case 107, and Willard Larkins of case 109.

The psychological staff proceeded to make an interesting suggestion about the future selection of subjects for radiation: the radiation team should assess patients' *attitudes* about vomiting and loss of control and their past vomiting histories. New "study personnel" should then be chosen accordingly. As in other facets of the project, it is not clear what this kind of selection would have had to do with cancer. We do not know whether screening rites of this kind ever took place, however, because the project suddenly came upon the "grievous times" of 1971–72 and reports on new subjects suddenly ceased.

Four irradiated patients, however, would remain unreported on in the annual DOD papers and would not become known until the release of the names of all subjects in 1997. Two of these patients appear as case numbers, without initials or dates of radiation, in *tables* published in the tenth report the year following the first public revelations. The last two subjects seem to have remained unknown outside the College of Medicine until the release of the hospital records, which purport to provide files for all those entered into the study.

None of these last four subjects died shortly after exposure, and as with the other longer-term survivors, it is difficult to know what exactly the effects were. They would certainly have suffered a serious ordeal of "treatment," often involving hospitalization they might otherwise not have had, as well as certain lingering effects; they were, in short, made more ill, in varying degrees, than they otherwise would have been. In the 1971 report, the doctors state that among patients who survived the acute radiation syndrome, "lassitude and anorexia persisted in some subjects for three or four months" (p. 9).

For reasons such as this, along with the consideration that virtually all the victims of the tests had been subjected to lethal risk, and that no one had been informed of this risk, I continued to feel that all the surviving families had a deep grievance against the researchers and should perhaps share and share alike in any monetary judgments. When asked my view of the matter, I always expressed this conviction to the families and attorneys, based on my study of the tests. This equal apportioning of remedies is, in fact, often the formula in class-action suits, and it was a share-and-share-alike basis on which the plaintiffs forged the original agreement with the researchers.

Yet in time it became a question of concern to the judge as to whether the experiences of the patients had been coequal *enough* that they could constitute a mandatory class for the purposes of settlement, especially in view of the objections of certain families to the agreement.

THE SETTLEMENT ISSUES will be examined in a chapter to come, but here we might ask what exactly had happened to the search for a radiation test for exposed soldiers, the indicator or "dosimeter," that is, which had been a major objective of the researchers all along but which seemed to lie continually just beyond their reach. The idea had been to provide a means whereby military personnel who had been exposed in a radiation attack could be quickly tested to see how much radiation they had absorbed and how ill they might become. Thus elaborate laboratory work continued throughout the project on the patients' urine, but to no avail.

The team also began charting another possible indicator: the intensity of nausea and vomiting itself just after exposure. But no pattern was discerned that could be closely related to the dose absorbed. Changes in the blood were also tracked for the hours and days immediately following radiation, but this too proved to be a recalcitrant index. Injury to the bone marrow was occurring in all the patients who received a significant dose of radiation, say the researchers in 1969, and the injuries are certainly dose-related, yet the changes did not reveal themselves soon enough or predictably enough to constitute the test the team was looking for. Some patients suffered, unaccountably, more than others at the same dose.[29]

But after all, the need, as the investigators saw it, for information on nuclear injury had not declined. In the contract signed with the DOD in 1969, we read of the ever-present need for vigilance against nuclear attack: "In spite of disarmament discussions, tensions may be increasing, as noted in current discussions concerning ABM defenses. In this present and continuing situation of crisis it is necessary to pursue with increased diligence the scientific investigations of acute radiation effects and the attendant treatment possibilities in the human being."

It may be that historians of the future will be more and more inclined to ask whether this concern of the Cincinnati researchers — and other Cold War investigators — for the country's national security is not reminiscent of the concerns of the doctors of the Third Reich tried at Nuremberg. One need hardly say that no mention is made in the Cincinnati reports of the Nuremberg Code as an ethical guide, though midway through the project the reports begin to cite the more generalized code later developed at Helsinki.

It is well known that during World War II the major defense of the Nazi doctors later tried at Nuremberg had been their concern for the military fate of their country. For the sake of German troops, they inflicted on captive people all kinds of battlefield-type injuries so they could learn how to treat or prevent them. They froze people to death. They killed them in sealed, pressured chambers that simulated high-altitude flying. They infected them with typhus, malaria, and jaundice — major diseases affecting the German army. They wounded people in all kinds of bizarre painful ways and deliberately infected the wounds. They poisoned them and studied their agonies as they died.

It is hard even to read of these deeds, the accounts, for instance, of the American prosecutor Telford Taylor in the opening statement of the trials on December 9, 1946. In our great zeal in the United States to divide ourselves irrevocably from everything that happened in Nazi Germany, we have generally refused even to consider that the Nuremberg Code could have any relevance for American doctors. Oral histories of American physicians looking back on World War II have become available, and they seem to indicate that many practitioners did not follow the proceedings of the Nuremberg doctors' trials and were hardly even curious about them.[30]

Citizens of the United States would in the years after the war try to bring to justice investigators conducting dangerous military research in this country, but with little success, as we shall see in a chapter to come.

As to protections for animals, it is hardly reassuring to read, in the absence of *human* guidelines in the early years of the project, that the Cincinnati research "has been conducted according to the principles enunciated in the 'Guide for Laboratory Animal Facilities and Care,' prepared by the National Academy of Sciences."

For five years this was the only guide mentioned in the reports, and thirty years later there would be baroque and labyrinthian discussions among members of Clinton's Advisory Commission as to what researchers working with the Defense Department should have been told, if anything, about the ethical standards expected. Should they have been informed that there had been a tribunal at Nuremberg and that American experimenters should not consider themselves exempt from the guidelines of the Nuremberg Code? Should the researchers under contract have had to show evidence of having been "trained" to conduct research humanely and ethically?

Somehow, the implication among the radiologists on the Commission was that if no one *was* instructed or trained or informed, then that was unfortunate, but that little fault on either side could then be established.[31]

We do not know of research by the Cincinnati team on animals, or why the animal disclaimer is written in, but it is obvious that in the U.S., as in the Germany of the thirties and forties, there have been groups vocal enough in their concern about the abuse of animals to gain the attention of experimenters. We look in vain for parallel concerns for humans, those considered to be of racial inferiority, for instance—in Cincinnati not Jews or Russians, Poles or Gypsies, but in the main black people, and simply the working poor, white and black, who were ill; and in other Cold War tests, military conscripts, Native American miners, prisoners, pregnant women, and mentally retarded children.

The Cincinnati team was performing experiments on human subjects in not only wide field radiation but in another procedure where animal studies were still being done. In the report for 1966 we are told that investigators are learning their techniques for storing the patients' bone marrow from experiments on beagles by researchers at the University of Rochester.[32]

In 1994 it was rather unnerving to hear a resident of Oak Ridge, being interviewed on the film Julian O'Halloran made for the BBC, describe the cages of irradiated mice that had once been lined up in the same corridors as the irradiated humans. This had been amazing to him, too, said Gary Litton, a songwriter in Nashville whose father had been irradiated at the Oak Ridge hospital in 1965. A physician also interviewed in the "Atomic City," Helen Vodopick, explained that the cages weren't supposed to be in that wing. "Oh well, the mice *should* have been in a different building," she said.

The chief radiologist at Oak Ridge, Clarence Lushbaugh, also became part of the BBC film. Lushbaugh had had close relations with Eugene Saenger for some years and first known Saenger when they were both in high school in Cincinnati. The two men came of age during the hyperkinetic period of atomic research before World War II, and both were intensely drawn to the relatively new fields of study developing. Saenger, as we have seen, did not leave Cincinnati General to join the war effort; he was a resident at the hospital from 1943 to 1946, and then during the war in Korea a major in the Army Medical Corps and chief of the Radioisotope Laboratory at Brooke Army Hospital in Texas.

Lushbaugh, for his part, made his way to Los Alamos; in the sixties the two became advisors to each other's military projects in Oak Ridge and Cincinnati.[33] Lushbaugh was outraged when the fifty-seven radiations at Oak Ridge were investigated by O'Halloran for "The Sacrifice Zone," and a tape of his voice on the telephone, hanging up on O'Halloran after a few brief exchanges, was played on the soundtrack of the film.

OAK RIDGE WAS ONE of a small group of hospitals irradiating cancer victims under grants from the DOD, as at UC. But like most of these hospitals, Oak Ridge irradiated fewer individuals than Cincinnati, and none, apparently, with colon or breast cancer or other solid tumors.

In one of the Advisory Committee discussions on Cincinnati in 1994, staff member Gary Stern cited a letter from the Oak Ridge Institute of Nuclear Studies explaining why researchers there were declining to do the work agreed to in Cincinnati. Stern said that ORINS "did not do any radio-resistant treatments or radio-resistant cancers." In 1966 the Atomic Energy Commission proposed that ORINS treat these cancers, but the researchers in Oak Ridge declined, saying that there was "so little chance of benefit to make it questionably ethical to treat them. Lesions that require moderate or high doses of local therapy for benefit, or that are actually resistant are not helped enough by total body radiation to justify the bone marrow depression that is induced. Of course, in one way these patients would make good subjects for research because their hematological responses are more nearly like those of normals than are the responses of patients with hematological disorders. . . ." [34]

The various hospital radiation studies, beginning with three limited trials under the Manhattan Project, "culminated," as Stern put it to the Advisory Committee, in the Cincinnati tests, the last of the DOD-funded studies and by far the most radical in terms of the radiation doses applied and the wholesale application of them to patients who were least likely to benefit, that is, those with localized, radioresistant tumors.

In the remaining hospitals engaging in large projects—the M. D. Anderson and Baylor hospitals in Houston—the maximum doses were considerably lower than at UC, but outcomes for the patients can certainly be assumed to have been serious. As things stand, the fates of most of those individuals are still unknown and are likely to remain so unless a search for surviving families is made and a lawsuit developed.

As in earlier exposures, the patients in Houston with radioresistant cancers were part of a larger pool of cancer types. Gary Stern tried repeatedly to make it clear to the Committee that, with respect to the general practice at DOD sites of using primarily patients with radiosensitive cancers, "the only exception was the University of Cincinnati." [35]

WHEN WE LOOK at medical complicity with the military in Houston, in the hospital at Oak Ridge, in Nashville, where pregnant women were given radioactive cocktails, and in the border town of Cincinnati, we might come to believe that conservative venues in or near the south had been considered choice sites for clandestine preparations for possible nuclear war. And, of course, another southern study sponsored by a government department, the Tuskegee syphilis experiments conducted by the Public Health Service in Alabama, ran concurrently with the government-sponsored radiation tests during the forties, fifties, and sixties.

On the other hand, it was primarily at the northern site of the University of Rochester where people were injected with plutonium; and other dangerous exposures occurred in such places as Nevada, Boston, Washington state, and Utah. Still, we cannot be sure that Cincinnati's reputation for hard-core conservatism and suppression of personal rights does not help explain the length and severity of the UC project. This reputation is on the whole well deserved and hardly needs explanation.

What is perhaps less known is that there is also an active left in Cincinnati always trying to assert itself against what are seen as the forces of violence and reaction. During the late years of the radiation project, the University of Cincinnati closed its doors for a full month at the end of the school year of 1969–70 because of explosive student demonstrations against the bombing of Cambodia during the Vietnam War.

Cincinnati has, in fact, seen its share of war resistance over the years. It has long been the home of a well-known community of Quaker pacifists and tax resisters and their followers, and of the well-known peace activist and hunger artist Maurice McCracken, a minister in a poor neighborhood downtown near the area where Jacob Heim grew up and where James Tidwell raised his nine children. McCracken died in 1997, but he had become greatly agitated about the radiation experiments at the local public university and more than supportive of efforts to help unravel the facts of the case.

A task force for opposition to U.S. military action in Central America and for solidarity with citizens in that part of the world has also been steadily active and well-organized in Cincinnati for over two decades; it has mounted strong challenges to Cincinnati's Procter & Gamble, for example, when this company refused to honor the struggle of Salvadorian coffee pickers, and to the ultra-wealthy Charles Lindner family and its Chiquita Brands operations in Honduras. Chiquita is a Cincinnati phenomenon and has been the frequent target in recent years of picketers at its downtown Cincinnati headquarters because of its displacement of local families on its Honduran estates. In 1997 a whole community of small homesteads was reported to have been bulldozed to the ground in Tachimichi.

A number of African American organizations are continuously active in Cincinnati and sometimes able to confront the power elite, and as we shall see in the next chapter, a mostly African American movement grew up around the UC hospital during the year following the early publicity around the radiations. As in many towns, African American groups have waged a constant battle against the operations of the local police department and the shooting of unarmed black males on the streets.

It can also be said that in Cincinnati's center city a tenacious group of poverty workers and neighborhood activists has operated for many years a large network of organizations to aid in low-income housing and people's needs of all kinds.

In October 1996, there took place a silent march of nearly two thousand people through the streets of the Over-the-Rhine section of Cincinnati's downtown. This was the funeral march for fallen homeless advocate Buddy Gray, who was shot to death by a mentally disturbed resident during a high-intensity hate campaign directed against him by supporters of downtown developers attempting to displace low-income residents.[36] "We Shall Not Be Moved" said one of the bright banners hung that afternoon from the upper floors of the rehabbed buildings along the march, and a placard on the street read "Stop the Ethnic Cleansing in Over-the-Rhine."[37]

Taking it all in all, Cincinnati has long been thought to be a backward place. Mark Twain once said that when the end of the world was announced, he would go at once to Cincinnati, where things always happened last.

Ohio had not had a state execution since 1963 until it put to death by lethal injection an individual named Wilford Berry in 1999. It now has nearly two hundred people on death row, and it is Cincinnati's Hamilton County that leads in the numbers of those waiting to die. On February 25, 1998, an article in the *Cincinnati Enquirer* stated outright that the office of the county prosecutor, Joseph Deters, who is also a member of the UC board of trustees, "is responsible for sending more men, per capita, to Ohio's death row than in any other county in the state."

(The *Enquirer* editors supported the execution of Wilford Berry, who had volunteered to be the first to die.)

Yet here too Ohio has had a counterhero of a kind, Governor Michael diSalle, who opposed the death penalty, commuted a number of sentences while he was in office, and after losing the governorship in 1962 —partly because of these commutations—wrote an expressive book about his conviction that killing by the state is wrong.[38]

But in general, violence of all kinds by the state and within state institutions is a feature of life in Ohio, as in most parts of the United States. The well-known tragedy at Kent State in northern Ohio occurred in the eventful spring of 1970—the calling out of the state National Guard, that is, to quell student protests over the bombing of Cambodia, and the shooting deaths of four of the protesters.

During this spring of 1970 six more citizens would be subjected to secret military radiations in the public university in Cincinnati, and two of these individuals would die within a month.

It is hard to contemplate all these events without recalling, once again, the words of Senator Mike Gravel, writing in 1972: "Life is cheap in the U. S. . . . ."[39]

WHEN EUGENE SAENGER WROTE, in 1958, to the Army's director of Nuclear Medicine about a request for funds for a radiation project, this officer, Lieutenant Colonel James Hartgering, wrote his superiors that on the basis of past research on dosimeters, he did not think anything productive would come of a new study at UC. But he added this: "There are so few radiologists willing to do total body radiation . . . that those that are should be encouraged more."[40]

This encouragement had been sustained, as we have seen, for over eleven years and had brought upon unknowing citizens of the city a small holocaust of injury and death.

10

The Experiments Must Cease

It isn't clear to me that we are properly constituted to reach a sensible, scientific conclusion as to whether people were harmed.
—DR. DUNCAN THOMAS, Advisory Committee on Human Radiation Experiments

The papers originally given me by Dr. Gall in the fall of 1971 consisted of the nine reports to the Defense Department which had been made at that time. A tenth report would follow during the year to come, but it remained largely unknown outside the College of Medicine until the lawsuit was filed in 1994 and the university released its back files.

This tenth and final report was composed some time after August 1972, following the cutting off of DOD support the previous spring. Anyone who reads the reports in sequence will know at once that something momentous had happened between the ninth and tenth submissions, and of course those intervening events were the public attack on the project by Kennedy and Gravel as "death-camp" style atrocities, and the Junior Faculty critique providing the missing details of the eleven years of the study and the early deaths of twenty-one individuals.

The tenth report begins in a way quite different from those that preceded it. "The purpose of these investigations has been to improve the treatment and general clinical management and if possible the length of survival of patients with advanced cancer." [1]

The earlier reports had of course patently focused on radiation injury; cancer research was seldom referred to. But here in 1972 the doctors simply record, about the voluminous injury studies of the past, that "investigations of biochemical, cytological and psychological tests have been reported elsewhere." But though they are now reporting on whole body radiation for cancer, they do not proceed to examine any individual cases or early deaths among their subjects. Instead they present three long tables grouping patients with three different forms of cancer—colon, lung, and breast—and assert that the average, or "median," survival of each of these three groups is better, or at least no worse, than that of other sets of patients with cancers similarly advanced, whom they say they have located at UC and elsewhere.

Some features of this report one hardly knows how to explain. The doctors write that "all patients gave informed consent in accordance with directives of the Faculty Research Committee of the University of Cincinnati College of Medicine and those of the National Institutes of Health" (p. 3). Considering what we now know of the severe and pitiable neglect of David Jungnickel after his radiation, of Louise Richmond and others, we wonder what can be meant by a sentence like the following: "The follow-up procedure is continuous during the lifetime of the patient" (p. 4). And we are also at a loss to explain how "fifty-six percent" of subjects can be said to have experienced the "palliation" the doctors say they were seeking for them.[2]

These findings were first composed as a paper for the American Roentgen Ray Society, meeting in Washington on October 2, 1972. In 1973 the same analysis was published as an article of some length in The American Journal of Roentgenology, Radium Therapy, and Nuclear Medicine.[3]

The authors note, among the outcomes for the subjects, that eight unidentified deaths were "possibly attributable to radiation," a conservative figure based, it would seem, on the fact that for eight patients who died early, tell-tale blood counts had already been recorded in the DOD profiles. It was, it seems, this 1972 statement about radiation deaths that Saenger intended to disavow in his testimony before the John Bryant committee in 1994, saying that he had come to consider that all patients had died of their disease.[4]

A peculiar aspect of the 1973 article is a comparison it makes between the individuals irradiated and twenty-four people screened for the project but not exposed. The doctors attempt to show in a statistical calculation that radiation did not shorten people's lives, but in fact it is easy to see that even though, according to the researchers themselves in their report of 1971, many of the untreated individuals had originally been excluded from the study because they were too ill, they actually did somewhat *better* than those irradiated.[5]

Four of twenty-four untreated subjects died within twenty to sixty days, and among the eighty-two patients actually treated, the doctors say, nineteen died within this same period (23 percent as against 17 percent for those not irradiated). The authors omit those within either set who died *within* twenty days—Jacob Heim, for instance, and Katie Dennis, Evelyn Jackson, Margaret Bacon—and it is not clear why the eight patients exposed during the final year of the project were also excluded. Though the doctors do not themselves draw such a conclusion, anyone looking over their figures will see that the less radiation received, the better a patient did.

In a meeting of the Advisory Committee on November 14, 1994, when radiologist Henry Royal seemed to be lending some credibility to the team's survival data, Duncan Thomas, a professor of preventive medicine at UCLA, jumped in to say, "Let me first of all dismiss Saenger's own comparisons because they're complete bullshit." Thomas went on to outline the rather obvious reasons why the concept of the untreated "control group" would not work when resorted to in this fashion, after the fact. "In my view," he says, "the only sensible comparison is the comparison which the junior faculty report attempted, but not particularly with state of the art methods, which is an internal comparison within the cohort under the assumption that allocation of radiation dose is independent of prognostic factors. Now that, of course, is also a leap of faith, but that's something for which—that's at least a testable hypothesis."[6]

The Committee, however, was not prepared to test any hypothesis that might lead them to confront specific instances of injury or death:

DR. THOMAS: I guess I do have some trepidation about whether or not this is an area we want to pursue. It isn't clear to me that we are properly constituted to reach a sensible, scientific conclusion as to whether people were harmed, i. e., had their lives shortened as a result of this and whether we want to open that even for the purpose of making remedies. . . .

I think we should think very carefully before we undertake such an analysis. (p. 44)

One of the documents I had sent to staff member Gary Stern, a five-page paper titled "Annotations on Certain Short Survivors of the Cincinnati Radiation Project," caused a brief episode of distress and confusion during the same discussion. I had drawn small portraits of some of the patients who died soon after radiation, as to what we knew about their blood counts and what we had learned about their daily lives and conditions before they were treated. Henry Royal objected to the presence of this document in the Committee packets:

> DR. ROYAL: Could I make one last comment and that is there's a document in the chart in the whole body section that mentions patients by name and has some personal information in it and I would hope that we have permission to—
> DR. FADEN: Okay, we missed it. We're going to apologize. We missed that so that will be—that should not have happened.
> MR. STERN: . . . many . . . of the patients' families have testified at the Cincinnati panel and named patients by name and I think, I believe that that document, all those correspond with patients who testified at the Cincinnati panel and just publicly disclosed the patient name and number. (pp. 44–45)

Ruth Faden, the Committee chair, seemed somewhat mollified by this, but when Ronald Neumann reported that the Committee did have portions of certain medical records, with assurances from attorneys that their clients had signed releases, she was disturbed again, saying that the records weren't "helpful or necessary" anyway. "We don't need them for our purposes. . . . It was just an oversight on our part. Thank you, Henry [Royal], for picking that up."

These exchanges would seem more than strange for anyone who did not know how it is that government examines itself; after all, families from Cincinnati had traveled to Washington more than once precisely to ask the Committee to study the cases of their family members who were irradiated.

BUT BACK IN 1972 the defenses of the radiation team, and the success of the College of Medicine in keeping the patients' identities a secret, served their purpose within the medical community and most of the reporting world. When the radiations ended, no more inquiries were made. Publicity ceased.[7]

I put away all my papers and the seven-page report I had drawn up. I had been sent by Edward Kennedy's office a hundred copies of this report as it had been entered by him into the *Congressional Record* alongside the article in the *Washington Post* that had detailed our findings. All of this fit on one long double-sided sheet of fine print, and I put this stack of single sheets away in a drawer in my dining room. Whenever the subject came up in the years to come, as once in a while it did, I sent the inquiring party this sheet. I wrote on it a note: "This is what really happened—if you care to know. It was not as the doctors maintained."

The College and a large platoon of its researchers had had a desperate brush with the reality of what had taken place, but in the end, fate had perhaps been kind. Though they had lost their funds and their project, they had escaped retribution in the courts or even serious censure by their peers. The victims and their families had been "protected"—they had learned nothing of what had taken place.

IT IS A GOOD THING, I feel, as I complete the medical section of this narrative to be folding away into a far cabinet of the room where I work the various medical records I have been studying. These are somber papers in more ways than one, and I know well that I could not have been a health worker, having to study such records every day and trying not to be personally affected by them.

I live among writings of an entirely different kind from these technical reports about the final passages of people's lives. Yet it is somehow odd to think that the writings I myself have read almost daily for most of my life—the stories and poems, sermons and dramas, that is, of the great body of belletristic writings of the past—have been writings which are themselves very often about the passing of individual lives and the eventual disappearance of all things in the world.

But as to the army of unwell combatants the radiation records describe, one word more ought perhaps to be said of these citizens who did not know they *were* combatants, who formed, as it were, an invisible brigade and fought for their lives in a battle against unknown assailants. Whatever happened to them at the ends of their lives, whatever they had to endure from the ravages upon their bodies, first of nature itself, and then of their own kind—as sorrowful as all that is, it is good to remember too that they were, for the greatest part of their lives, as their children and other relations have explained a good many times, simply normal people with jobs and families and their own special life interests, with problems and predilections of all kinds, we can be sure.

One hopes, of course, that they had their share of pleasure in life, that they succeeded, in spite of everything—the caste system most of them lived in, for instance—in getting the better of their circumstances from time to time, as all of us hope to do. And indeed there is the image of Lula Tarlton riding trains to far-off places, a little grandchild by the hand; of James Tidwell rearing up in church with a good streaming prayer. John Webster on his back steps after work, strumming his blues guitar. Maude Jacobs playing with her kids up and down the house, laughing, carrying on with them. She was a great tease, they say.

We naturally do not want to remember only the glooms and sorrows of life if we can possibly help it. The ninety individuals of these tests were victims but they were not *just* victims. Mary Ann Houchins seemed to speak for many when she said, asking the judge to approve the settlement and let people get on with their lives, that she did not want to remember her Uncle Johnny simply as a victim of government fraud or as he was in his last illness but as she had known him over his healthy years.

Kurt Vonnegut, who grew up in Indianapolis, a two-hour drive from Cincinnati, wrote his novel *Slaughterhouse Five* during the period we are discussing. This book is about a fantasy land where all the moments of people's lives exist at the same time and people can travel backward and forward at will; they can *live* at any time in any moment of their lives. In this magical land even death is not final but simply another "moment" in the ever-revolving circle of a person's life. For everyone there are always "happy moments" they can visit again whenever "bad moments" oppress them.

VONNEGUT'S BOOK, as has been noted already, is also about the awesome reality of World War II and the bombing and near-destruction of Dresden by U.S. planes at the end of the war. In Dresden the American prisoners of war took refuge in what had been an underground animal slaughterhouse. Vonnegut himself took refuge there and lived to tell the story. He wanted to tell it, he said, because he did not believe the fire-bombing of Dresden should have taken place or that war is necessary. This is a book that speaks back against war and violence of all kinds. And it is well to remember that the years of the 1960s, when Vonnegut wrote, were fight-back years in the U.S. in more ways than one.

As to the fifty-six African Americans subjected, along with thirty-four whites, to battleground-like injuries by their government, it is one of the somber anomalies of the Cincinnati tests that these events came during the massive struggle of black people in the south to win their full rights as U.S. citizens. Along with Tuskegee, where *all* the victims were African Americans, what the Cincinnati blacks were afflicted with stands as a living memorial to the kinds of abuse black people had been enduring for two centuries and more, and the reason why the struggle against U.S. apartheid had to take place.

In short, two-thirds of those irradiated were black, and the federal judge who in 1995 ruled against immunity for the researchers took under consideration the claim—among others—that the rights of minorities to equal protection had been violated. Her ruling strongly suggested that when the full facts were ascertained, it might be found that if there had not been available to the Cincinnati doctors a hospital predominantly African American, the project might not have been conceived there, or conceived at all.[8]

Indeed, to enter the doors of General Hospital of that day, and to a considerable extent even today, was to enter an overwhelmingly black venue. Not only were the patients mostly black, but the facility was maintained by a staff that was 95 percent African American.[9]

IT IS A SOCIAL PARADOX, in a way, that in 1960, the year of James Tidwell's irradiation and death and of injuries to seven other black patients, four years had elapsed since the Montgomery Bus Boycott, which had ended in victory 381 days after it began. Doris Baker, whose grandmother was irradiated in 1962, had had a brush with the movement in Alabama as a teenager, when she frightened her family in Tuscaloosa one day by declining to sit in the back of a bus.

During the month of Tidwell's final ordeal in 1960, Martin Luther King Jr. was jailed in Atlanta during a sit-in at Rich's Department Store and then transferred to a maximum security prison. (Presidential nominee John F. Kennedy telephoned Mrs. King to express his concern.) One of King's great speeches would be spoken a few years later at the massive March on Washington of 1963. "I have a dream" was its tense and poetic refrain, touching back to the recurring lines of the old black spirituals and the famous dream poem of Langston Hughes: "What happens to a dream deferred? Does it dry up like a raisin in the sun? Or fester like a sore—and then run?" Does the dream "just sag," Hughes asks, "like a heavy load?" Or—in the line that would be remembered for many years—"*does it explode?*"

This poem of 1951 had become well known among black people, and seemed to have prefigured the explosion touched off in Montgomery in 1955. In the years afterward, African Americans sat-in at lunch counters and movie theaters. They marched and sang and prayed at courthouses and in the streets, were clubbed and hosed and jailed, and when released, went back into the streets again. They began trying to vote. They attempted to integrate schools and libraries, hotels, pools. They presented themselves to the registrars of white colleges.

As it happens, it was the year after the Cincinnati radiations began and the African American woman Evelyn Jackson died ten days after her exposure, that Fannie Lou Hamer left her farm in Mississippi because of death threats against her for attempting to vote. Hamer moved into her sister's house in town to help organize the voting campaign. In 1963 she would endure a savage beating in a county jail in Winona, Mississippi, but her work would go on and she would become a hero and martyr of the struggle. (Years later honors would come to her even from the Mississippi legislature.)[10]

In Cincinnati black people and white people were going down into Tennessee and working for months at a time in the work camps and voter registration drives.[11]

By the time Louise Richmond had become ill, moved back to Cincinnati to be with her family, entered the hospital in 1968 for treatment for her cancer, and suffered the injuries brought on by three hundred rads of lower body exposure, King was marching in the tense parade in Knoxville led by garbagemen trying to start a union. A few months later he would be shot to death in Memphis. It was a few years later—in 1970—that Philip Daniels was taken off his job as a janitor in the hospital, placed in the cancer ward, given an enormous dose of radiation over his whole body, and died thirty-one days later.

These were the events that formed the social background of the Cincinnati tests. Of course political polarization was a staple of the times. McCarthyism was not long dead, fear of Communism and nuclear war was still everywhere engendered, the English were building their own bomb, and war machines continued to face off against each other in the Cold War, in Cuba, and then in the shooting war in Vietnam.

BY 1967 MY OWN FAMILY had moved to Cincinnati from Georgia, as I have explained, and I had begun teaching modern literature on the main campus of UC, completely ignorant, of course, of what was taking place in our hospital across the way.

There had been "race riots" in Cincinnati the summer we arrived, and the major road leading north out of downtown into our neighborhood had the look of an abandoned war zone for several miles.

In the fall of 1968 the United Black Association at UC staged a major protest on campus and made a number of "un-negotiable demands." One of these was for courses in black literature. Like most schools, UC had no black faculty. (It had very few women, black or white; the English Department had hired its first woman professor the year before I arrived.) In any case, I agreed to develop and help teach new courses in black literature. Faculty did not seem entirely sure there *was* any black writing worth studying, but when I went to work on this project, I was soon shocked at my own ignorance of what African Americans had done. "Black people have lived as a nation within a nation," I wrote my colleagues, "and so of course there exists a culture and a literature among blacks that is separate from that of whites and little known to whites."

Black students themselves had been very few and far between at UC and been distinctly unwelcome as English majors, but now we suddenly had a fair number of African Americans in our classrooms. I remember that as for my own classes, especially in the new field of black lit, I felt we were having a very good time of it. This was the heyday of genuine engagement and debate on campuses.

When we succeeded in starting up a Black Studies Department a year or two later, I ceased to teach black literature, but like many teachers I continued over the years to include in my courses the works of African Americans. I virtually always attached to my syllabus Richard Wright's book of short novels about Mississippi, *Uncle Tom's Children*, and units on black poetry. The Hughes poem "Harlem" quoted above, with its prophetic lines about the explosions that may come when dreams are deferred, has a resonance that never fails, but I remember that reading this poem with classes in 1994 was an electric experience, as publicity began to rage again around the abuse of African Americans on our own campus.

We were reading, too, the lyrics of the old religious songs of the plantations, works that once led Richard Wright to say that "the Negro is a Negro even in his religion," and that "his consciousness of being a rejected American seeps into his worship, his prayers" [12] — as we find in this handsome little slave song:

If I had-a my way,
I'd tear this building down.
Great God, then, if I had-a my way
If I had-a my way, little children,
If I had-a my way,
I'd tear this building down. . . .

We read "Joshua fit the battle of Jericho" and marveled when — in the poem at least— "the walls come tumbling down." There is plenty to admire and enjoy among the great grieving poems and stories of African American artists down through the years, those of Howard University poet Sterling Brown, for instance, who is known best for his lyrical verse "You gotta walk that lonesome highway" and for blunt terse lines like these:

They don't come [at us] by ones
They don't come by twos
But they come by tens
They got the judges
They got the lawyers
They got the law

They don't come by ones
They got the sheriffs
They got the deputies
    They don't come by twos
They got the shotguns
They got the rope
    We get the justice
    In the end
And they come by tens. . . .[13]

DURING THESE YEARS, in any case, black people and common citizens all over the country were going to work for themselves, and in Cincinnati in 1972, in the same hospital where the military experiments had taken place, and partly as a result of the partial revelations about them in 1971 and '72, a popular movement grew up that gave local African Americans and low-income whites a chance to vent their frustrations about the abuse they were suffering in this public institution.

This crusade named itself the People's Health Movement, and it attempted to organize the public hospital in Cincinnati on a different basis than it had ever been organized on before and almost succeeded. The movement launched a campaign to radically alter by referendum the ruling board of the hospital.

As I have been writing this chapter, I have pulled out from records of the past an old file of yellowed artifacts of this crusade around the hospital. I find bulletins and position papers, photocopied booklets with original cartoons, news clippings, flyers and agendas, letters to the editor, including a long one of my own headed "General Hospital's Future." I find correspondence of various kinds involving the Junior Faculty Association, and colorful hand-drawn posters. Many of these materials should be preserved, I reflect, in proper frames and hung where people can examine them at their leisure and learn this particular history of people's struggle. The People's Health Movement campaign was the kind of grassroots action whose memory is always in danger of being lost, especially in the interior reaches of the country, where it seems that much of life goes unrecorded and that all too often we see, in history lessons in schools and in public media of all kinds, a transfiguration, or even outright suppression, of popular protests against the existing order.

The workers in the People's Health Movement were largely people who had jobs in the hospital and were also users of the hospital, though a certain number of doctors and nurses joined in, along with progressive people in the general community.

The petition campaign to get a hospital amendment on the ballot needed 12,254 signatures, and by the fall of 1973, 16,085 had been collected. "We, the undersigned electors of the City of Cincinnati," read the petitions, "in accordance with the provisions . . . of the Ohio Constitution . . . hereby petition . . . Council . . . to provide for submission to the electors . . . the question of amending the Charter of the City of Cincinnati. . . ." On the new hospital board proposed there would be, not simply the members of the UC board of trustees serving as a hospital board as well, but fifteen new members, six appointed by various authorities and nine *elected* by the city at large.

The hope was, among the PHM people, that they could elect workers at the hospital to the hospital board. (That was a radical idea even in the early seventies, and it would be an even more radical idea today, but surely common sense tells us that it is for the good of all if the whole range of workers within an institution have something to say about its operation.)

Then the moment of crisis arrived. The new statute was printed on the November ballot for the city of Cincinnati of 1973, and on election day people voted on it yes or no, but their votes were never counted.

Ballots must be printed far in advance, and by the time of election day the forces that opposed the new board had discovered ways to invalidate enough signatures on the petitions to declare the referendum null and void. Some of the signers, they said, had used pencil rather than pen; some of their addresses did not match the addresses on their voter registration cards; some of their words or letters were illegible. Only 9,342 signers, they ruled, were valid signers. This, of course, is the time-honored way of pressing the delete key on grassroots initiatives that threaten entrenched interests.

The chairwoman of the People's Health Movement was Yvonne Mayes, a young black woman who worked in the laundry at the hospital. "These tactics come as no surprise," Mayes told one of the local papers. "We know Council does not want this issue on the ballot." She said she was asking for the right at least to *see* the petitions that had been invalidated.[14]

My own family and friends were among the many people who circulated the petitions and attended the large dramatic meetings of the movement, and the Junior Faculty Association had also taken as a priority for the school year the aiding and abetting of the hospital campaign. At UC we had an African American serving as our Vice President of Metropolitan Affairs, and I find an old letter of mine, as president of the JFA that year, writing to this man, Charles Johnson, about our procedures for a debate he was moderating for us on the amendment. We had speakers pro and con, including members of the PHM and representatives of the medical school.

Our feeling then, and mine today, is that struggles such as this have to take place. Generally—they fail. But they pave the way for others that come afterward. We felt, of course, that what had happened to the PHM petitions did not represent the kind of "democracy" most Americans want to have. (Or that if this *was* democracy, we had better have something else.)

The campaign to change the hospital through the vote had been destroyed, and yet a great scare had been thrown into the ruling engines of the town. The university and its business allies, who made—and make today—large profits servicing the hospital, had put some of those profits to work. They had hired a local advertising agency to lead a massive campaign to defeat the proposal.[15] The *Cincinnati Post*, a major paper during these particular years, cooperated by publishing a series of detailed articles defending the hospital by a reporter named Polk Laffoon. These pieces would in time be issued by the paper as a book with the title *General Hospital* (1974). This work depicted the head doctors as selfless, dedicated, overworked men who labored for little reward because they cared about the place so much.

But the PHM contended, in *their* literature, that what the medical men cared about was their careers as physicians and researchers and their incomes, not about their patients or about the 1450 workers who kept the plant going for a few dollars an hour. Top pay for most categories of workers was $3.50 an hour, from a low of $2.25.

Of the rank and file workers, 95 percent were black and 75 percent were women. They cooked the food that everybody in the hospital ate, and washed the dishes, stacked the trays, mopped the floors. They moved patients from floor to floor. They did the laundry. They loaded supplies and put them on shelves and took them *off* shelves. They cut the grass. On the wards themselves the black workers did all *that* work, and the PHM charged that speed-up was always to be reckoned with. "Sometimes, because there aren't enough workers, or when workers are absent or on vacation, the patients themselves, if they are able, must get their own linen, change their beds, or give themselves a bath."

The predominantly female work force labored for very little reward and with almost no hope of advancing themselves. "For most of us," said the PHM, "if you go into the General as a maid, you leave as a maid." Work five years, or fifty years, you are still a maid, it was said. If you went in as a "unit helper," generally you left as a "unit helper." Inflation was at 10 percent in those years, and the year before the campaign, the workers had received a raise of 3.5 percent. Their jobs were hard and humiliating, and they said that young doctors and medical students treated the black help like people who did not have normal intelligence and did not know how to do anything.

One three-page position paper of the movement was titled "Worker Conditions at CGH" and another "Patient Conditions." One handout was called "Radiation Research or How the University Tricks Us into Serving Their Interests" and another "The War Machine and the University of Cincinnati." If we in the JFA had had trouble circulating to the city and campus elite and the local media our report on radiation injuries and deaths, we had *no* trouble with the PHM. Our findings were repeated in graphic detail on the movement fliers. "General Hospital is a hospital of poor and black people who are not only getting second class health care, but being used daily for study and research purposes by the University of Cincinnati Medical School," one handout concluded. At the bottom of another, one could read, "It was not so long ago that another country was experimenting on human beings, and we know what that led to!"

The conditions in the outpatient clinics were a special focus of the anger of the PHM. There were fifty-seven different clinics, providing practice and "raw material" for the various specialties, but patients were said to be caught in an endless runaround, sent from clinic to clinic with no communication between them:

> The doctor in ob/gyn may not know anything about how the doctor in Gastric Clinic has treated you or why. Some of the clinics are still in the dark tunnels and halls of the hospital. But even when they are remodeled, treatment of patients doesn't change. People are used as teaching "material" and hardly treated as people who have sense and feelings. We wait all day, first to sign in for a financial interview, then again at each clinic. Doctors are cold, impersonal, maybe interested in our illness but not our health. We often leave without knowing what is wrong, what the treatment is, or why we're getting it.[16]

Even Polk Laffoon had to accede to some of these arguments. Among the many doctors he became acquainted with, as he followed the staff on their rounds and into the conferences and disputes in their offices, was one who was a serious critic of the institution. This was James Agna, head of the outpatient clinics, or Ambulatory Care, as it was called. Agna, in fact, was resigning in disgust. The clinics should be the most important part of the hospital, he said, since they served the most people, but they were severely neglected. The young doctors there might be trying hard to keep up with things, but the head physicians rarely came around to help or consult, and the various backup services for lab work and so on often did not respond. Disorder, long waits, and confusion of all kinds awaited most people who tried to get help. Clinic visits were not free; they were eighteen dollars each, unless you knew how to apply for financial help and could qualify.

The assault of the People's Health Movement on this institution and the radiation travail of the year before were wounding experiences for the professionals under attack, as is made clear in the study by Laffoon. Many doctors were extremely perturbed by what was being said and written about the General. They felt themselves to be misunderstood. Laffoon drew compelling portraits of the working days of the doctors and of each crisis as it arose on the wards and in the department offices—the budget and hiring crunches, for instance, as they constantly afflicted department heads.

Laffoon wrote of an ugly crisis in the radioisotope lab run by Eugene

Saenger. Early one morning, when Jerry Wiot, the head of radiology, walked into his office, a memorandum from Saenger to the entire staff awaited him. "To all general Hospital services and clinics," the memo began. "Funds are no longer available . . . and services . . . are being suspended as of Monday, April 7." The exception would be for services paid for in advance, Saenger wrote. "It is a bombshell," writes Laffoon, and though Wiot was sympathetic to Saenger's problem with funds, he was "also sure this is the wrong way to handle it." [17]

We read that Saenger's lab "did approximately five thousand 'imaging studies' per year of patients' brains, livers and lungs, and to a lesser extent, kidneys, adrenals and spleens. Here patients are fed one of Saenger's famous 'hot cocktails'—a radioactive material that can be chemically altered to be absorbed by the organ under study—and photographed by a gamma camera." The lab is a mysterious place, writes Laffoon, "grungy in the far reaches of the H. Pavilion tunnel (Saenger's secretary was mugged there not long ago), and filled with arcane talk of thyroid uptakes, red cell survivals and in-vitro blood tests." [18]

There follows a rather heroic portrait of Saenger and his original "one-room lab" back in the forties and fifties, when isotopes were "about as obscure as space capsules," and then his pioneering work building up his sprawling basement complex of fifty people and elaborate equipment.

Neither in this portrait of Eugene Saenger nor in that of Edward Silberstein in a later chapter does Laffoon make any reference to the radiations for the DOD that had still been taking place just a year or two before he wrote; nor does he describe any one of the many other human experiments always in progress in the hospital.

Silberstein is shown by Laffoon making rounds with students one day:

A reputedly brilliant man who specializes in radioisotopes, he teaches with compassion and competence, but often makes students uneasy. He asks them a lot of questions, not always nicely, and unlike most attendings, insists that they give a summary of each patient's marital status, children and lifestyle before getting into the disease. He wants the patients to be recognized as individuals. "Silberstein comes on really strong and puts you on your guard," one student said. "Other attendings might ask the same questions, but in a nicer way." Still, they respect his knowledge and the care he takes with them.[19]

Laffoon goes on to describe a curious incident on this day of Silberstein's rounds with students. A long-time patient with mental problems had been refusing to cooperate, and Silberstein took the occasion to denounce loudly this individual to all within hearing, as if she were not present.

Laffoon was a canny observer within the limited field of observation he had apparently set himself, and the reader gets a searing picture of what daily life was like for professionals in the public hospitals of the day. As I reread in 1997 this small volume, I wondered if I could discover just how it had come about, why—exactly—there had been no mention of the radiation ordeal within the College of Medicine and its hospital, or indeed of any human research. I was interested in knowing, too, what Laffoon might now be feeling about the new publicity around the DOD experiments, which he had so scrupulously failed even to acknowledge in his book. I wondered where life had led such a writer, and whether he would feel, today, that he could speak frankly about these matters of the past.

One day I called a "Polk Laffoon" listed in the Cincinnati directory. This turned out to be Laffoon's father, a courteous man who had time to talk about his son's career and then to tell me how to reach him in Miami, Florida. He said his son did not write any more, and he thought that was a pity. He reminded me of two other special series for the *Post* Laffoon had done, one on the tornado that struck a suburb of Cincinnati back in the seventies and the other a study of Cincinnati neighborhoods.

I did reach Laffoon in Miami one afternoon, but he did not wish to respond to any inquiries about *General Hospital*. "That was a long time ago," he said; "I don't remember very much about it."[20] He did tell me about his present employment; he is Vice President of Corporate Relations with Knight-Ridder Newspapers headquartered in Miami.

When I broached the subject of the radiation tests at General Hospital, he said that though he believed he was at the *Post* in 1971–72, he did not remember any such tests. (Over twenty-five reports were published by the *Post* in that period, mostly defenses of the project by Senator Robert Taft and others.) Laffoon had mentioned both Edward Gall and

Clifford Grulee in his book but had declined to say *why* they had been replaced, after the halting of the radiations; he says now he does not remember these two men. He does not remember anyone at all in radiology except the head of the department, Jerome Wiot. Laffoon says he did not ask any questions about human research in the hospital because he did not know enough about it to inquire.

This is a blank—but it bears out for me that in some quarters the denial of the whole radiation travail is almost as strong today as it was in 1972.

Yet it was a young reporter at the same paper, Nick Miller, who in 1994 declined to engage in the communal act of denial of the past. His editors must have come to feel that the story was distant enough by that time that it could be told, and might even be regarded as a welcome assault on a people's institution, one that needed, not humane reform, but privatization.[21]

But as we saw in the early chapters of this book, the press nationwide has been slow, even today, to acknowledge the deliberate exposures of the Cold War, and the most revealing reports have appeared, not in the U.S., but in England and Japan.

It was not a surprise that a history of the University of Cincinnati, penned in 1995 by a journalist heading the UC public relations department, Greg Hand, and a school archivist, Kevin Grace, should not even refer to the full body radiations at UC, or to the People's Health Movement that worked to change the hospital after the tests first came to light.[22]

A FEW WORDS NOW about the further activities of the Junior Faculty Association. In the years that immediately followed the events around General Hospital, this group took stands on various issues on campus. In late 1973 we moved to challenge UC's policy of keeping strictly private the incomes of faculty and administrators. After six months of negotiations with the university around the ways salary information of various kinds might be made public, none of which seemed to us satisfactory, we prepared to file a lawsuit. We believed that in court the state information act would easily settle the question in our favor and bring about full disclosure. The suit was to be filed on a Monday at twelve o'clock noon. At ten o'clock that day the provost of the university, Robert O'Neill, agreed to issue a complete printout of annual pay at the university and place it in the main library (where it continues to be made available each year).

Faculty had been receiving little or no yearly increase, and when they saw what administrators were taking for themselves, the union fever that had already broken out rose several degrees. Strong leaders emerged, and within a year the faculty had the votes needed to form a union under the American Association of University Professors. The first contract resulted in a historic strike and large increases for faculty across the board. Powerful leadership from labor-minded faculty throughout the UC campuses has been sustained, and the union has remained one of the strongest in the state.

The JFA, as its members either left the university or graduated from the junior faculty by way of tenure and promotion, soon vanished without a trace. It might be said that history was changing its course and for many years groups like this one were deemed to be phenomena society could do without.

ABOUT A DECADE after the events described above, Eugene Saenger retired from UC and received many honors. In 1987, a feature article about the de Hevesy award appeared in a university bulletin with these opening paragraphs:

> Eugene L. Saenger, world renowned expert in radiation accidents, has been honored by the Society of Nuclear Medicine for his pioneering work in his field.
>
> Saenger, director of the Eugene L. Saenger Radioisotope Laboratory at the UC Medical Center, received the 28th Georg Charles de Hevesy Nuclear Medicine Pioneer Award June 2 at the SNM's annual meeting in Toronto.
>
> Saenger's interests range from radiation injury to nuclear medicine efficacy. He and his colleagues did much of the groundwork for radiation protection, accident management and dosimetry. . . .

"Saenger Honored for Pioneering Efforts" is the title of this pleasant report in UC This Week for June 12, 1987.

In 1994, six months after he became a defendant in the lawsuit, James. G. Kereiakes was also the recipient of a high honor at UC. Kereiakes was the medical physicist who, during the eleven years of the radiation project, calculated for each patient the air doses needed to bring about the absorption—in effect, the injury—the doctors wanted to achieve. The Daniel Drake Medal awarded to Kereiakes in the fall of 1994 was described in the UC bulletin as "the highest honor bestowed by the UC College of Medicine on former students or current or past faculty members." Back in 1988 Kereiakes had received the highest *national* honor in radiology, the Gold Medal, from the Radiological Society of North America.[23]

III

The Legal Story

11

A Civil Action

I was still just a punk . . . and wanting badly to do civil rights.
—Attorney LISA MEEKS, July 1997

In the late fall of 1993, an event took place in the offices of Attorney
Robert Newman that would have a considerable impact on the development of the lawsuit against the doctors. Newman's firm acquired a
young woman attorney who would find this kind of action exactly to her
liking. She would work hard on the case and compose most of the early
briefs, pleadings that would anchor the case securely enough in law—
and in common sense—to sustain its fundamental arguments during
the years of legal storms that followed.

When I first spoke with Newman about a lawsuit concerning the
radiations, in February 1994, I of course had no idea that a few months
earlier an attorney especially interested in civil rights had been sworn
to the bar in the state capitol and was proving to be an apt learner of her
new job at Kircher, Robinson, Newman, and Welch. This new associate,
Lisa Meeks, had already served a year's tutorial with the firm as a law
clerk while still in school at Northern Kentucky University, just across
the Ohio River from Cincinnati.

But the radiation case would be the first significant civil rights case
Meeks would work on where she could sign her own name on the complaint just under the signature of Robert Newman. "I was still just a
punk," she told me later. "I was just starting out and wanting badly to

do civil rights, and it was amazing that this case, this largest of all civil rights cases you could have, should have come along at just that time — and that I would be able to work on it." [1]

Meeks was a little older than most new law graduates and a person with an oddly multifarious past. One reason she had decided on law school, after almost becoming a music historian, was that she had become interested in the legal struggles of gays and lesbians.

Meeks is a small sturdy woman, spectacled, studious looking, with a pale Celtic complexion and short curly red hair, an individual hard to miss among large, dark-suited males in a courtroom. She had been hired by the firm the very day she had come in to be interviewed, hoping to clerk with the group and then stay on. When one of the partners had asked her how she had known about the firm, she had said without equivocation that she had learned about it through her involvement in the local gay and lesbian organization Stonewall. [2]

Bob Newman had told her that day about the kinds of cases he handled and what he liked to do and asked her what she wanted to do. She said quite plainly, "I want to do what you do." She was very clear about that. "I couldn't possibly have found a better guide to break me in to the kind of work I was looking for," she says. [3] "What I am doing is a magnificent opportunity, especially for someone who's just a new kid on the block."

When the radiation case came along, Newman took up certain papers from his desk and walked down the hall to see Meeks. "Do you want to get involved in this?" he asked, and she said, "*God* yes!" She helped write the first brief that same week and would eventually read extensively in the literature on human experiments and the related constitutional issues, and begin to conjure up the more elaborate pleadings that would be filed in the months to come, including the crucial reply to the researchers' motion to be dismissed from the suit as individual defendants.

Newman had posited the original events as violations of the victims' civil rights, but he and Meeks had to ask themselves this: what portions of the Constitution best protect citizens from the kind of assault these individuals had suffered? In short, what exactly were the constitutional grounds of the case to be?

Meeks and Newman worked the issue between them day after day.

It was an intense dialectic, she says, sometimes exhilarating. She had begun to work closely with Newman on other civil rights cases, but the case against the doctors was another matter entirely. For one thing, she feels it was a qualified immunity case of almost epic proportions, and the challenge was all the greater because of the distance in time from the original events to the present.

Beyond that, she and the firm had to coordinate their work with a large class-action firm from out of state that had succeeded in claiming a set of surviving families, as well as with other attorneys in town; and they had to confront, on the other side, a heavy roster of well-known lawyers from prestigious Cincinnati firms. Each of the thirteen individual defendants from UC had retained his own counsel—or hers, as the case may be, as there was one woman defendant—and the two government doctors had yet another attorney. Then there were the legal departments of the defendant university itself and of the city of Cincinnati, and in time, counsel for the Department of Justice and for the Defense Nuclear Agency.

There were at times as many as twenty-eight attorneys in court. "You go to the hearing," Meeks said, "and—good lord a-mighty! . . . look at all those *suits* up there." Meeks amazed herself at times reflecting on the travails of coordinating all the lawyers for the defense. "I bet it was a true nightmare," she said, "and think how much it *costs* to fill up one whole side of a courtroom with all those attorneys."

Meeks had interviewed with some of the larger firms in town before she had learned about Newman, but when they had asked her what her interests were, what she hoped to be doing as an attorney, and she had made her reply, she says the interviews had gone quickly down the drain.

IN TIME LISA MEEKS and I became acquainted, and as I was beginning the final chapters of this volume, she came to my house one afternoon after work to talk things over. We sat on my back porch and played with the cats and ate tuna sandwiches, and we ruminated and reflected on the case for over three hours.

I wanted to understand something of Meeks's perspectives on the law in general, and I asked her to tell me a little bit about her other work in civil rights. By this time, she had become closely involved in a statewide suit of Newman's against the Ohio prisons. The firm was defending a prisoner in the state prison in Lebanon who was severely mentally ill and not getting treatment or help of any kind. Their suit against the state—*Dunn v. [Governor George] Voinovich*—had in fact just prevailed when we talked, thanks in large part to Robert Newman's success in gaining the cooperation of the prison system itself. By the time Meeks and I had our conversation, policies were being put in place in Ohio to change radically the way mentally ill inmates would be treated. The firm had shown that, according to case law and under the Eighth Amendment, which forbids "cruel and unusual punishment," it was illegal for a prison to display "deliberate indifference to a serious medical need" of an inmate. Newman had convinced the state of Ohio to enter into a consent decree providing for a comprehensive system of mental health care that would dramatically improve prisoners' lives. In due time "the Ohio plan" would become well-known as the first of its kind to ensure such care.[4]

Meeks was also representing the family of a woman who had just died in a horrifying way in the county jail, bleeding to death because of an ectopic pregnancy, in spite of urgent calls for help from other women on the floor. When she had been sent to the infirmary, this woman had not been able to walk, and when placed in a wheelchair had fallen piteously forward. But she had been sent back to her cell with two tablets of Tylenol. She had murmured, "Don't let me die in here—*not in here . . .*," but when she was finally taken away to a hospital, she was acutely ill and had died the next day. The hope Meeks had was that a class-action suit could be developed on behalf of all inmates who would need medical care in the Hamilton County Justice Center.

First Amendment cases were especially to Meeks's liking, and she had also been helping Newman represent a high school boy who had been forbidden to wear his Ku Klux Klan shirt to school. The trouble was that other students were wearing *their* political shirts, picturing such figures as Malcolm X, and so it clearly wasn't fair. It is obvious to Meeks that people have to be allowed to express what they think even if we do not like what they express. "Otherwise," she says, "look—I can't march in the Gay Pride parade." She and Newman had succeeded in blocking a summary judgment from the court against the student who was bringing the suit.

Meeks grew up in Memphis, went to a small Southern Baptist college in Jackson, Tennessee, and moved to Cincinnati to attend the College Conservatory of Music at UC on a piano scholarship. At the university it was the studious side of the music world that had more and more engaged her. She was working on her master's thesis in music history when this part of her life seemed suddenly to collapse upon her. She had transcribed an Italian Renaissance choral part book and needed only to attach some prose to her transcription when she realized she could not go on with this manner of work and left the Conservatory.

But after a few years, study and research, hard intellectual endeavor, would become her life again, in law school in Kentucky and then as an attorney—but this time it would be mental endeavor with the social meaning she had been looking for.

In Cincinnati, as in other towns, there is only a small group of attorneys who do civil rights law. Meeks says it is grueling work, it takes painful study, and that you're always going up against the people who seem to have all the power. She is happy with the fact that Newman will tackle hard cases that others will not—challenges to major institutions, for instance.

But is it possible to make a living from civil rights? I asked Meeks, and she said, "Some people do. . . . Yes, I think you can." She thought about this a bit. "In our firm we also do some personal injury and some medical malpractice, and these are your cash crops. They help pay for the other good things you want to do. And when you do win a civil rights case, you know you will get fees and costs. The judge will have some discretion, but you will be paid."

The firm had recently won a malpractice suit against a doctor who failed to perform a routine test that would have saved a woman's baby in the womb. The damages were large, and the firm received a third of the final award.

MEEKS LIKES to do her most concentrated work on Sundays when the offices of the firm are mostly silent and uninhabited. At the time we spoke, as the radiation settlement was progressing, Meeks and her younger sister, a student at UC, were fixing up an old frame house in a working-class neighborhood of Cincinnati; but on certain Sundays

Meeks would get into her blue jeans and Keds and go back downtown. Writing the radiation briefs, she spent a number of such Sundays up at her desk on the twenty-fifth floor of the Kroger building.

Up there, she said, she could hear nothing when the offices were closed but the dim whir of the computers. At the big windows she could look out over the city skyline and think restfully about her case. As it happens, she could spot from her office the towers of UC—the white tower of red-brick McMicken Hall, for instance, where English and history teachers are quartered—and the spires of the medical campus itself. She could see the hospital where the events she was describing in her briefs took place.

When I asked Meeks why it was she who had written the early radiation briefs instead of Newman, she said that she thought Newman had just given in to her "insatiable desire" to perform this kind of composition. "Digging and studying and then writing up what I find is what I like to do. I like to write and to see what I have done there on the page." But Meeks insists the development of the case remained throughout a collaborative effort. In time four firms filed suits, representing the various plaintiffs identified by Laura Schneider and eventually by attorneys and the public outlining of the case in the media.

None of these firms wanted to give over their families to the others, and so things were tense in the beginning, but as the case progressed there was plenty to do, and Meeks and Newman came to feel that a group of strong-willed attorneys who had not known each other learned to work together to good effect.

At the first hearing, however, the members of the team were divided as to what to do about the federal judge assigned to the case. Judge Carl Rubin was well-known in Cincinnati as a highly conservative individual. He had known Eugene Saenger socially and had also been involved in work with the University of Cincinnati. Newman felt that Rubin was not sympathetic to civil rights cases and informed him that his clients would not waive the conflict of interest issue. The other attorneys did not favor this move since they felt Rubin could be counted on to certify the case as a class action. But the case was rerolled in the clerk's office to Judge Sandra Beckwith. "One of my colleagues said, 'Who's he?'" Newman recalls, but the presence of this relatively new woman judge would turn out to be a fateful turning in the long road of legal combat that followed.

After the closing of the case in 1999, Newman would look back on the joint endeavors of the attorneys with satisfaction:

> Our team of lawyers had a shaky start, but after five years we became friends, which is rare in cases where several lawyers are thrown into the same stew.
>
> Robert Nelson, an incredibly able lawyer, guided us skillfully through the maze of class action law that nobody else understood. David Thompson wrote several sections of our winning briefs. Gary Lewis was our expert on municipal liability. David Kamp and Mike Alexander made invaluable contributions at the end, which made settlement possible.
>
> Of course, I hardly need to describe the work of Lisa Meeks . . . who among other things was a kind of den mother who settled our disputes over sentence structure, footnotes, the ordering of arguments, and so on.
>
> But the person who put the most time in on the case was Jennifer Thomas, the paralegal who kept track of the documents, the people, the deadlines and all the complaints.[5]

The case required, then, a committeelike approach that was a further test of Meeks's resourcefulness. Her part, at times, and as Newman suggests, was simply to keep the collaboration going. As the critical Memorandum in Opposition to the Motion to Dismiss was developing, it was up to her to keep a core draft circulating among the group. The skeleton and large sections of this brief she wrote, but others read and edited and suggested and sent over from time to time passages of their own.[6]

At times she and Newman saw things somewhat differently. She wanted to "barrel in," as she put it, on the due process violations, but Newman had a fundamental instinct that the case was one about denial of access to the courts and of the patients' rights to privacy. In sum, the argument was that the victims and their families had had, at the time of the radiations, no means of challenging any wrong they had been done, since they had not known *what* had been done nor how they had been injured. No one could complain or ask for remedy or redress because no one knew enough even to demur, and thus fundamental civil rights had been denied. The Due Process Clause of the Fourteenth Amendment provides that no state shall "deprive a person of life, liberty, or property without due process of law."

A number of claims against the researchers were detailed in the original filing of the suit and then in the Memorandum asking Judge Beckwith to find against the doctors' plea for qualified immunity as public employees. The victims, said Newman and Meeks and associates, had been denied a whole compendium of civil rights under the U.S. Constitution. They had been deceived, and thus denied "due process" both substantive and procedural; they had been denied the right of access to the courts, the right to privacy, to bodily integrity, and to make decisions about their own bodies—and, for the minorities, the right to equal protection under the law. The doctors were said to have "perpetrated a fraud" upon the victims in order to study injuries on an "atomic battlefield." To put it another way, they had subjected the patients to the "abnormally dangerous activity" courts had found to be a violation of civil rights in the past.[7]

As to the individual liability of the researchers named, it was repeatedly insisted that a minimal responsibility of each one, regardless of his particular role in the project, was to decline to collude in afflicting injuries on patients but in fact to *protect* these patients by making known to them what was being done:

> At all times relevant herein, Defendants were acting under color of law, jointly and in concert with each other . . . [yet] each Defendant had the duty and opportunity to protect the Plaintiffs from the unlawful actions of the other Defendants but each Defendant intentionally and/or recklessly and/or knowingly . . . failed and refused to perform such duty, thereby directly and proximately causing the injuries to Plaintiffs as alleged herein. (p. 33)

THE DOCTORS FOUGHT this battle over their immunity very hard; for them it was the crucial moment of the case. Their briefs contended that the cases the plaintiffs attempted to use as precedents were *not* precedents, that the doctors had not known in the sixties they might be violating anyone's civil rights. Public officials must be protected, they argued, from constant suits and harassment. They cited a court opinion from 1945 to the effect that "an accommodation for reasonable error exists because officials should not err on the side of caution because they fear being sued."[8] The plaintiffs, said the defendants, could not "create Constitutional rights where none exist":

> A careful review of the essential allegations of the Complaint discloses that Plaintiffs bring claims on behalf of patients who were voluntary consumers of medical services, all of whom suffered from inoperable cancer during the period 1960–1972. The Individual Defendants are a broad group of physicians and specialists from other disciplines, working in cooperation with one of the nation's leading medical schools, the University of Cincinnati College of Medicine. Plaintiffs concede that the persons whom they represent agreed to receive radiation treatments and do not allege that the Defendants physically restrained them in any way. Rather, the Individual Defendants are accused of providing inaccurate information about the radiation treatments which these patients agreed to receive in an effort to be spared certain death from inoperable cancer.[9]

The charge that they were "somehow not practicing medicine," say the defendants, is simply "ludicrous." And they argue that voluntary consumers of medical services did not have, as of 1972, an established constitutional right to be informed of all the possible risks of treatment.[10]

If the doctors' motion to dismiss had succeeded, the plaintiffs would have been left to battle simply with the university, the city, and the federal government, the "entities," as Meeks refers to them. But the case would have shrunk and turned rather pale. "There's not much 'gut' in a case when the individuals actually working the levers and turning the knobs are missing," Meeks said. A contest of this kind is not often won, she noted. "Qualified immunity is a powerful tool—and especially where you have conduct occurring at a time when you may not have much case law that describes it."[11]

This lack of close parallels in law was, in fact, one of the strangest aspects of the entire action. For after all, as Meeks explained, "You have to allege whatever you allege with *particularity*." The right not to be used by public employees in just the way these individuals had been used had to be established through similar cases of the past. And there were very few that provided a reasonable match. That part, Meeks said, was "scary."

This state of affairs painted, indeed, a bizarre color upon the case. It seemed to me passing strange that because acts as menacing as these seemed to have seldom, if ever, occurred in the United States before, this should in itself make the case difficult to try. It seemed a very curious catch-22. Was what had happened so bad that it had no precedent at all anyone could point to — except in the German prison camps — and was therefore all right? Not actionable in U.S. courts?

During the UC radiations, as already observed, experimenters in Alabama were withholding life-saving medicines from black men with syphilis. The Tuskegee project was still in progress when the UC tests ended and still largely unknown outside the Public Health Service; it had left no tracings on American law. Nor had the plutonium injections of the forties, for instance. The eighteen individuals injected with this radioactive substance under the direct guidance of the U.S. Army's Manhattan Project had not learned, at the time of the Cincinnati tests, that they had been "guinea-pigged," had certainly not appeared in the courts. (As in Cincinnati, it was only when the identities of the plutonium victims had been established through the detection work of independent parties, many years later, that legal action had begun.)

In the early rounds of the Cincinnati case, the defense of the University of Cincinnati was laid out in highly abstruse terms by Lee Fisher, the state attorney general, and his local associates. The university had been a municipal institution until 1977, when it had become a state school and its assets were transferred to the state of Ohio. Thus, ran this argument, the present-day University of Cincinnati had no responsibility whatever for anything that had taken place in the *defunct* university of the past.[12] Cincinnati General Hospital itself had been owned by the city "at all times relevant to this litigation," and the executive and administrative control of the hospital had been "vested in the Board of Directors of the [now defunct] Municipal University" — appointed by the mayor of the city (p. 34). Thus, the city and the federal government it contracted with, through its university of the past and its hospital, were the responsible parties:

The radiation research which is the subject of this litigation was at all times conducted by the Municipal University and its agents in accordance with the requirements of its contract with the Defense Atomic Support Agency of the United States of America, in accordance with federal government standards, and subject to the oversight of the federal government, which supervised, ratified and approved the research conducted under said contract. (p. 36)

What is more, it was said, none of these layers of authority were relevant anyway, since all the public entities in question were immune from suit under the Eleventh Amendment.

Yet UC would eventually contribute in good measure to the settlement, like the city and the U.S. government, and its legal bills for 1994 alone would mount to over $200,000. It would eventually try to prevent a memorial plaque from even *mentioning* the radiation project, or listing the victims by name, and it would succeed in placing the plaque in a little used backyard of the hospital.

A defense around the statute of limitations was intensely argued by the city of Cincinnati. The injuries to the patients, said the city, were not "concealed," and thus the clock on the statute of limitations had long since run its course and the case become moot. The families had known that deaths were occurring and could have sought at the time the causes of death. They had not exercised the "due diligence" the law requires.

Had the families of Lula Tarlton, of Katie Dennis and Philip Daniels, of Margaret Bacon and James Tidwell and Maude Jacobs simply not been "diligent" enough in ferreting out the real motives behind the radiations?

In the Memorandum in Reply, the plaintiffs wrote that the doctors appeared to believe that they had had no constraints whatever upon their conduct but could use in any way they wished any patient they could find. This pleading conceded that the framers of the Constitution had not contemplated the occurrence of such acts as the doctors had committed, and so had not provided a specific protection against them. Did that mean, though, that there *were* no legal constraints upon these "exotic and harmful and sometimes fatal experiments upon unsuspecting and helpless patients" for the sake of the nation's military planners?

"What is material and controlling," this brief argues, "is that the constitutional right to bodily integrity has always been respected and must be so respected here." [13]

In a sentence that would obviously resonate with the court at the hearing on these motions the following October, we read this: "The allegations of this case involve the most fundamental responsibility of organized government, i. e., protecting the life and well-being of its citizens, and involve the most extreme deprivation in which a government can engage, i. e., the taking of life" (p. 1). The brief goes on to argue, in very plain language, that if the court were to dismiss the researchers from the suit, it would be granting protection to any public doctor in any conduct whatever, "including the systematic murder of patients" (p. 10).

A case originating in New York state, *Barrett v. United States* (2d Cir., 1986), turned out to be of considerable interest to Lisa Meeks as this brief developed. In 1953 a young man at a state mental hospital died after being injected five times with a mescaline drug. His mother brought suit against the hospital for negligence and wrongful death, and was awarded $18,000. But no one in the family knew until twenty years later that it had been the U.S. government that had supplied the drug—in order to study its mental effects on troops. The family then brought another suit. The federal defendants were not dismissed on the basis of qualified immunity, and because of the original and continuing deception, the right of the deceased man's family to sue for damages many years after the event was upheld.[14]

IT HAS SOMETIMES been asked why the Cincinnati case was not patently a medical malpractice case. The defendants, in fact, argued that it was just that, if it was anything. They contended that if the families had any cause of action at all, it was under state law in state courts. The plaintiffs pointed out that such actions had become a possibility only when families had learned from others what the doctors themselves had so studiously concealed: ". . . it is only after more than a quarter-century of silence and deception that the true story of the experiments in the basement of General Hospital have at last come to light."

State claims were in fact included in the plaintiffs' complaint, since a federal court can consider such claims in cases where related federal charges may be dismissed, and yet a state claim of wrongful death is expected to be made within two years of the event. The defendants would later be rebuked by the judge in their insistence that only state law could be applied. "The Defendants unwittingly assist Plaintiffs in their cause," she wrote, supporting the plaintiffs' claim that fraudulent concealment for many years had left them with no option but appealing to the federal courts—on the basis, that is, in part, of having been barred by this long deception from their access to the state of Ohio.[15]

As to the privacy violation, readers of the Memorandum in question are reminded that Judge Louis Brandeis, in a dissenting opinion in a 1928 case, had described the constitutional right of privacy as "the right to be let alone—the most comprehensive of rights and the right most valued by civilized men" (p. 42).

THE MEMORANDUM of the plaintiffs also repeats the claim that African Americans had been singled out as the group at which the experiments had been "predominantly directed." Of course there are a great many cases on record that have derived from the equal-protection clause of the Fourteenth Amendment. As far back as 1885, a Chinese American named Yick Wo had been denied a license to operate a "wooden laundry" in California. A court found that in fact all the Chinese applicants had been denied licenses and that it was not the city license statute itself that was discriminatory but the unequal application of it.[16] The plaintiffs suggested that among the numberless "progeny" of Yick Wo—that is, the minority individuals who have been singled out for unfair treatment and have taken their case to court—could be added now the fifty-six African Americans in Cincinnati injured by radiation in their public hospital, twelve of whom died within about a month of being irradiated, along with nine whites.

The only claim of the plaintiffs that the court would strictly dismiss was the charge that the doctors had violated the victims' rights under the Price-Anderson Act, which indemnifies citizens injured by a "nuclear incident" brought on by public officials, a concept sometimes quite broadly interpreted but not broadly enough, in the eyes of the

Sixth Circuit, to encompass the use of a radiation machine in a hospital, even if deliberately used to inflict injuries on patients.

IT WAS IN THE COMPLEX and comprehensive Memorandum I have been discussing, composed by Meeks and her colleagues in September 1994, that we find the first mention, in the ever-lengthening papers of this action, of the Nuremberg Code.

On page twenty-three of this sixty-seven-page Memorandum we read that "an additional irony of the case at bar must be noted." The brief goes on to describe the 1947 trials of the Nazi doctors in Nuremberg, reminding the court that this Tribunal was led by American prosecutors and that the code it created stated unequivocally that in human experiments the "voluntary consent of the human subject is absolutely essential."

The ruling of Judge Beckwith the following January would take up and greatly embellish this passage on the relevance for the Cincinnati tests of the code that grew out of Nuremberg. In sum, it did not prove possible for the court to set aside the parallels of the case in front of it with the acts of the Nuremberg doctors.

IN THE EIGHTY-EIGHT-PAGE "Opinion and Order" of Judge Sandra Beckwith of January 1995, ruling against immunity for the Cincinnati doctors, she included, as we shall see in the chapter that follows, not a passing reference or two but seven pages on Cincinnati and the Nuremberg Code.

It might be interesting to consider for a moment what a departure this was from court opinions of the past. Very few U.S. rulings on actions involving human experiments, whether for or against the investigators named, have mentioned Nuremberg at all, and as of 1995 only one had cited the Code in a decision where a doctor was found liable.

These facts are clearly put forth in an essay by legal scholar George Annas of the Boston University School of Public Health. This essay appears in a volume called *The Nazi Doctors and the Nuremberg Code* (1992), edited by Annas and his colleague Michael Grodin, and sets forth the record of U.S. rulings over the years that have referenced in any way the Nuremberg Code.

Annas explains his view that the Nuremberg Code is "the most complete and authoritative statement of the law of informed consent to human experimentation" and that there is no reason that it cannot be applied in both civil and criminal cases in the U.S. by courts at all levels.[17] He then goes on to show that it has, in actuality, been applied but rarely. To begin with, few court cases of *any* kind involving people used in experiments have been tried over the course of U.S. law. (Those who know the Cincinnati case may suspect that most people used in experiments never discover that they *are* used.)

During World War II, the United States was testing malaria treatments on prisoners, the retarded, and the mentally ill, and in time the polio vaccine on retarded children, and all of this was generally seen as reasonable and appropriate.[18] In the years that followed the war, the U.S. medical community consistently declined to consider that there could be any connection between human research in this country and the Nazi atrocities, and as Annas explains, various other medical codes began to be formulated.

The most influential of these was the Declaration of Helsinki, adopted in 1964 by the World Medical Association, a group that formed in Britain in 1946 as a deterrent to medical war crimes. The Cincinnati team began to assert their adherence to it in 1966, the only *human* guideline referred to throughout the project, along with guides to the use of animals. Annas cites, on Helsinki, a perspicacious statement made at an international conference in 1973 by another well-known scholar in the field of human research, Jay Katz of Yale University:

> Do not place too much reliance on codes of ethics, such as the Declaration of Helsinki. That would be dangerous. Codes are deceptive documents to which all of us probably could subscribe in principle; but if you study them carefully, you will find that they are painfully vague. They do not inform us well about actual decisions which investigators have to make day after day. The Declaration of Helsinki, analogous to a legal statute, requires opportunities for interpretation; only then could it become a viable document.[19]

As for the world-famous code composed at Nuremberg, the first use of it in a U. S. court also came in 1973, when Michigan doctors wanted to perform experimental psychosurgery on the brain of an inmate in a state hospital. This individual had been considered a criminal sexual psychopath for seventeen years, and he and his parents had signed a detailed consent form. But a suit was filed opposing the surgery by a public interest group, and a panel of judges in a Wayne County Circuit Court (*Kaimowitz v. Michigan Department of Mental Health*) found that an involuntarily confined individual could not legally give his consent to such a procedure. "In the Nuremberg Judgment, the elements of what must guide us in decision are found," wrote the court. No element of force or fraud or duress should be present in true consent, they said; it must be "a totally voluntary one." [20]

A 1980 case outlined by Annas, *Pierce v. Ortho Pharmaceutical Corporation*, is also of interest. A woman researcher working for a drug company in New Jersey was discharged because she objected to the development of a new drug for diarrhea that she felt would be dangerous to test on children and the elderly. In the opinion of the New Jersey Supreme Court, cited by Annas, the doctor was found, on various grounds, to have no case for wrongful discharge. "Chaos would result if a single doctor engaged in research were allowed to determine, according to his or her individual conscience, whether a project should continue," the court said. The Nuremberg Code was brought into play in this case by a dissenting justice, who set forth the text of several principles of the Code and noted that under the Code investigators must satisfy themselves that an experiment is safe.[21]

In 1981 the first of several decisions was made that "seemed to justify," in Annas's words, "brutal experimentation if it was needed to fight the cold war" (p. 209). In *Jaffee v. United States*, a soldier who later died of cancer was one of the men ordered in 1953 to stand in a Nevada field, unprotected, while a nuclear device was exploded. A suit was brought. The U.S. Court of Appeals threw out the case, ruling that the Supreme Court had established that soldiers injured in the course of duty could not sue the government for compensation. Dissenting judges complained strongly that exposing to dangerous radiation so many "atomic soldiers," as these men came to be called, was a "violation of human rights on a massive scale," and that such actions violated every known human rights code, including the Code of Nuremberg.[22]

In 1994 Clinton's Advisory Committee did not see the situation nearly so clearly as that but found the whole Nevada issue a "difficult" one and could not quite tell if a "human experiment" could be said to be involved there or not.[23]

George Annas also reviews the case of the Navajo uranium miners. The Public Health Service studied a group of miners from 1949 to 1960 to see how they would be affected by their exposure to uranium, without telling them why they were being monitored or helping them understand the risks being studied. But when suit was brought, a federal court in Arizona decided that public officials in this case were performing "discretionary acts" associated with their work and in the interest of national security.[24]

The final lower court case citing Nuremberg involved a deep-diving experiment. The experiment had been agreed to by a diver who then suffered injuries he had not expected and brought suit (*Whitlock v. Duke University*, 1986). Though the court cited Nuremberg as authoritative on the consent issue, it found that the known risks had been properly explained.[25]

In the fifties, large-scale biological warfare experiments had been sponsored by the CIA in collusion with researchers at over eighty institutions. As Annas explains, many individuals suffered from these tests and at least two subjects died. In 1984 the tests were defended by the Supreme Court as necessary for the national defense, and the Nuremberg Code was not referred to.

This leads us to the single case in which the Nuremberg Code has been cited by justices on the Supreme Court, though once more in dissent. An Army soldier named James Stanley was given LSD in 1958 without his knowledge, simply to test its effects, and the drug seriously affected his mind. Many years later the Army inadvertently notified Stanley of his use in the test, and he brought suit.

In 1987 the Supreme Court split 5 to 4 against Stanley, and Justice Antonin Scalia wrote the majority opinion defending the Army's need for proper discipline and decision making. Justice Sandra Day O'Connor wrote a strong dissent, citing the Nuremberg Code quite forcibly—an opinion later referenced by Judge Beckwith in Cincinnati—and Justice William Brennan wrote the dissent for the remaining justices, also citing at length the Nuremberg Code. Brennan wrote that any immunity military officials might claim in such a case should be qualified, not absolute—should depend, that is, on the facts of the individual case—and also that soldiers should not have to defend a Constitution "indifferent to their essential human dignity." [26]

Annas provides a note about Desert Storm. During that war, the Department of Defense, in association with the FDA, used unapproved drugs and vaccines on U.S. soldiers. These practices have now been supported by the U.S. judiciary. The defense of the country is paramount, says our highest court. If there is a mystery and a paradox here, when we consider that the Nazi doctors could also claim they were defending their country, it is a paradox our Supreme Court seems not to have been troubled by.

Annas reminds us that the Nuremberg Code describes experiments that were not directed at the subjects' own illnesses, and that in contrast, such human research cases as have arrived in U.S. courts have often been, not of this nontherapeutic kind, but experiments in new treatments, where Nuremberg is even less likely than otherwise to be considered material.

OF COURSE THE LINES dividing these two kinds of research are not by any means always clear. The doctors in Cincinnati were claiming to be doing therapeutic research, but as we have seen throughout this narrative, there are many different kinds of evidence that treatment for cancer was not their purpose. Single-dose, wide-field radiation for cancerous tumors ceased to be administered once military funds were withdrawn, nor is there a record of any treatments of this kind before the DOD grant was received.

Yet the defendants have never ceased to insist that they were simply trying to help people who were ill. Even as they negotiated a settlement with the families of the people they had exposed, they continued to maintain this position and offered no apologies, admissions, or regrets. The pleadings of their attorneys do not explain *why* the researchers were agreeing to settle, even though they believed that no charge against them could be sustained. Their briefs remind the court that "cancer is the second leading cause of death in America after heart disease" and that the defendants had been engaged in "the fight against cancer" for decades. They say the DOD funds were never used for patient treatment but only for the auxiliary study of radiation "effects." [27]

THE DECISIONS of U.S. courts described above form, in any case, the resistant and unpromising context of Sandra Beckwith's ruling against the Cincinnati investigators on January 11, 1995. The "discretionary functions" of public doctors at work had been very expansively defined by the courts, especially where the U.S. military was involved. In general it seemed that individuals used in research could be treated almost any way anyone wished to treat them, as long as what was done was felt to be in the national interest.

Judge Beckwith, however, as we shall see in the pages that follow, did not hold these views about the sanctity of military research.

12

An Angry Judge

This rookie judge just stepped up to the plate, out of nowhere, and hit a home run. —Attorney ROBERT NEWMAN, January 1995

The comprehensive and expressive essay that constitutes Judge Beckwith's Opinion and Order of January 11, 1995, was read by those of us involved with awe and considerable surprise. Lisa Meeks said that on the morning she found it in the mound of express mail at Kircher, Robinson et al. she read it immediately and that doing so was "almost like a religious experience." [1]

It was a ruling that was not in the least expected. Meeks said she had thought the judge "would give us a little here and them a little there and *maybe* eke out enough constitutional grounds for the case to stay alive." Robert Newman was also surprised. He said, "This rookie judge just stepped up to the plate, out of nowhere, and hit a home run. . . ."

Indeed this document of eighty-eight pages seemed to be a gift for common justice, and one need hardly say that in the U.S. today we are not accustomed to very many such gifts. It seemed clear that the plaintiffs had the whole factual record of the case on their side, but we did not know whether or not any individual in authority in the country would acknowledge these facts for what they were.

The full opinion as I myself studied it a few days later seemed to me much more a speaking and feeling document than I would have thought a legal order could be. The details of Beckwith's arguments against immunity for the doctors unfold almost like an absorbing story, and one hears all the while somehow, no matter how studied and formalistic the prose may seem in certain passages, the personal voice of a deeply reflecting writer, one who has no merely casual interest in what she is setting down. Judge Beckwith wrote of "an outrageous tale of government perfidy" and of allegations so "inflammatory and compelling" that it had been difficult to examine them objectively. She wrote that it was "inconceivable to the Court that the individual and Bivens Defendants, when allegedly planning to perform radiation experiments on unwitting subjects, were not moved to pause or rethink their procedures in light of the forceful dictates of the Nuremberg Tribunal and the several medical organizations." [2]

At the opening of the hearing of 1997 on the settlement agreement reached by the two sides, Beckwith would state from the bench, "This is a singular case in terms of having public interest, and the court is interested in that." This assertion was a simple one, on the face of it, and almost an understatement in view of what she had already written, yet her quiet enunciation that day of this fundamental idea had a force that held the whole courtroom in suspension for some moments and seemed to frame the case anew—to thrust all parties up once more against the seriousness of what they were about. Many judges, as I understand it, would not have wished to call attention to this aspect of the case or to acknowledge the public attention that was surrounding it, as Beckwith had, in fact, already done in the first sentence of her ruling of 1995.

But her opening paragraphs should be cited in full:

The Complaint in this much-publicized matter alleges that the Defendants engaged in the design and implementation of experiments from 1960 to 1972 to study the effects of massive doses of radiation on human beings in preparation for a possible nuclear war. The experiments utilized terminal cancer patients who were not informed of the existence or purpose of the experiments. The Complaint alleges that most of the patients selected were African-American and, in the vernacular of the time, charity patients. The Complaint further alleges that the various Defendants actively concealed the nature, purpose, and consequences of the experiments. The allegations of the Complaint make out an outrageous tale of government perfidy in dealing with some of its most vulnerable citizens. The allegations are inflammatory and compelling, creating a milieu in which it is difficult to objectively examine the allegations for legal sufficiency or to apply a view of constitutional rights unilluminated by the legal evolution that has taken place since 1972. . . .

[But] the Court has ignored all factual disputes in arriving at the respective conclusions. It has adhered to the fundamental tenets provided by the case law as enunciated by the United States Supreme Court with little recourse to other precedents. The questions to be resolved are as follows: (1) Can the Plaintiffs prove any set of facts in support of their respective claims? (2) If so . . . were the constitutional rights, which Plaintiffs allege were violated, clearly established at the time of the events at issue, so as to overcome the individual Defendants' claim of a qualified immunity defense? . . . .

In brief . . . the Court concludes that the Defendants have not established that the Plaintiffs can prove no set of facts that would support their claims. . . . Moreover, the Court is satisfied for the purposes of these motions that the contours of Plaintiffs' constitutional rights as regards those claims were sufficiently developed at the time of the events in question to afford a reasonable public official notice that the acts would likely violate Plaintiffs' constitutional rights.

The Court therefore, will DENY the individual . . . Defendants' motions to dismiss. . . .

We have already noted Beckwith's assertion that the researchers could not be considered immune from suit as public physicians for the reason that they "were not acting as physicians" when they carried out the radiation project but as "scientists interested in nothing more than assembling cold data for use by the Department of Defense" (p. 38). She stated her views on this issue quite plainly indeed: "The Court never authorizes government officials, regardless of their specific responsibilities, to arbitrarily deprive ordinary citizens of their liberty and life" (p. 39). Using a passage from an opinion of years earlier, she wrote that "every human being of adult years and sound mind has a right to determine what shall be done with his own body"; the invasion of bodily integrity that was being alleged, she said, had had for the victims "extreme consequences, among them the most permanent of all possible consequences."[3] This last line seems, of course, deeply ironical, in a literary kind of way, in its deliberate understatement of what had taken place. Beckwith does not use the simple word *death*, as she does in other passages, but refers in this oblique and striking way to that *consequence* which is, of all consequences, the most final.

SANDRA BECKWITH IS a long-time resident of the conservative town of Cincinnati on the Ohio. Her law degree was earned at the same university that was defending itself and its medical professors in this case. After she left UC in 1968, she joined her father in the practice of trial law in Cincinnati and remained in his office for eight years.

When she wrote the 1995 opinion, Beckwith was serving her third year on the federal bench, an appointee of George Bush, and the first woman judge in the United States district court for southern Ohio. She had served twelve years as a judge in local courts, the first woman on the municipal court and then the first on the court of common pleas. Three years before her appointment to the federal bench, she had been elected a county commissioner, running as a Republican. When the radiation complaint came to her court in 1994, she was in her early fifties, a slender blonde woman who did not stride with rapid and military bearing into the hall, as some judges do in Cincinnati, but at the bailiff's call slipped rather modestly into her place, at first almost unseen.

For the general observer, at least, nothing in Beckwith's background quite explains why we should have had from her the kind of ruling she made, with its engaged protest against actions leveled by figures of authority at common citizens of the lower orders, people generally regarded as of small significance in the world. It may be, of course, that a woman judge, of whatever persuasion, may bring to her work something of her own struggle for empowerment in a profession where authority and power have long been the prerogatives of men.

In any case, Beckwith's ruling constituted, along with a learned exposition of constitutional rights and case law, a cogent history lesson, as it were. She took it upon herself to tell, as if for the first time, what personal rights people are assumed to have in this country and the ways in which these rights have been written into our laws over the years. She drew a rounded lesson in civil rights, a rounded lesson in the Nuremberg trials, in the views of John Locke, and in the origin of the now-common phrase "to shock the conscience," first enunciated by Justice Frankfurter in 1952.

Beckwith was, of course, also peering sharply into the ways that lay ahead for this case, and towards the inevitable appeal of her opinion to the Sixth Circuit Court and then beyond, quite possibly, to the Supreme Court.[4] The cases she cites from the past are abundant and compelling. We had seen during the earliest hearings that the attorneys for both plaintiffs and defendants, all men except Lisa Meeks, were having considerable difficulty keeping abreast of Beckwith's control of legal precedent.

In the ruling in question, she concurred in the use Meeks had made of the Barrett case in New York State—*Barrett v. United States* (2nd Cir. 1988)—where it had been found twenty-three years after the fact that state officials had no claim to qualified immunity when they secretly tested mind-altering drugs on an inmate in an asylum. They were found to be acting beyond the bounds of the powers delegated to them, Beckwith asserts, and she writes that Barrett "is both factually and legally analogous" to the Cincinnati case.[5]

She also gives great weight to Justice Sandra Day O'Connor's fervid dissent in the Supreme Court decision against James Stanley, the soldier who had been given LSD by the Army without his knowledge, in order to study the effects the drug might have on U.S. troops. Though the Supreme Court found against Stanley in a 5-4 decision, Beckwith wrote that with regard to Cincinnati, "because Plaintiffs in this case are not [like Stanley] military personnel, the Court is convinced that Justice O'Connor's dissent in Stanley controls."[6]

A large number of other precedents are clearly outlined. Regarding the haunting question for the plaintiffs as to what parallels could be found for such acts as the doctors had committed, Beckwith displays a sentence from a past opinion that shakes apart the strange contention that if an act has not happened before, and already been found to be against our laws as our Constitution conceives them, then such a thing may happen without penalty. Judge Posner in New York State, writing in

1990, had declared himself no advocate of such a view. Beckwith cites Posner's assertion that "there has never been a . . . case accusing welfare officials of selling foster children into slavery; but it does not follow that if such a case arose, the officials would be immune from damages liability." [7]

Beckwith strokes and massages for several pages the case that shocked the conscience of Justice Frankfurter in 1952. The Supreme Court had found, in *Rochin v. California*, that even a suspected felon had the right not to have his body invaded by state officials—in this case police—without due process. "Simply put, Rochin was the red flag," she wrote, that the defendants "failed to heed" when they forcibly invaded the bodies of citizens in Cincinnati, or "allegedly selected unwitting cancer patients to be the subjects of the Human Radiation Experiments." [8]

ABOUT NUREMBERG we read in this Opinion and Order of 1995 some rather startling pages. It had proven "impossible," wrote Judge Beckwith, "for the Court to ignore the historical context in which the Human Radiation Experiments were conducted." She remarks on the "succession of criminal trials" the U.S. and its allies conducted after World War II, and describes the trial of the twenty-three Nazi doctors and its legal framework. She identifies the four judges hearing the case and reminds readers that they were "all Americans appointed by President Truman."

Beckwith seems to have become particularly interested in comparing the defenses of the Cincinnati researchers with those of the Third Reich doctors. As to standards for experimentation, she writes that in Nuremberg the "lack of a universally accepted principle for carrying out human experimentation was the central issue pressed by the defendant physicians throughout their testimony," and she summarizes five "ethical arguments" presented by these defendants. The first of these concerns the need in time of war for medical information:

Research is necessary in times of national emergency. Military and civilian survival may depend on the scientific and medical knowledge derived from human experimentation. Extreme circumstances demand extreme action.

The German doctors also argued, Beckwith writes, that at times "it is necessary to tolerate a lesser evil, the killing of some, to achieve a greater good, the saving of many."

She cites at length the first provision of the trial's "final judgement," the statement that became known as the "Nuremberg Code":

> *The voluntary consent of the human subject is absolutely essential.* This means that the person involved should have legal capacity to give consent; should be so situated as to be able to exercise free power of choice without the intervention of any element of force, fraud, deceit, duress, overreaching or other ulterior form of constraint or coercion and should have sufficient knowledge and comprehension of the elements of the subject matter involved as to enable him to make an understanding and enlightened decision. This latter element requires that before the acceptance of an affirmative decision by the experimental subject there should be made known to him the nature, duration, and purpose of the experiment; the method and means by which it is to be conducted; all inconveniences and hazards reasonably to be expected; and the effects upon his health and person which may possibly come from his participation in the experiment.
>
> The duty and responsibility for ascertaining the quality of the consent rests upon each individual who initiates, directs, or engages in the experiment. It is a personal duty and responsibility which may not be delegated to another with impunity. (p. 55)

From a legal point of view, the question of consent is of course a crucial one, and the whole issue of "voluntariness" loomed large in the Beckwith opinion.

The Code developed at Nuremberg had become "part of the law of humanity," said the judge, and "even if it were not afforded precedential weight in the courts of the United States," it could not be "readily dismissed in this case." The defendants, she said, must have been aware of this Code and related guidelines, and it was here that she wrote of her puzzlement that the researchers had not been moved "to pause or rethink their procedures in light of the forceful dictates of the Nuremberg Tribunal. . . ." (p. 58).

Unlike the Advisory Committee, Judge Beckwith had no trouble finding that there had been clear acknowledgment, by the time of the Cincinnati radiations, of the validity of the Code for U.S. researchers; she cites a 1953 memorandum from the Secretary of Defense, the so-called "Wilson memo," directed at the Army, Navy, and Air Force. She viewed this memo as "a mirror of the Nuremberg Code." She mentions strictures of the World Medical Association and the "rigid safeguards" developed during the fifties at the National Institutes of Health, also based on Nuremberg (p. 56).

The memorandum from Secretary of Defense Charles Wilson and other interesting documents of this kind would appear in the historical sections of the final Advisory Committee report, and yet physicians on the Committee argued that in assessing the deeds of the Cincinnati doctors, it had to be taken into account that they had not been notified of any government guidelines against the use of uninformed subjects. In the roundtable discussion on Cincinnati in 1994, staff physician Ronald Neumann put it this way: ". . . although I think it's clear that . . . Nuremberg Code was supposed to apply to DOD and its contractors, we have at least reasonable evidence in the case of Dr. Saenger in Cincinnati that no instruction was given to contractors. He and his attorney have no records that were ever found in their extensive search of the Cincinnati files that suggest that there was any forwarding of regulations or educational materials or instructional materials of any sort vis-a-vis how one is to do clinical research or human research, at least in the context of a government contract in that period of time." [9]

Among the Nuremberg parallels, it might be pointed out that the court could also have considered the degree of collusion within the two wider medical communities. The Nazi investigators, as cruel as their experiments were, discussed them openly at the time with other German scientists. One of the doctors on trial had presented a paper on "Prevention and Treatment of Freezing" in Nuremberg itself, at a medical conference in 1942, and another on "Warming Up—After Freezing to the Danger Point." These are titles with an innocent air about them, but for this research captive women and men had been subjected to all manner of torturous ordeals of cold—left naked, for instance, outside in subfreezing weather for as long as fourteen hours.

To study injuries and to learn to heal them seems on the face of it to be a humane idea—if you do not have to *inflict* these injuries first in order to study them. "Radiation Effects in Man: Manifestations and

Therapeutic Efforts" was the generic title of the final five UC reports; the article of 1969 in the *Archives of General Psychiatry* was headed "Total and Half Body Irradiation and Its Effect on Cognitive and Emotional Processes." [10] The Cincinnati investigators have consistently maintained that their own tests could hardly have been anything other than reasonable and proper since they had not been "secret" but had been described to other radiologists and scientists in the journals of the day. (To know this is not, of course, to be reassured about the moral vision of either U.S. medical research itself or its publishing guild.)

Altogether, Beckwith's ruling was a firm denial of the defendants' contention that they had not used people against their will or exceeded their authority as public doctors:

> If the Constitution were held to permit the acts alleged in this case, the document would be revealed to contain a gaping hole. This is so in part because the alleged conduct is so outrageous in and of itself, and also because a constitution inadequate to deal with such outrageous conduct would be too feeble in method and doctrine to deal with a very great amount of equally outrageous activity. Indeed, virtually all of the rights that we as a nation hold sacred would be subject to the arbitrary whim of government. (pp. 40–41)

The judge reminds readers that in centuries past kings and leaders were immune from legal challenges to their authority from ordinary people — "sovereign immunity" was their sword and shield against accountability for their acts (p. 20). But today, after all, we are not saddled, she says, with the old dictum that "the king can do no wrong."

WHAT OF THE fifty-six African Americans in the tests and the claim that their right to equal protection had been denied?

The judge considered this question closely. She reminded the parties to the suit that to find discrimination a court must find that a difference between the races was made and that it was made "with intent." The doctors claimed first of all, as we have seen, that no one was coerced into treatment, that the patients were free to leave the hospital at any time and in other words, as Beckwith puts in, "carried the key to the hospital exit" (p. 31). They also asserted that they used no more black patients than would normally be found in Cincinnati General Hospital and that the plaintiffs would have to show that *within the tests* African Americans were treated differently.

The judge replied that "defense counsel's universe is simply too small," and that only with "diligent discovery" could it be determined what universe existed *from which the subjects could have been drawn*. She observed that if, for instance, it should be found that in the sixties black people had only one hospital they could use, they could hardly have been considered to be making voluntary use of that hospital. Her view of the matter suggested that if only one hospital had patients who were predominantly black (in a city that was less than one-third black), it might be found in a trial that doctors who used this hospital for dangerous experiments were guilty of discrimination.

The doctors, on the other hand, would certainly have replied to such a charge that they were using the only research and university-operated hospital in town, and that if the patients there had been predominantly white, they would have been used in the same way. Of course we were to have a settlement out of court, and we do not know what the outcome of this dialectic would have been.

In certain lesser causes of action put forth by the plaintiffs, Beckwith accepted the views of the defendants, and in a number of ways showed herself willing to consider closely their replies to their antagonists.[11]

WHEN THIS OPINION of the U.S. district court was issued, there broke out, we can be sure, a crackling fusillade of reaction in certain legal offices in Cincinnati and in the suites and corridors and homes of the medical people of the town. The researchers had not spoken out for themselves and had not thought they needed to, but now in thirteen local firms in high-rise suites, austere and expensive, with their commanding views of one bend or another of the Ohio River and its riverfront sports palaces and its bridges and barges and thick marine life of all kinds, its wooded banks beyond—defendant doctors and medical professors sat edgily, it must be assumed, in the mahogany offices of their chosen solicitors, or spoke warily to them on long distance phone. There was, no doubt, a somewhat different temper than before at the university as well, on its own now stockbrokered, smartly managed hilltops; in the rooms of the city solicitors; and in the executive offices of the hospital.

An appeal of Beckwith's ruling would soon be filed in the Sixth Circuit, but before many months had elapsed, there had also begun to be rumors of settlement.

By December of 1996 formal negotiations were being held in the chambers of an officer of the Sixth Circuit in Cincinnati. Five meetings took place during that winter and spring and a tentative agreement was produced. The negotiators for the defendants were Leo Breslin, an attorney representing certain insurance companies, and Alphonse Gerhardstein, counsel for defendant Robert Kunkel, one of the project psychiatrists. Gerhardstein is an attorney well-known to Robert Newman and often associated, as Newman is, with civil rights cases. For him to face Newman across such a table was a new experience for the two men, and perhaps putting Gerhardstein forth in this way was thought by the defendants to be a strategic move.

Newman had the assistance of the local attorneys already mentioned, David Thompson and Gary Lewis, and at times Robert Nelson of Leif, Cabraser, and Heimann of San Francisco, each of them representing a set of surviving families.

The plaintiffs put the number eight million dollars on the table, and in time it was countered by 1.75 million. When a standstill was reached at four million, Newman made a decision to query his clients, and a large meeting was held in the basement hall of a progressive church near the university.[12] To this meeting people piled in rather effusively, far more families than we had seen in the gatherings of the past. Doris Baker and other family activists set up a table in the front of the room and helped conduct the activities. Newman expressed the view that in all candor he did not think there was more money to be had than the four million being offered, and though it was not clear why he felt this sum to be the limit of reparations, his view of the matter was not directly challenged.

But on two questions there was excited discussion. What were the remedies other than money that might be won? Would the doctors apologize? Would they submit to statements and questions from the families in an open forum? Would they in any way whatever face their accusers? "We want them to look us in the eye and tell us why they did what they did" was a feeling we heard more than once that day.

There was also anxious discussion about how a settlement might be distributed. Would everyone be included? Newman did not seem entirely certain about that. A few members made highly agitated statements about what their short surviving victims had suffered and said they were not in favor of a share-and-share-alike system, but in this meeting and in the others to come, the overwhelming majority did favor such a system, even among families whose family member had died early. Some members, both white and black, spoke quietly and persuasively about the need to proceed harmoniously and with all due speed, to resolve the matter and put it behind them.

People did not openly voice the view that the money offered was not enough. No one said, *This does not represent serious compensation for what we have been through, then and now, and it is not a serious penalty for what was done.* Yet it would turn out that privately a few members of the group did have strong reservations about the settlement sum.

The following July the still-simmering agreement suddenly became public through what appeared to be a leak to the press. It was said that a family member working in Washington, D. C., had contacted Paul Barton, a Gannett correspondent there, with information about the negotiations and that in the face of a stream of inquiries, the two teams had quickly conferenced and drawn up a written pact that could be released. But not everyone involved remembers the same train of events.

The public unveiling of the settlement that followed seemed to mark the end of a long travail, and possibly it did mark the end of any residual trust, in the public mind, in the claims of the researchers.

BUT A LEGAL ACTION that had had a smooth start in the context of a massive and mostly accurate public campaign, of careful and comprehensive pleadings presided over in large part by Lisa Meeks, of Judge Beckwith's authoritative ruling against immunity for the doctors, then the meeting of minds of the two sides as to a settlement—all of this soon fell into a state of considerable confusion.

It is a commonplace, no doubt, among litigants to say that a legal action may assume—usually does assume—a life of its own, and this action declined to settle down respectfully into the seemly vessel of gentlemanly agreement being shaped for it by the local attorneys.

Motions were filed by the two teams—now acting as a united front before the court—to support the agreement they had forged. But before the judge could act on these motions, events took place that would alter quite considerably the course of the proceedings. That is, a group of attorneys from outside the city appeared in the night, as it were—out of nowhere, as some felt, a marauding band—to challenge the pact that had been drawn up.

One of the objecting attorneys, Cooper Brown, had become acquainted early on with Gwendon Plair, the family member working in Washington, D.C., and it seems that Brown had been put in touch with two other dissident families as well: the daughter and other relations of Willie Williams, who had died in 1970 twenty-two days after his radiation, and the children of Maude Jacobs, now in their forties, fifties, and sixties, who said they did not care how many years it might take for the litigation to resolve itself, they would not accept so slight a penalty for the doctors as they felt the proposed settlement represented.

I had, of course, come to know this family rather well, and I understood why they felt as they did. I even felt to some degree implicated in this dissent of theirs, because I had from almost the beginning of the campaign outlined to journalists in various places the special tragedy of a mother taking care of young children at home and then being swept into the hospital one day for a "treatment" that would end her life. When asked for families to contact, I had consistently named the children of Maude Jacobs as among the most knowledgeable witnesses to what had taken place; they did not seem to have forgotten a moment of their mother's last travail and death. Other individuals had had their lives affected just as radically, but many of these victims had been elderly people who now had few close relations to tell the tale, and some had no families at all yet known to us.

THE ATTORNEYS FOR the objecting families filed their first brief opposing the settlement on December 16, 1996, and the following February a two-day hearing on the proposed agreement took place before Judge Beckwith. It proved to be an event full of legal drama and conflict and did not turn out particularly well for the now united front of plaintiffs and defendants.

In the packed courtroom on that first day, I counted twenty-one attorneys—all of them males except Lisa Meeks, all appearing of course before a woman judge. This number included the five counselors for the objectors—large, somehow rather impressive men, it seemed to me, perhaps simply because they were mostly unknown to us and came in a posture of invasion and attack. Two of these attorneys practiced law in Philadelphia, and another in Houston, Texas,[13] and they were accompanied by Cooper Brown, the attorney from Takoma Park, Maryland, and a local associate, John Metz. Two of these counselors, Daniel Berger of Philadelphia and Cooper Brown, had come from a fresh radiation kill, so to speak, in Rochester, New York, the first of the radiation cases to be resolved. The federal government had settled on November 26 the claims brought against it by the plutonium families.

Berger identified himself as "co-counsel of record" for a group of the plutonium families, that is, for three multiparty University of Rochester suits that formed part of the 4.8 million dollar settlement with the government. In a personal affidavit, Berger argued that the Cincinnati case was a far worse case. The patients injected with plutonium had suffered "no acute toxic effects," he said, so that in spite of the settlement that had eventually evolved, serious questions had been raised by the defense "as to the bodily injury component of compensable harm but also as to any compensation based upon pain and suffering." The Cincinnati case was a different matter entirely, he said, and victims were "exposed to high level radiation which was expected to produce, and did produce, acute radiation poisoning."[14]

The Berger affidavit was in some respects a compelling one and would have been even more persuasive, perhaps, if he had acknowledged a significant difference between the plutonium and Cincinnati experiments. In the plutonium experiment researchers for the government had been trying to learn how plutonium was excreted from the body in order to protect nuclear workers. Researchers wanted to control the dose taken in, in much the same way in which the UC researchers would later control the airborne radiation their subjects would receive from a machine.

But in the plutonium experiment the government itself had set up the study, hired the contractors, and supplied the radioactive material. So it could be argued that the U.S. government had a clearer liability than at UC, where there had been uncovered no evidence that government officers initiated the trials, chose the personnel, provided the Cobalt-60 machine, or, in short, exercised the same kind of practical control.

Nevertheless, there had been federal on-site visits to UC, and we can read about them in the investigators' 1971 report to the DOD: "Valuable interchange of ideas has been stimulated by visitors from Department of Defense laboratories who give our staff a more practical insight into military problems than we might otherwise have." We learn that these visits led to cooperation between UC and nearby Air Force bases, and also that conferences led by Colonel E. J. Huycke of the Defense Nuclear Agency had been attended by UC researchers.[15] No discovery to investigate such matters further had been granted to the plaintiffs by the court.

But from the beginning of the suit, two United States contract officers who had worked with UC had been named as defendants, as had the university and the city of Cincinnati. None of these entities had been dismissed, and in fact all three were contributing to the proposed settlement. At that point a million dollars was coming from the federal government and half a million each from the city and the university. Yet all were at the same time forcefully asserting their immunity from suit and disclaiming any responsibility.

The university's motion to be dismissed from the action stated that it was protected by law from suit and was strictly "a voluntary defendant." [16] The judge had declined to act on this motion while the settlement was still before the court, and on a similar motion from the city.[17] But her orders had not appeared to rule out the possibility, at least, of eventual judgments at trial against the government entities.

Still, to establish claims against the U.S. government, in particular, is always a complex and arduous undertaking; we have had a glimpse, in the Nuremberg-like cases already outlined, of the way in which American courts have tended to regard such claims. The plaintiffs themselves, in their brief in support of the settlement, reminded the court that the government is a party at any given time to thousands upon thousands of contracts around the country and that law had established that it could not be held responsible for the actions of the countless individuals who operate under these contracts.[18]

Both plaintiffs and defendants argued that in the Cincinnati case the government had not exercised any direct authority as to the planning or implementation of the tests and thus was not a "deep pocket" to be drawn upon in a settlement or a trial. The government itself took the same position, needless to say, and we have records, within the legal filings, of correspondence from government attorneys attesting to the fact that they had received multiple requests for indemnification from the defendants and had denied all such requests from either the individuals or the university.[19]

But again, one need not necessarily share the government's own view of its distance from the Cincinnati tests. I had always assumed that a department of government where medical officers had received detailed annual reports from contracting doctors over a period of eleven years, on the subject of military preparedness and weaponry, would have been at least *as* able as an assistant professor of English to see in the countless analyses, tables, and patient profiles attached the plain truth that people were being injured in exposures they thought were treatments for cancer. Visits to the UC "laboratories," to use the doctors' term, *were* made; contracts renewed. (The backgrounds of the decades-long military interest in radiation injury had been explained, in part, by staff scholars of the Advisory Committee in 1995; and this story of the long struggle beginning in the thirties and forties to discover what happens to people exposed to radioactivity would eventually be told in far greater detail by Eileen Welsome in *The Plutonium Files* of 1999.)

What was being proffered, we learned, by the U.S. government in support of the Cincinnati settlement was, first, the monetary contribution, and then, an apology to the families, or so it seemed. The proponents included this apology as part of the injunctive relief, but when Judge Beckwith directed questions on this issue to the government attorney, she was unsatisfied with his reply. "We are prepared to issue an apology," said U.S. Attorney Stephen Doyle, "when this case is resolved." But could the United States, asked the judge, "produce language and signatories" to such an apology at a final hearing to approve or not approve the settlement? The reply was equivocal. The attorney could "recommend" to his superiors, he said, that this be done.[20]

Here the defendants were compelled to reverse themselves on the major legal defense they had been making for several years. They were obliged to argue that like the federal government, the city of Cincinnati and the university itself would have strong defenses in a trial, just as they were asserting, and probable immunity from having to indemnify researchers who—even if they were found to be liable as claimed—would also be judged not to have been simply carrying out their normal duties but acting on their own, and that, in short, their various superiors would not be responsible and no large sums of money would become available to the surviving families.

Anyone who reads the UC disclosures of March 1, 1994, will have a rather different view of this matter. If the analysis that has been made in the present volume has had any point at all, it has been to document fully the widespread collusion in this project by governments at several levels, an institution existing in the public interest, and a broad band of the medical community.

As for the university itself, it had been a fact of the case ever since the opening of the back files of the College of Medicine in 1994 that the administration of the College had been frequently warned by its own review committees that the radiation tests were dangerous and that their medical purpose was — at best — unclear. The director of the Medical Center was himself, as we have seen, a sometime participant. The pathologist Edward Gall had assessed for the team the falling blood counts that had presaged for certain patients their early deaths from injury to the bone marrow and the massive uncontrolled infections that ensued.

If a hospital or a university is ever liable for anything, it was hard for some of us to see why these entities would not be liable in this case.

It was almost amusing — if anything about these tragic events could be amusing — to imagine the three governmental defendants dancing nimbly around each other and coolly asserting their total immunity from suit while at the same time acting intently behind the scenes to cope with their possible vulnerability.

THE OBJECTORS' FIRST MOTION against the settlement had argued that the proponents had not offered "a single piece of evidence relating to the nature of the alleged injuries suffered herein," nor made "any judgment — informed or otherwise — of the value of the injury claims." [21] The objectors did not assent to the view that the case against the various defendants would be difficult to try:

The type of alleged misconduct — if proved at trial to a jury — is unprecedented in the annals of American jurisprudence. The recent disclosures of a broad based program [within the U.S. military] of biomedical research on radiation health effects, including extensive human experimentation under the nation's nuclear weapons program — if true — is certainly "conduct which shocks the conscience" of civil society. It is suggestive of some of the worst fears about advanced industrial society, when science and technology get out of control and their pursuit is divorced from humanistic values. . . . the Total Body Irradiation Program . . . was apparently one of the most egregious instances of human radiation experimentation — and the Cincinnati TBI among the worst, if not the worst, of the TBI programs. It was commenced relatively late when the perpetrators should have known better . . . and involved primarily poor, sick and elderly African Americans whose participation was allegedly the product of total fraud, including being undertaken under the cloak of experimental medical treatment but where it was known to have no therapeutic benefit; it was extremely dangerous and many of the victims apparently died from the exposures. . . . [Thus] it seems likely that a jury would find liability and impose damages to the fullest extent of the law on these defendants under these circumstances.[22]

Thus was a duel joined that would occupy everyone involved for several years and lead to two turbulent events in Judge Beckwith's courtroom.

13

The Case Closed

I feel in my heart that all is going to be well for us. God be with us all, because I truly hope that something good comes from all the work that has been done. —DORIS BAKER, leader of radiation families, February 1997

The objecting attorneys did not care, either, for the plaintiffs' much-repeated assertion that money in this case was not the issue, that the action was an action in civil rights, more concerned with such remedies as the raising of a memorial plaque. "It is not the pursuit of money, it is the pursuit of the truth that is the moving force of this litigation," they had read in the major settlement brief of the plaintiffs,[1] and in a personal affidavit on the settlement Bob Newman had seemed to underscore this view of the matter.[2]

Indeed, most of the family members testifying at the hearing in February 1997 and submitting affidavits seemed genuinely to subscribe to this view and these feelings. They might be "as mad as all get-out," as one witness put it, but generally speaking, they wanted the case to end, so that whatever was coming to them could come and they could take satisfaction from having pursued the course of justice and from the correction of history they had helped bring about.

The Kentucky mountain woman whose mother-in-law, Mary Hampton Singleton, had died in the hospital twenty-five days after her radiation said from the witness chair plainly and softly, "It's no matter what we get. That part don't matter." Georgiana Burch, whose aunt was not seriously ill when she was irradiated and had recovered from her injuries and lived on for eleven years, spoke, as many did, for resolution. "Right today!" she said, "I should be home with my husband. He has had heart surgery and I should be home with him. So you see—a lot of us need to close this case." Members spoke of the pain of living through the deaths of family members once more. By now, one witness said, it was as if the victims were "waiting to be buried again." Many plaintiffs were "getting up in years"; they wished the end to come, to live to see whatever award they might be entitled to, and to have their lives settle down again.[3]

Time was passing. Since the legal action had begun, not only the husband of Georgiana Burch but Catherine Hager's husband Bob had suffered a heart attack; Lilian Pagano had also been ill, and no doubt many others; family leader Doris Baker had been hospitalized with a severe asthma attack that she attributed to stress over the case; Katie Crews had developed high blood pressure.

Even so, the phrase we were hearing so often from the proponents of the settlement—*This case is not about money*—had been announced a few times too often for the comfort of some of us in the courtroom. For of course much of life is about money and inescapably so; the lives of attorneys, of doctors and judges, of professors of English, of government officials are certainly in part, and sometimes in large part, about money, and to ask these generally not very well-off families to forswear any concern for material compensation for what they had been through, first with their families back in the sixties, and then during three years and more of legal combat in the nineties, was not gratifying, to say the least.

Even among the families approving the settlement, some clearly did not feel that money was beside the point and held the view that in the best of all possible worlds larger damages from the researchers would have been exacted, since the money penalty seemed to be the only real penalty that could be imposed. "While I now support the settlement, I am not fully satisfied," said a man named Charles Davis, whose father had had a large dose of radiation two weeks before Christmas in 1965. "I believe an award of $100,000 per victim would be more fair and appropriate," Davis continued. Leon Thomas said the money award was *needed* as a "token of guilt."

Elise Feldstrup and her brother Stephen Strohm wrote that since "the parties involved refused to accept personal and moral responsibility for their actions, it is only by means of a monetary settlement that we can achieve some sort of responsibility from these parties." It was also a "right and fair atonement," they said, for the suffering inflicted; they were also concerned that hospital patients in the future be protected, that in Cincinnati true consent be required to be sought by experimenting doctors, and that the consent standards be "reinforced legally" and "on the record." [4]

For some observers it seemed obvious that if the plaintiffs had had in the beginning a case that was not about money, it would have enjoined the institutions to take certain serious and specific steps to assure the court of their respect for the constitutional rights of research subjects, and to immediately divest themselves of all remnants of research that could not be performed on truly consenting individuals. The case had originally been conceived as one about fraud and victimization—and serious compensation. Newman had stated as much at the press conference in 1994 announcing the suit and had posited a quite large sum to be sought as damages. Defense attorney Alphonse Gerhardstein, however, was now explaining to the court, about the importance of the non-monetary relief, that "Civil rights cases are usually brought for public purposes . . . and this is a civil rights case."

And in short, because the settlement fund might not appear to the judge or to certain families to be a highly significant sum and had to cover the survivors of over sixty families, the plaintiffs were now uniting with the defendants, in this winter of 1997, to insist that it was not so much money, but the nonmoney remedies, the "injunctive relief," that was the crux of the matter. They did so in part, no doubt, because the case had taken on the appearance of an extremely onerous and expensive undertaking, but they also had a strong conviction that to proceed towards trial in the highly conservative Sixth Circuit would risk the overturning of Beckwith's historic decision of 1995.

The objectors, of course, disagreed with this view of the matter, as to the remedy that ought to be sought. The case had been *filed* as a money tort case, they said, not to enjoin the College of Medicine or the city or the Defense Department to do any particular thing—so how was it that the proponents could now say that the case was not about money?

It was an action that might be worth billions of dollars, they maintained. "We say that the institutions in this case are liable," they said, and they brought forth case law to support such a contention. The city of Cincinnati still claimed to own the hospital, they said, and was challenging the university's right to turn it over to a private agent. The insurance companies, they averred, were liable for what might be very large compensatory damages—even to the extent of their net worth, which the plaintiffs had not looked into; no one had considered their true "capacity to pay a judgment." With the exception of Nationwide, the policies of these companies had not been made available. Aetna, for one, said the objectors, "had wanted a seat at the table" and must have felt it had liability. There were "deep pockets aplenty in this case," it was said, and during a break in the proceedings, one of the younger family members whispered to friends in the aisle, "If these doctors don't have deep pockets, maybe they had better change their trousers." [5]

Yet as it would turn out, the objectors themselves would not succeed in bringing into play, in negotiations on behalf of their own clients, the large sums they claimed were at issue.

The defendants hotly contested all the assertions of the objectors about possible damages and argued that a trial would have an uncertain outcome and that the costs would be "staggering." There would be *hundreds* of depositions, they said.[6] On the first afternoon of the hearing, they also staged a three-hour presentation to show that the doctors were guilty of nothing and had acted strictly with "therapeutic intent."

These arguments for the defense were couched in the same highly generalized discourse they had deployed all along, as far back as 1971 and '72, and then in the unpublished paper "Ethics on Trial," authored by Saenger and Silberstein. As in the past, we still had no comment from the defendants on the crucial issue of immune system destruction, no reference to the injuries of the many patients who had died within weeks after their radiations.

Indeed, the doctors did not comment on individual cases except once: they did not decline to reply on one point to earlier contentions of David Egilman, who had written that patients were not treated for their acute nausea and vomiting after exposure and had later apologized to the

Advisory Committee for overlooking data to the contrary for certain individuals.[7] In the course of the defendants' presentation, records were produced showing that two of the three patients represented by objecting families were among those given the drug compazine for nausea.[8] But again, with neither of these patients, "Patient Jacobs" nor "Patient [Willie] Williams," was there any comment on their early deaths after treatment.

It was on this occasion that we viewed the video talks by Bernard Aron, speaking as a Jewish doctor with painful emotions about the Holocaust (and about its medical atrocities, we presume); by Harold Perry, speaking as a minority physician hardly likely to do injury to other blacks; and by Eugene Saenger. But again, none of the three doctors provided any details about his personal involvement in the project or any explanation for the outcomes of the patients under his care.

We have noticed already the stern cross-examination by the defendants of objector Lilian Pagano as to the nature of her mother's illness and final days. Pagano told the court that her mother, Maude Jacobs, had taught her the Pledge of Allegiance and that she could say it before she went to the first grade; and after all, she said, this pledge assured Americans of "justice for all—not just for a few." When attorney Leo Breslin cross-examined Pagano, he said, "Don't you want justice for the doctors too?" Pagano bristled and chafed at this—and at the absence of the defendants in court except on the video screen. "Why don't these doctors come out and show themselves?" she cried.

Pagano and I had talked on the telephone from time to time about the settlement, and she had said the monetary award was trivial and not a fit penalty for the researchers. I understood this view very well and respected it, but said that the law being what it was—and the financial balance of power being what it was—I was not sure that anything more could be achieved.

To abjure the settlement now, in any case, and try to proceed to trial would wreak havoc, I felt, on many lives, and I was somewhat surprised that Pagano herself, a woman in her sixties not in very good health, would wish to proceed, given all that that would entail. But the whole family, as we have seen, were united against the settlement and liked to say that they did not care how many years it might take to indict the doctors, they would persist as long as any of them lived. As I have explained, Pagano was one of seven living children of Maude Jacobs, each of whom would receive, according to the agreement proposed, no more, it appeared, than seven or eight thousand dollars, a fact that possibly contributed to their sense that the money involved was not a proper award nor a serious penalty.

I recall that during Pagano's cross-examination one line of questioning was especially disturbing. Alphonse Gerhardstein was taking his turn at trying to discredit Pagano's memory of her mother's mental turbulence and pain after her treatment, and then of her death twenty-five days later, and he attempted to tear down her depiction of Jacobs's acute illness directly after exposure, compazine or no. Wasn't Jacobs ill from cancer? he asked, and he tried hard to confuse the daughter's narration about those weeks before her mother's death. He did not succeed in this, but his attempt seemed to me ignoble and unethical, because he would have had to know that Jacobs suffered directly from the radiation, acutely, and then never recovered from the damage to her blood.[9] Gerhardstein was representing defendant Robert Kunkel, a UC professor and psychiatrist who had been involved in the psychological studies of victims just after their radiations.

At the end of the day up on the eighth floor of the Potter Stewart United States Courthouse, Gerhardstein and I happened to ride down on the elevator together, and I remarked on what I felt was his savage questioning of Pagano, who after all was telling nothing but the actual truth of Jacobs's last weeks as they had been narrated by the doctors themselves.

Gerhardstein might read, I suggested, when he returned to his office, the medical summary for Jacobs in the doctors' own reports, and he would see there what he might have known on this afternoon, if he did not know it: that this woman became acutely ill and mentally deranged just after her radiation and then died of it three weeks later with her immune system destroyed and her blood counts down to virtually nothing. I recounted the figures for Jacobs's white blood counts. Gerhardstein appeared to be somewhat perturbed by what he heard, though of course I do not know what exactly his feelings were.[10]

But as to Pagano's questioning and the postures of the defendants, they had not hesitated, in their motion on the settlement, to make more than clear their general contempt for the objecting families:

The defendants deny that any of the actions taken in connection with the study violated any of the patients' legal or constitutional rights, but nonetheless, following months of talks mediated by the Sixth Circ. Conf. Att., they agreed to a settlement of the case.

The problem facing this Court is that the objectors believe this case is only about money. They have bolted because they don't like the size of their potential cut. Plaintiffs' class counsel have pursued a much more comprehensive strategy, seeking accountability to all study patients through an injunction in addition to a monetary recovery.[11]

But the injunctive relief was no relief at all, the objectors maintained, and they were particularly derisive about the object proposed for commemorating the victims. A bona fide memorial monument would of course have been something of value—but this was not to be. What had been negotiated was a wall "plaque" about the size of a small poster, twelve inches by twenty-five, and no one would know what it was *for*. In short, we were to have an unidentified plaque with nothing etched upon it but the initials of the victims and the words *In Memoriam*; the radiation project itself would not be named. No location was specified; for all we knew, it would be installed in a broom closet of the hospital or in a restroom.

The judge too appeared to be contemptuous of this plaque from the beginning; she asked pointedly of James Wesner, General Counsel at UC, why such a memorial was not to record the full names of the victims. The reply of my university—the same university that had awarded Sandra Beckwith her law degree and afforded her the opportunity to accost it in this way—was this: that the researchers felt that a listing of actual names would be damaging to their careers.[12]

WHAT, IT WAS ASKED by the objectors, was the value of the other scattered items of relief? For the hospital to promise to release the full records of all those irradiated—even those not identified by surviving families—was not, they said, a bona fide injunction; this disclosure would certainly have to be made anyway before any legal resolution could take place. As to the promise of the school to abide by all relevant codes and guidelines for human research, this assurance, the objectors observed, was couched in language that was perfunctory and vague, and no court monitoring of such a promise was even being proposed.

It was also pointed out that neither from the doctors and the College of Medicine, nor from the university itself, was there to be an apology to the families, even of a limited and unincriminating kind.

It could certainly be argued that worst of all, in a way—among the remedies that *would* be granted—was the provision of a one-hour consultation for each of the families with a physician provided by the university; this doctor would explain the effects of the radiation on the victim. This concession seemed to be worth hardly a laugh, at best a healthy sneer, and that was in fact the way the objectors responded to this particularly unfortunate element of "relief."

In Bob Newman's personal affidavit, we had read that this case had been brought "to right a historical wrong." It was not a "mass tort case," he said, not primarily about money.[13] Yet what *was* the wrong that was being righted? We find in the plaintiffs' settlement briefs a drawing away from many of the basic facts of the experiments—in order to show that the agreement was reasonable and that little monetary relief would stand to be gained in a trial. Newman had told me before the hearing that the proceedings would seem to an observer like myself strange and unsatisfying now that the opposing sides had to form their united front before the court, but that that was the way things worked, and that in exchange for settling the case, the losing side, so to speak, is typically afforded the right to proclaim their innocence unchallenged—and, presumably, to have their way in court with the facts of the case.

For one unversed in the curiosities and contradictions of law, all this was not a little disagreeable. If this was a historic case, a civil rights case, an action in the public interest, why did it also make sense to undermine the facts of the experiments as the public had come to know them through the comprehensive public airing we had had for over three years? Was it necessary to leave unchallenged in court the defendants' contentions that "therapeutic intent" was indeed, as had been alleged all along, the motive for these experiments and that they were in fact conducted to provide "palliation" for people with a dread disease?

Many observers of courtrooms have concluded, no doubt, that the law is mainly about the law; it is not necessarily—perhaps not often in fact—about fairness or our common concerns as citizens, who wish to engage, some of the time at least, in the pursuit of our own happiness undisturbed.

WE HAD HAD, nevertheless, a successful suit in the sense that we had achieved a powerful "landmark ruling," as Robert Newman termed it, on the unconstitutionality of dangerous human research. This ruling had been followed by the long-sought capitulation of the doctors, their institutions, and the U.S. government—a public capitulation quite different from a discreet malpractice pact that few would know about, and one to which the defendants had been driven, at least in part, by the mass publicity the case had engendered.

As odd in a way as it seems, given the normal day-to-day interests of the giant media companies of our time, only rarely focused on the victimization of common citizens—and for the complex reasons outlined in this book—we had had a trial in the press and a comprehensive one at that, based clearly on the early records of the case, the university disclosures of 1994, and the materials and testimonies generated by the public hearings and the Advisory Committee. (It was important that Robert Newman and his associates had not discouraged the families from telling their stories to the press.)

It began to come clear that this public reenactment, so to speak, might be the only large reconstruction we would have of the events that had transpired in the basement of our hospital. Indeed the media exploration of the envelope of events around the tests was still evolving even as we sat watching the proceedings that winter—on our mahogany benches in the austere, dark-paneled courtroom of the Potter Stewart Federal Courthouse.

A radio team making programs for the BBC, led again by John Slater, had come back to Cincinnati a few weeks beforehand to partake of our settlement drama. They had worked up the new developments with my help over at the Blue Gibbon restaurant in Paddock Hills, and then Slater and his producer Peter Hoare had gone out to collect new interviews. They had not been able to remain in town for the hearing, though, and I had helped arrange for the assistance of Jay Hanselman, a young anchorman from WNKU, the public radio station across the river at Northern Kentucky University.

Hanselman was present for much of the proceedings, and he and I conferred, whispering at times in the hallway just outside the room, about the personages of the play in progress and the whereabouts of the individuals he needed to talk to—mostly certain family members on both sides of the settlement, but also the lead attorneys. Hanselman would send off his tapes to Slater in Birmingham, England, and would also write brief stories of his own for local consumption on NKU radio. (We did not expect to hear any such news emanating from the public station of UC.)

Other television and print reporters came in and out of the room during these two days, and journalists from outside called in. At home I received, as I have reported, a call from Senior Editor Gwen Tompkins for a weekend show of National Public Radio, and I was able to describe to Scott Simon in considerable detail the fundamental facts of the experiments and the events of the hearing.[14] Tompkins asked me, as did others during the years of this affair, what was happening in my own life at the university. She had wondered, said she, with some bemusement, whether or not she would be able to reach me through UC. Twice since 1994 I had in fact been called up by the university on charges of unprofessional conduct, for offenses said to be unrelated, of course, to my activities around this case. These were claims that could lead to suspension or dismissal, under an article of our AAUP contract; in both cases, however, the charges had in time been allowed to lapse. Robert Newman had come to my defense, as had the board of our faculty union.[15]

In any case, the public campaign some of us were still at work on— Doris Baker, for instance, and the Massachusetts physician David Egilman—was progressing, and seemed, again, all the more imperative if the essential truths of the matter were to become fully known. When I write the word *truths*, I mean by this, as always in this narrative, the incontrovertible facts as readily available in the researchers' reports to the DOD and their publications, and then in the new documents of the nineties sketched above—the 1994 releases from the back files of the College of Medicine, the written data collected from family members, and the records from the hospital itself.

LITIGATION, HOWEVER, has a logic of its own, and in 1997 the legal briefs of the attorneys for both the doctors and the families were full of unwarranted assertions of all kinds, or at least so it seemed to me.

The plaintiffs themselves had come to feel, they said, that the crucial issue of consent was a confused one and might not fly a straight path in a trial. It was noted that there were a number of different consent forms (when there had been any at all), some more informative than others, and that the doctors were also claiming "verbal communications" with the patients.

Yet anyone who examines the written forms will see at once that none of them revealed the most serious risk, that is, death from destruction of the immune system within forty days.[16] Surely, I felt, a trial court or a jury would be able to understand that if this somber risk of the exposures *had* been revealed, no one would have agreed to be irradiated and there would have been no experiments.

As for "verbal communications," there are occasional handwritten notations in hospital records about what the patient is being told about the coming treatment, but again, no notation that I have seen describes a "communication" in which the lethal risk is said to have been explained. We find, for instance, a notation in the hand of Edward Silberstein about his conversation with Margaret Bacon, whose death would come six days after her exposure and her bone marrow operations:

> I have talked to this pleasant, elderly Negro widow, reviewed her chart, and discussed whole body radiation with her. She understands what it can do and that it will not cure. She has agreed to this treatment. Please call me at 4282 about the preparations.[17]

Altogether it is hard to see why in a trial the consent issue would be difficult or confused.

Some families, it was also said, would be shown, if the case proceeded through the courts, to have known about the debate on the radiations during the seventies, and so for them the statute of limitations would have long since run its course. But again, no one who read the local papers in 1971 and '72 could have read of the specific charges of the Junior Faculty Association, the only group attempting to make known the basic figures on the doses given, the deaths occurring shortly afterwards, and the exact nature of the consent process.

In 1972 three patients, it is true, were notified by the doctors that they were among the individuals being anonymously referred to in the unspecific press reports of the time. These three individuals were interviewed by Edward Silberstein with the idea of demonstrating to Senator Kennedy, who was asking to talk to victims himself, that the patients and their families were satisfied with the way they had been treated and trusted their doctors not to have used them as "guinea pigs."[18] But in fact while Silberstein does reveal to the patients during these interviews some limited information about the military factor, nothing is confided about the injuries being sustained.

In the plaintiff briefs we also read that "some few numbers of patients" had been helped, not hurt, by the exposures, and that the sole survivor, Donna White Cristy, "owed her life" to the radiation, a claim also put forth—for the first time—by the defendants.[19] Yet we also find a conclusion by the plaintiffs that Cristy alone, as the one surviving victim, might be entitled in a trial to large "compensatory damages."

The first claim may require a word of explanation. When Cristy was irradiated, she was ten years old, suffering from Ewing's sarcoma, a form of bone cancer. She is a twin, and to protect her blood after her radiation, she was infused with healthy marrow that had been aspirated from the chest of her twin sister. The doctors denoted this transplant as a "Take," the first fully successful transplant and one of only five that succeeded over the whole course of the project, of thirteen attempts made.

We can assume that the procedure itself would have been a risky and uncertain one for both donor and recipient. Four of the five subjects where transplants had been attempted before Cristy's had failed, and the fifth denoted as a "possible partial take." Of the seven subjects who had transplants *after* Cristy's, three still went wrong. The retired African American teacher Margaret Bacon, died, as we have seen, from a complication of the transplant operation itself; Philip Daniels, the worker who had been on the job in General Hospital when he had been taken into the research, died in spite of his transplant on day thirty-one (and was designated by the doctors as a "No take"). Even in the final year of the tests, one of the two transplants, that of Rose Strohm, was notated as "doubtful," since an error had been made in assessing her blood status before her aspiration and reinfusion.

These then were the risks entailed in this experimental procedure, offered only to high-dose patients and during the final half of the project. In short, the prospects for a successful transplant for Donna White

Cristy in 1969 seem to have been dim, and yet she had been given the dangerous dose of two hundred rads of whole body radiation, in a single exposure. Of the adults receiving this dose, barely half had survived for over a month.

Still, the three children with bone cancer may have been more appropriate subjects for full body radiation than the adults with solid tumors, and they may well have been sent over to the UC team by doctors down the block at Children's Hospital in hopes of helping a sick child with an advanced treatment, or to protect a cancer-*free* child from a recurrence. The Children's doctors may not have known about the military connection or how the exposures would be administered — that is, in one continuous dose. Judge Beckwith did not agree to the discovery process that would have illuminated such issues.

IT WILL HAVE BEEN SEEN quite plainly, I expect, that as in many such actions, there was considerable disharmony between the plaintiffs' claims as stated in the early briefs and the positions announced after coming to terms with the defendants.

One could read in Newman's settlement affidavit, for instance, only one pointed statement about the injuries suffered. This statement comes from the physician consulting for the plaintiffs, Joel Tepper, a specialist in nuclear medicine and chairman of the Department of Radiation Oncology at the University of North Carolina. "The experimenters should have known," he wrote, "that death could result from this experimentation and they should have known that it was unethical and immoral to perform these experiments if there was not appropriate informed consent."[20]

The settlement sum agreed upon was not huge, but at least one could be gratified by the fact that — with regard to the class plaintiffs at least — it would go mostly to the families themselves and would not be swallowed up by the costs and fees of the attorneys. As early as June 1995 Newman had succeeded in convincing the other three firms representing families at that time to cap their combined fees and costs at one million dollars.

Money issues of various kinds were paramount, however, for the objectors, as we have seen, and on July 27, 1999, they would ask the court to authorize a disbursement for their own fees and costs — for far more limited labors—of $810,275.26. (It may be difficult to make such calculations, but it was noted by some that the original settlement sum had been earning interest for several years and that that money could be said, in effect, to have been transferred, along with a portion of the principal, to the coffers of the objectors.)

Within the war of motions both before and after the hearing there was a pitched battle over the question of what damages might be assessed in a trial and who would pay such damages, issues a court must take into account in approving a mandatory settlement for a class of plaintiffs. For some of us, a strange new catch-22 seemed to present itself: if the actions of doctors are bad *enough*, even their insurers and their institutions may not have to back them up, and there may be little remuneration that can be won by the victims or their families. Where doctors' acts are found to be intentional, damages may be designated as "punitive," said the proponents, and insurance companies not required to pay. Far better for individuals trying to recover something for injuries sustained if the perpetrators have acted simply in negligence. Better, too, where money awards are concerned, and in a federal case at least, if the defendants have brought on their victims not acute illness or death, but long-term disability and pain.

Wrongful death, argued the proponents of the settlement, is a claim that must be heard in a state court, and in Ohio (along with many other states) the rigid statute of limitations is two years, even if there is fraudulent concealment and the victims have not been able to discover what happened to them for many years.

In short, the fundamental argument of the proponents was that *if* further litigation led to a trial, and *if* a jury found for the plaintiffs, and *if* they awarded damages, those damages might well be of the punitive kind that only the individual defendants could be assessed. Their ability to pay would almost surely be found to be quite limited, and by law individuals being sued cannot be driven to bankruptcy.

The defendants themselves were saying, in effect, this: "We did not do anything wrong, but if we did, it would be hard to prove in a trial, and even if it were proved, it would be hard to collect any serious damages from us."

Plaintiff attorney David Thompson summed up the position of the class members this way:

There is not a plaintiff's lawyer in the country who would not be delighted to have the case depicted by the Objecting Parties here—a compelling case with defendants who basically have no defenses, no immunities and bottomless pockets. Reality is harsher, however, and the case far more complicated than the Objecting Parties assert.[21]

The presence of the objectors, though, had brought about an extended courtroom drama around this case for the first time, and a group of family members, those approving and not approving the settlement, had had a chance to express themselves in court. Journalists and other onlookers were able to hear a rounded tale of injury and death from Maude Jacobs's daughter Lilian Pagano. Pagano knew exactly what she meant and what she had seen of her mother's last days and could not be discredited. Judge Beckwith listened to her story with what appeared to be unwavering interest and concentration.

The court had also received written affidavits from thirty-one families, some of which were noticed above. "This settlement will tell others that we are all created equal and must be treated the same—and humanly," said Leon Thomas. "We could all use money!" he said, but he added that once he had learned what had happened to the whole group, he had wanted more than anything else "to get after the person or persons that caused this to happen and see that no one else would ever be treated this way again." Thomas went on to say, "I will never forget my mother, nor will I ever forget this tragic event, but it is time to put this behind us."[22]

Many others felt the same way. Charles Davis reported that it had been his father who had been "a victim of the atrocity known as the whole body radiation experiments at General Hospital." Such acts, he said, "would have been an atrocity no matter where they happened. But it is hard and painful to believe this atrocity happened in the United States of America and was sponsored by our government." It had been shown, he went on, that in the U.S., just as elsewhere, there were "unprincipled people who take advantage of other human beings, who violate basic human rights . . . to gain fame and fortune for themselves." But he and his family could not "change history," he said, and though they thought a much larger settlement would have been fairer, they did not want to go on to a trial.

James Wilson said his mother Necie "was used as a guinea pig and then discarded." The hospital records had no date of death for her, and it had been one of those reported in the *Enquirer* as unknown. "What hurts most," Wilson wrote, "is that General Hospital did not even know that she had died. I guess there was no follow up." He expressed keen resentment that the doctors had sent his father a bill for his mother's care, in spite of what they had been doing, an act that seemed especially "insulting and unfair." The hospital and the doctors, he said, "knew all of the problems she would have and yet they allowed it to happen. . . . It really hurts to know that she suffered for nothing." Still, Wilson was asking the judge to approve the settlement. "I know Judge Beckwith is a fair judge. I also know she has compassion for the law and people. She proved that when she said the radiation experiments violated the law, the Constitution and the victims' human rights."

Another daughter of a victim mother, Zettie Smith, said that "the persons responsible for this terrible act are finally responding to our requests . . . and I hope something as cruel as this never happens to anyone on this earth again."

A woman I did not know named Lottie B. Wallace discussed her own travails since the revelations. "Since learning my mother was a victim, I have thought and worried a lot about everything that happened to her, and I have had a stroke. I really believe my stroke was due, in part, to my thoughts and worries about my mom and the suffering she went through because she trusted the doctors to do what was right for her, and they didn't."

Doubts were often expressed about the intentions of the university. "I hope," said Nancy Crawford, "the University people are being truthful when they say this will not be repeated. . . . No amount of money can really make me comfortable when I think of my brother or anyone else being experimented on."

A man named Charles Stone was admirably succinct. He wrote only two sentences: "This was a tragic event," he wrote, "and I want it never to be forgotten. However, I agree to the settlement because I think it is the best result we can expect."

A woman from Kentucky, Mary Ann Houchins, spoke up feelingly for her Uncle Johnny, a victim of the last year of the project who died on day sixty-nine after his radiation. "It is one thing," she said, "to lose a family member through natural disease, but quite another to find out that the excruciating pain and suffering he went through was brought on by someone deciding that his life was expendable." Houchins rehearsed the news coverage, hearings, and other events the suit had helped bring about, and said she felt gratified by the tremendous exposure the case had had and felt it would help prevent such things from happening again. But now, she said, "we want only to find peace of mind for the injustice done to our family . . . and to put this tragic part of our lives behind us."

Doris Baker, the penetrating African American woman who had attempted to organize the families, and succeeded up to a point, took the stand and found herself on this day in a melancholy mood. Baker was often unwell, struggling with a severe malady of the lung, and her means for living were meager. She had not always been financially able to carry out the tasks she set for herself. Various individuals, in and out of town, along with certain national groups studying radiation had helped fund her trips to Oak Ridge, Washington, D.C., Albuquerque, and southern Louisiana, so she could meet other victims of the Cold War exposures.

Baker was a strong figure to me throughout the ordeal of revelation and publicity, of legal moves and countermoves, and the disturbing swayings back and forth of the Advisory Committee in Washington. Her mood was sometimes sad and shaken, and one might discover her to be, on any given day, in a near trance of otherworldly religious feeling. But at other times her reactions were fierce and pointed and as worldly wise as they could be. Wherever families were gathered for meetings, press conferences, and hearings, she could be seen among them in richly colored guise, often in wide hats and sweeping capes. She would often rise suddenly in a meeting with a rather grand authority and a decisive logic of comment or rebuttal that could not be gainsaid.

But Baker had become deeply disturbed by the division among the Cincinnati families over the settlement. Everyone had started out together, she said, and it had been her hope that the families would still be united at the end. "We had to fight many hurdles," she wrote in her affidavit, "to get where we are now. I myself had to go through this fight because of what they did to my great grandmother. I *had* to fight, and I went hungry some days to save money to pay for research material, and

for transportation to hearings out of town." She repeated these senti-
ments in court, saying she knew full well that the long chronicle of ups
and downs in the campaign had taken their toll on people. "Our hearts
are heavy," she said. "I for one can't take much more . . . but I feel in
my heart that all is going to be well for us. God be with us all, because I
truly hope that something good comes from all the work that has been
done." [23]

In the courtroom during the hearing there were hugs and handshakes
all around; the gatherings of this group had come to seem a little like a
family reunion. Of course some families—the family of James Tidwell,
for example—appeared on every occasion; others might come around
only rarely or simply when they could get off work. There were always
people I myself was glad to see again and new families I wanted to meet
and learn from.

I spoke at times with the attorneys, and once to one of the counselors
for the objectors, on the subject of the final days of Maude Jacobs. I also
spoke, when I had to, to the lead counsel for the defendants, Joseph
Parker, a slight dapper man with a low-key soft-voiced style. Parker
seems to pride himself on civility and grace under pressure, and when
we met during the hearing, he would bend toward me smilingly and
greet me softly by name. *How are you today, Professor Stephens?* The idea,
of course, was to state in effect, *We all know we are civilized people here, able
to contend over such a matter as this without discomfiting each other and having
feelings about things. . . . We are the sort of people who can do that, aren't we?*

I hope I am not that sort of person, and I replied only perfunctorily to
such greetings. At one time during the proceedings, the objectors read
from the JFA report, and when they did so, Parker rose to his feet. "Your
Honor," he said, as if to brush this matter peevishly aside, "you need to
know that that report is not by a physician. It is by an Assistant Professor of English." He sat down just as summarily, as if that were all that
need ever be said on the subject. But rebukes such as this had become
commonplace and are of course part and parcel of any legal conflict. I
assume Parker knew full well what I know about this report: that it told
the simple truth about what had happened, that the report was accurate
in 1972 and was accurate in 1997, and if it had not been, I myself, and
my colleagues among the junior faculty, would have been the subjects
of a suit brought by the doctors.[24]

Are ordinary people to be disbarred from the study of medicine and science? Should we ask if doctors and lawyers should be barred from the study of literature? Many physicians have, in fact, contributed to literary studies, and among authors themselves Chekhov, for instance, was a doctor, as was Somerset Maugham, and among Americans, Walker Percy and the poet William Carlos Williams.

IN 1972, AS I HAVE explained, I had written about people I did not know and did not expect to know as individuals. In the report I drew up, I identified them by their initials and the case numbers the doctors had given them. Those of us interested in the project at that time could not find attorneys to assist in a lawsuit or local media to help us press the case, and we did not try to uncover names and families. Looking back, it seems clear that we should have. As I have written, I myself thought of those irradiated as invisible victims of the Cold War, an army of unknown soldiers "fighting," as it were, in darkness — in ignorance of all that was taking place and the role they had been assigned in the secret defense of the country.

But in the courtroom that winter of 1997 I could sit among the children and grandchildren, the nieces and nephews, brothers and sisters of these once-unknown people. I sat as they did, gazing intently forward upon the morality play being enacted before us, and listening once more to the accounts they themselves rose to tell of the times gone by in which their people had been "guinea-pigged."

AT THE END of a long day of testimony, I stood with reporter Jay Hanselman inside the massive glass doors of the federal courthouse. It was six o'clock, and the chill February twilight was gathering on the cascade of marble steps outside. Hanselman needed, for the BBC, a final reflection on the day's events, and I looked at some dim notes in my hand and tried to oblige. In the empty hallway where we stood, the lights were being lowered and a thickly stuffed mail cart was being rolled with a light clatter down the hallway. It was cold and noisy on the steps outside, as after-work traffic blew and blustered down the city street, and we had been granted by the security men a few final minutes inside.

I spoke on Hanselman's tape of the painful avalanche of patent untruths we had heard that day from the defendants, through their attorneys and their video addresses, and of how disturbing the need for these deceptions must have been for the researchers themselves. Yet the truth in this case had prevailed, I felt, in spite of everything. When people go up against the system, they don't usually expect to win. But here was a case where they had, I said. The families and their advocates had gone up against two major systems of the country—the war department of our government and a U.S. medical community virtually united against them—and had prevailed.

We felt that and knew that again on this final day of the hearing.

John Slater had asked me on his tapings in Cincinnati what I thought the general feeling was, in the community, about the settlement and the effectual capitulation of the researchers. Were people shocked? Were they surprised? Of course I did not really know, but I felt that not very many people would be greatly surprised—certainly not African Americans, for instance—by anything a war machine might do in any country when it felt it was beset by enemies. What seemed to me to have been a surprise to people, I said, was the broad collusion with the military of civilian physicians, in Cincinnati and across the country, a collusion that was continuing in many quarters right up to the present day. That, I gathered, was the strange and disturbing part—but a phenomenon, after all, that people needed to confront, a somber segment of U.S. history that all of us needed to study and learn from.

WHEN THE JUDGE'S ruling against the settlement was issued six months later, there was considerable alarm, needless to say, among the attorneys who had forged the agreement. Judge Beckwith was not happy about much of anything that had been agreed upon by the two sides. She was unhappy not to have been informed of the ability of the individual defendants to pay claims. She was unhappy about the analysis of the injuries suffered and the prospect for damages in a trial, and she was very unhappy about the memorial plaque.

She denied preliminary approval of the agreement, but gave the proponents a month to try to improve their situation.

New briefs were rapidly filed by members of the plaintiff team, by the defendants, and by the objectors; and within another three months, a new ruling by Beckwith appeared.

This time the judge lent her provisional approval to the refurbished agreement, but her doubts about it were by no means entirely dispelled. She insisted, in fact, that this concession was provisional only, for the sake of opening the remaining records and allowing those families who were still unknown to be sought.

The injuries to the patients that the plaintiffs and defendants were now discounting she did *not* discount. She had heard enough to convince her, it seemed, from the comprehensive briefs of Lisa Meeks and others, the pleadings of the objectors, the hearing testimonies, and perhaps the public revelations themselves, that in a trial compensatory damages might be large. Even accepting, she wrote, for the time being, the proponents' analysis of the injuries that might be compensable, "the Court is not convinced that the award to each individual plaintiff would necessarily be small." She granted that in a trial awards would be based on the "subjective injuries" the surviving families had sustained, but wrote that "juries could award amounts ranging from pennies to hundreds of thousands, or even millions, of dollars in compensatory damages." [25]

She accepted, she wrote, "for present purposes" the argument that punitive damages could be awarded only against the individual defendants and that thus "a limited fund" might exist that would—according to the legal rules for setting up a class—allow for its certification and a mandatory settlement, where no families could opt out and pursue their own suits. Still, on this issue she reserved a final decision:

> The settlement proponents first ask the Court to conclude that the individual Defendants have limited funds from which to satisfy judgments. The Court cannot reach that conclusion from the current record in this case. The evidence concerning the individual Defendants' financial situations is incomplete and does not prove that their ability to satisfy judgments is limited. Because they, as proponents of the settlement, have placed their financial situations in issue, they are obliged to provide competent evidence, in addition to their own assertions of impecuniosity, to support their assertion that a limited fund exists. Before the Court will certify a class pursuant to Rule 23(b)(1), the record will contain such evidence. [26]

Neither did Judge Beckwith agree that the case was "not about money" but about injunctive relief, and she was not prepared to certify the class on that basis, that is, according to the rules for civil rights certifications. She conceded, though, that for the families, the proposed plaque and other injunctive relief "did appear to have some value." The plaque would be somewhat larger than originally proposed, and a location for it in a yard of the hospital had been agreed upon. It would affix the full names of the victims, but it appeared that no reference would be made to the experiments—no explanation for the existence of such a plaque except for the words *In Memoriam*.

Beckwith's ruling appeared to come from a judge who did not much like the pact that had been agreed on but who knew that a collapsed settlement might, in the long run, be even more unfair to the families and would not serve the public interest.

In the absence of a class settlement, suits by individual family members, she wrote, "would consume substantial resources, both of the Court and of the litigants. Moreover, many years would inevitably pass before all individual claims were resolved. The proposed settlement offers each member of the proposed class a significant monetary payment, other relief, and the added benefit of finality and a certain, favorable outcome."

If litigation proceeded, many obstacles would have to be overcome, beginning with the defendants' appeal, already before the Sixth Circuit, of her own ruling against qualified immunity for the doctors, and then with other "dispositive issues." The absence of informed consent would have to be established without the testimony of the victims. The injuries to the families would be, as she had noted, "largely subjective." In short, the plaintiffs' task, she said, would be "burdensome," and so "for those reasons, and others not expressed, the Court concludes that the proposed settlement is *within the range* of fair, reasonable, and adequate settlements of this action." [27]

I had come to admire the logic and language of Beckwith's rulings, and this order was composed with the grace I had become accustomed to. I felt that this judge was one who knew that words do matter. She does not waste them, and yet she is not cryptic and mysterious either: she explains herself. In good writing, even complex writing, readers have a sense of space and amplitude around them and easygoing progress down an unfettered path — or so says an English teacher — and I felt that these writerly traits shone through in these important documents.

IN MARCH 1998, a year after the events described above, a new hearing on the settlement took place. The objectors had been granted the right to take depositions from the defendants as to their assets, and we heard detailed testimony about the doctors' ability to pay claims. The assets of the defendants were said by the objectors to be in the neighborhood of twenty-nine million dollars, not the eleven million their original balance sheets had purported to show.

Joseph Parker, however, had various arguments to assert against the view that any such sums as those might be available to pay judgments in a trial. The larger figure included pension funds, for instance, that the researchers would soon be compelled by law to start drawing upon. Their average age, he said, was seventy-one. Several defendants had residences in Florida and might not be required to transmit funds to Ohio. If the present settlement did not succeed and sixty-seven individual lawsuits were launched, he argued, many years would elapse before their resolution, and much of the money in question might in the interim have been disbursed or have reverted to the defendants' estates.

Alphonse Gerhardstein again attempted to convince the court that in a trial there would be no compelling evidence against the investigators. He said that the defendants' team had sat down and studied a set of individual cases very hard, and with the best will in the world could not find any way to distinguish between injuries from radiation and injuries from cancer.

Yet Judge Beckwith found herself still unable, at the end of two days of testimony, to grant final approval to the settlement. She strongly recommended that all three sides commit themselves within ten days to further negotiations, and this they did.

It was in this way that the objectors gained "a place at the table." It became known that after a few meetings they and the defendants were meeting without the "class plaintiffs" and attempting to shape a pact of their own. If they succeeded, the class plaintiffs would be left with certain discouraging options. Should they continue asking the judge to approve one enlarged settlement for all, with no one able to opt out? If the dissenters *could* opt out and cut their own deal, should the class plaintiffs forswear settlement altogether and try to move toward trial, or even individual suits? Or should they simply write a close to the whole matter by accepting lesser awards than the objectors?

Many of us interested in this case found it hard to understand how the court could legitimate a class settlement that would allow a group of disaffected families to go off into a separate corner with the defendants and negotiate larger awards for themselves.

In time a large family meeting was held one Saturday morning in a room in the Kroger building. Robert Newman had struggled against the possibility of separate pacts for over a year. It was angering, demeaning, and unfair. On May 11, 1998, he had sent out the following letter to his clients:

Dear Friends:

Several settlement meetings have taken place since we last met in court. Recently, the objectors have been meeting separately with the defendants in the case in the office of the Sixth Circuit Mediator. Nothing concrete has been proposed, although there has been a suggestion of the format of a settlement whereby the objectors are allowed to opt out and a separate fund of money would be created for them and for their attorneys. Under this format, some of the money will be taken from our existing settlement and transferred to the objectors' fund and the likelihood is that the objectors would end up getting more money than those who are presently in our class.

I have advised the Sixth Circuit Mediator, the Defendants and the Objectors that we would oppose any method of settlement whereby unequal shares were given to families of the victims of the radiation experiment. I have said this because since day one there has been near unanimity that we should have an equal division of any settlement. Please let me know if you are still in agreement with this principle. If, on the other hand, you would be satisfied with having your family awarded $40,000 to $45,000 and did not care if some of the objectors might receive more money, let me know if you have that preference.

It would be best if you dropped me a note in the mail to let me know because I'm in court a fair amount these days.

Newman was also contesting the right of objecting attorneys to qualify for attorneys' fees, and he was charging that they had contacted at least one family already being represented. A month after writing the letter above, he sent an angry brief to the court:

> This case is foundering on lawyer greed. A proposed $4.26 million settlement was reached and agreed to by a near unanimous vote of the then plaintiff class members. With the entry of the counsel for the objectors into this case, following their solicitation of objectors, and their proclaiming that millions of dollars are to be had for those who hold out, the present settlement or even some reasonable modification of it is seriously threatened. The 45%, then 40%, contingency fee agreements obtained by objectors' counsel without taking into account that $4.26 million already had been negotiated is a fair enough indication that unreasonable claims for attorneys' fees may be preventing a settlement that would otherwise be acceptable to all class members.[28]

But many unavailing months had followed these communications, and now a bristling wall of hard facts had to be faced. Partly because of certain new legal impediments surrounding class certifications, it was becoming clear that the judge was not going to set up a mandatory class with no allowance for dissenters or "opters out." In any case, the objectors had in some way to be dealt with, since there loomed the inescapable reality that the defendants might walk away from any settlement that did not involve each and every known family. They would not be willing to face the possibility that a dissenting family that declined to be included might eventually launch an appeal of any settlement made or an action of their own.

By this time the objecting attorneys had captured not only three clients from the original class set—the families of Maude Jacobs, Willie Williams, and Beatrice Plair—but nine new families located through their own search.

The defendants now had to satisfy both parties, and they were not willing to try to do so by providing more money for all, but only for those who were posing the gravest threat. The objecting attorneys were felt to have the means to try the case and thus to be antagonists who had to be dealt with. Or at least that is what we were learning in the course of the family meeting called by Newman.

Newman had invited to this event an officer of the court, Mediator

Robert Rack, to explain to the assembled families the entire harrowing situation for what it was, and why the judge might be prepared to sanction two separate pacts.

Robert Rack seemed manifestly a troubled man. He had had many years in the work of mediation, he said, but no case in his career had caused him so much grief. "I take this one home with me," he said. It seemed to have come to constitute his own *Bleak House.* The negotiations went on and on and dogged his days and slept with him at night. He could not forget them or resolve them. Close to a year had elapsed since the three teams had been at work and the whole triangle become so snarled.

What the families had to face, it seemed, was that if they did *not* sign on to the original unenlarged agreement still open to them, the whole matter might stew on for years without resolution or trial. Eventually nothing might be left but individual suits, and some families might never receive anything at all. Some might be considered to have lesser causes of action than others and find no one to press their case.

It was too late to default. It seemed that no *new* objectors were now likely to be accepted, to share in the separate fund already developing.

Newman, for his part, now wished to put an end to things and to encourage the class families to sign the original agreement. Most of those present felt resigned to this new aggravation in a case that would not go away. But some declared their firm resistance to unequal awards. *This is the work of the devil,* they seemed to say, and at least one individual left the room in disgust.

Doris Baker herself felt betrayed. She felt she had worked, above all, for a united front among the families, betokened, as much as by anything else, by equal shares of any settlement. For some months after this family meeting, she and at least two other individuals withheld their approval.

But various private meetings were held with Newman over the ensuing months, and finally the remaining family representatives inscribed their names with the rest. Newman had succeeded in having the court set aside $65,000 for Recognition Awards for class plaintiffs who had worked hardest for the lawsuit, and the three withholders would in time all be recognized by the court for special endeavors.[29]

On May 4, 1999, a final—final-*final*—hearing took place in Judge

Beckwith's court. A little over five years had elapsed since the action had commenced. Two hundred and thirty-two filings had been made, a hundred and forty-four of them during the three years of the settlement disputes.

In court, there was now a common front, if not a very spirited one, of all three legal teams. Everyone rose to thank everyone else, as if no matters of injury and death had ever been at issue in this case (for we are all good civilized people after all), and in conclusion the judge announced to the room at large her intent to accept without further ado the new dispensation—which would involve one settlement between the defendants and the class plaintiffs, and a separate agreement with the twelve objecting families.

It was not made known at the time what monetary relief the objecting families would receive. In time I would learn from the probate documents for the victims' estates that each objecting family was receiving an award of $85,318.72, to be divided among legal heirs, and each class family $50,978.45. Attorneys' fees had already been separately disbursed from the top of each settlement fund, except for the fees of the lawyers for probate (for Newman's clients, at least, generally about two thousand dollars).

As for the final costs borne by the defendants, we do not know what this figure was, since we cannot know, for instance, what was paid to the long roll-call of attorneys for the defense. It could not have been a small sum.

Nor do we know how such sums were covered and how much, if anything, was exacted from the doctors themselves.

BUT WHAT WAS the overall effect of the intervention of the objecting attorneys?

Their appearance in the case had brought about acute conflict in court and a modest simulation of the trial that would not take place. But for those families who had fought the case from the beginning and become in time simply tired of the struggle, it was a poor bargain. They were the poorer monetarily, and the legal tensions finally puzzled and exhausted them—along with the continuing anguish of revelation about what had once transpired in the tomblike depths of Cincinnati General Hospital.

One of those who died of heart trouble before she could receive a settlement was Madge Spanagel, whose husband Mike, the ad salesman for television, had died in 1967, thirty-one days after his radiation. One of the younger members of an objecting family, Greg Plair, had died of cancer. No doubt others among the many families involved had passed away during the long ordeal of settlement, without knowing the final result or receiving any award; and we cannot know, of course, all the other psychic and physical ills suffered during these years of conflict.

In terms of the penalties inflicted upon the thirteen UC researchers named in the suit, the objectors had impelled them to augment—up to a point—the funds that had to be gathered to settle the case and pay for their defense, and had prolonged by several years their travail of litigation, the uncertainty of outcome, and their exposure in the press.

IN THE COURSE of the settlement talks, the memorial plaque had been slightly improved, and at the end the families were divided as to whether it was a satisfactory acknowledgment of all that had taken place. Many families refused even to visit its location, they found it so repugnant, but a group of objecting families decided to regard it as a victory and held a commemorative service at the site.

This plaque is not by any means a highly conspicuous one; it measures twenty-six by twenty-six inches and sits on a low stone base in a seldom-visited backyard of the hospital, in a grassy plot among the high back walls of various old buildings that once constituted General Hospital. This object does not, at least, deal in initials; the long-unknown soldiers of these secret military tests have regained at long last their full names. These are the only explanatory words that appear: *In Memoriam: Radiation Effects Study 1960–1972.*

As to the researchers, we do not read on the plaque that commemorates their project the famous exhortation of Shelley's once-powerful Ozymandias, whose stone head came to lie in the sand beside his broken statue—*Look on my works, ye mighty, and despair!*— but perhaps an ironical line of that kind would not have been amiss.

Robert Newman felt in the end that the real memorial in the Cincinnati case, more important than any material plaque, was the powerful 1995 ruling by Judge Beckwith that might have been lost if the settlement had failed. "In the end," he said, "the question was how best to honor the plaintiffs' mothers and fathers. The consensus was to preserve the legal and moral precedent we had achieved—the *invisible* monument to all our endeavors *In Re: Cincinnati Radiation Litigation,* 874 F. Supp. 796 (1995)." [30]

Still, many families felt that there should also have been a more prominent memorial and a message for posterity true to the full tragedy of what had taken place. At one time, it was believed that a more public memorial might be raised simply by the efforts of the families and their supporters, perhaps on land near—if not *on*— the hospital grounds and in some such style as this:

> The Cincinnati citizens listed below were the innocent victims of human radiation experiments in this hospital from 1960 to 1972.
>
> Their names are placed here so that all may remember their injuries and afflictions, and their unwitting sacrifice in a project sponsored by the U.S. Department of Defense and carried out by professors in the University of Cincinnati College of Medicine.
>
> This plaque has been installed following the settlement of a legal action brought by the victims' families against the doctors who conducted the experiments, the government officers who coordinated it, and the owners and operators of the hospital.
>
> The settlement agreement provides for monetary awards to the families and other remedies and was approved by Judge Sandra Beckwith of the United States District Court, Southern District of Ohio, on May 4, 1999.

Appendices

Appendix 1

TABLE OF CINCINNATI RADIATIONS*

No.	Name	Age	Race	Dose	Date rad.	Death	Cancer
004	John Worthy	67	B	50TBR	5/24/60	8/5/60	tonsil
006	Al Thompson	67	W	54TBR	7/4/60	7/14/62	rectum
007	James Tidwell	62	B	100TBR	10/28/60	11/29/60	intestinal
008	Cora Hicks	60	B	100TBR	11/8/60	2/7/61	breast
009	Bule Bentley	67	B	16TBR(2×)	11/11/60	1/23/62	lymph
010	Lula Tarlton	66	B	100TBR	12/4/60	1/22/61	breast
011	Zonnie Westerfield	52	W	100TBR	2/9/61	12/29/61	brain
013	Roosevelt Datcher	49	B	50TBR(3×)	5/19/61	9/9/61	skin
015	John Davis	61	B	100TBR	5/18/61	9/16/61	rectum
017	Mary Pasley	39	B	100TBR	5/18/61	4/16/67	tongue
018	Herman Gramman	67	W	200TBR	11/5/61	8/30/62	esophagus
020	Gertrude Newell	69	B	200TBR	4/22/62	10/24/64	rectum
021	John Edgar Webster	74	W	200TBR	4/28/62	6/3/62	bowel
022	Evelyn Jackson	48	B	150TBR	5/11/62	5/21/62	breast
023	Booker T. Law	49	B	200TBR	5/15/62	2/25/64	colon
024	Ellen E. Conyers	39	B	200TBR	6/10/62	12/21/62	cervix
025	John Henry Wells	64	B	150TBR	9/25/62	10/28/62	lung
026	Franklin Bunch	29	W	100TBR	2/9/63	11/17/64	lymph
027	David Jungnickel	17	W	150TBR	2/23/63	11/8/64	bone
029	Flonnie Belle Wells	63	W	150TBR	3/14/63	8/15/63	breast

* Aside from my own studies, this table draws on data provided by attorneys Newman and Meeks, and with regard to certain lines, a chart created by Tim Bonfield of the *Cincinnati Enquirer* from similar materials.

No.	Name	Age	Race	Dose	Date rad.	Death	Cancer
030	Jeff Dennis	54	B	100TBR	6/6/63	12/23/63	stomach
031	Mary Laws	81	B	100TBR	6/16/63	9/5/64	breast
033	Albert Johnson	64	B	100TBR	7/7/63	10/1/63	colon
035	Margaret Ruff	53	B	150TBR	10/27/63	3/5/66	breast
036	Sylvester Harvey	64	B	100TBR	11/24/63	7/20/64	colon
037	William Rucker	64	B	150TBR	12/15/63	2/6/64	esophagus
038	William Blunt	73	B	25TBR	3/22/64	n. r.	sinus
040	America Jackson	82	B	100TBR	4/26/64	n. r.	breast
041	Sil Watkins	63	B	50TBR	4/26/64	5/5/64	stomach
042	Geneva Snow	42	W	150TBR	5/4/64	1/21/65	cervix
043	Jacob Heim	45	W	100PBR	10/16/64	10/31/64	stomach
044	Beatrice Plair	53	B	100TBR	11/7/64	5/23/65	lung
045	Maude Jacobs	49	W	150TBR	11/7/64	12/2/64	breast
047	Frank Weyler	57	W	150PBR	2/20/65	7/17/65	colon
049	James Rice	75	B	200PBR	4/24/65	10/10/65	rectal
050	Leo Wessel	80	W	200PBR	4/24/65	11/7/65	rectal
051	John Joseph Mitchell	66	W	150TBR	5/1/65	7/14/65	lung
052	John Wynne	60	W	200PBR	5/1/65	7/31/65	colon
053	Louis Romine	66	W	200TBR	5/8/65	6/5/65	lung
055	Lillie Wright	57	B	200PBR	9/18/65	2/13/66	breast
056	John Byers	53	B	100PBR	9/18/65	10/26/65	lymph
057	Clara Johnson	55	B	100TBR	10/2/65	7/20/77	ovary
058	Estella Goodwin	47	B	50TBR	10/16/65	1/4/66	cervix
059	Reed Taylor	42	W	150TBR	10/16/65	11/17/65	renal
060	Carolyn Brown	49	B	150TBR	11/6/65	12/6/65	breast
061	Mary Linder	64	B	50TBR	11/20/65	3/13/66	liver
062	Charles Davis	60	B	150TBR	12/6/65	n. r.	colon
063	John Yaegel	38	W	300PBR	2/25/66	n. r.	lymph
064	Rosa Hayes	54	B	300PBR	4/2/66	n. r.	colon
065	Lela Austin	84	B	200PBR	4/16/66	n. r.	liver
066	Willie Hutchison	63	B	200PBR	6/11/66	1/10/67	rectal
067	Amelia Jackson	52	B	100PBR	10/13/66	3/25/67	colon
068	Willie Thomas	76	B	150PBR	10/27/66	12/22/66	cervix
070	Frank Hale	62	B	150TBR	3/2/67	5/9/67	n. r.
072	Lillian Roehm	62	W	300PBR	8/4/67	4/10/71	lymph
075	Nina Cline	60	W	200PBR	10/31/67	12/28/68	ovary
077	Grey Spanagel	63	W	200TBR	11/7/67	12/9/67	sinus
078	Lee Hoskins	55	B	200TBR	12/5/67	2/4/68	lung

No.	Name	Age	Race	Dose	Date rad.	Death	Cancer
079	Necie Wilson	50	W	100TBR	12/12/67	5/4/68	breast
081	Irene Shuff	52	W	100TBR	1/16/68	2/9/68	lung
082	Louise Richmond	49	B	300PBR	2/6/68	3/11/68	colon
083	Edna Pape	78	W	100TBR	9/4/68	5/26/69	breast
084,097	Elijah Cohens	65	B	300PBR	11/7/68	8/7/70	lung
086	Marie Johnson	57	W	100TBR	2/25/69	3/18/69	lung
087	Donna White Cristy	10	W	200TBR	2/17/69	living	bone
088	Katie Dennis	53	B	150TBR	4/9/69	4/16/69	lung
089	Edna Anders	71	W	200PBR	4/28/69	5/14/69	breast
090	Margaret Bacon	80	B	150TBR	6/4/69	6/10/69	lung
091	Genevieve Stone	62	W	200TBR	7/2/69	8/23/69	colon
092	Willa Rivers	69	B	150PBR	7/16/69	n. r.	colon
093	Terry Holmes	9	W	150TBR	9/17/69	6/22/76	bone
094	Minnie Mae Johnson	67	B	150PBR	10/22/69	10/11/70	lung
095,104	Amanda Cartright	58	B	200TBR	11/5/69	n. r.	colon
096	Albert Smith	43	B	100TBR	12/2/69	n. r.	colon
098,103	Ruth Stanford	45	B	200TBR	1/27/70	n. r.	colon
099	Philip Daniels	47	B	250TBR	3/3/70	4/3/70	pancreas
100	J.D.	76	B	300PBR	3/17/70	n. r.	colon
101	Marshall Harper	76	B	257PBR	4/21/70	n. r.	colon
102	Willie Williams	49	B	200PBR	4/28/70	5/20/70	lung
105	Pat Gebel III	13	W	100TBR	9/22/70	4/2/74	bone
106	Mary Singleton	58	W	300PBR	11/10/70	12/5/70	colon
107	Rose Strohm	58	W	200TBR	12/15/70	3/14/71	colon
108	Adelphia Snell	66	W	300PBR	1/27/71	1/20/73	colon
109	Willard Larkins	54	W	300PBR	3/24/71	6/12/71	colon
110	John Stillwell	51	W	300PBR	4/14/71	6/27/71	skin
111	Maggie Mitchell	52	B	200TBR	5/19/71	n. r.	colon

This represents the best information available at this time. TBR: total body radiation. PBR: partial body radiation. n. r.: not recorded. The only subject known to be living is Donna White Cristy (087). At least three subjects were irradiated twice and have two case numbers. Subjects 009 and 013 were irradiated in divided doses.

Data is incomplete for the final four subjects known: William Russia (112), Parthenia Marshall (113), John Dillard (114); Dillard was almost surely irradiated twice and is also "J.D." (100); Herbert Walker (115)

Appendix 2

Hearing Testimony of Eugene Saenger

[Author's Note: Omitted from this written testimony are the opening Summary and the Appendices. The Summary is identical to the lettered points of the Introduction.]

Statement of Eugene L. Saenger, M.D.
Before the House Judiciary Committee
Subcommittee on Administrative Law and Governmental Relations
April 11, 1994
Cincinnati, Ohio

I am Eugene L Saenger, M.D. of Cincinnati. It is a privilege for me to speak before this distinguished sub-committee of the Judiciary Committee of the U.S. House of Representatives to present a summary of our work on the treatment of far advanced cancer and the effect of wide field radiation therapy, work which I was privileged to direct and the results of which I am proud. The participation and support of the highly qualified physicians, allied scientists and associated health professionals is gratefully acknowledged. My Curriculum Vitae is attached. (See Appendix I.)

I am a graduate of Walnut Hills High School, Harvard College, 1938, cum laude and University of Cincinnati College of Medicine 1942. My training in Radiology was at Cincinnati General Hospital completed in 1945. I am a Diplomate of the American Board of Radiology and the American Board of Nuclear Medicine.

My major appointments at University of Cincinnati College of Medicine include rising from Assistant Professor of Radiology to Professor of Radiology from 1949–1987 and Professor Emeritus since then. I was the founder and director of (what continues today) the Eugene L. Saenger Radioisotope Laboratory from 1950 to 1987. I was Radiology Therapist at Children's Hospital from 1947 to 1987.

I have given over 40 guest and invited lectures in the U.S. and elsewhere. I have received the De Hevesy Nuclear Pioneer Award of the Society of Nuclear Medicine and the Gold Medal of the Radiological Society of North America and the Daniel Drake Award of the University of Cincinnati College of Medicine, these being the highest honors of these organizations.

My consultant appointments to my government encompass both domestic and international service, and include among others requests from the Department of Justice; Department of Energy; Environmental Protection Agency; Department of Health and Human Services; National Institutes of Health; Department of Defense; Food and Drug Administration: International Atomic Energy Agency; Oak Ridge Affiliated Universities; Surgeon General of the Air Force; the U.S. Public Health Service and numerous government administered hospitals. Additionally, I was proud to serve my country as an officer in the United States Army, attaining the rank of Major prior to my honorable discharge.

My principal appointments at the University of Cincinnati College of Medicine range from Assistant Professor of Radiology in 1949 rising to Professor, and from 1987, the rank of Professor Emeritus. I am a member of 29 medical and scientific societies and the Founding President of the Society for Medical Decision Making. In addition to being an honorary member of the National Council on Radiation Protection and Measurement (NCRP), I delivered the Sixth Lauriston Taylor Lecture—the highest honor of this organization. The NCRP is an organization chartered by Congress that develops recommendations for radiation safety used by Federal Agencies for protection of the public.

With my colleagues, I am the author of 187 publications in the scientific literature, the majority being in refereed journals.

I. Introduction

Several important points are presented summarizing our work:

A. One purpose of the study was the treatment of patients with far advanced cancer for whom the goal was the relief of pain, shrinkage of cancer and improvement in well being.

B. A second purpose was to study the systemic effects of radiation on the patient.

C. Treatment was given only if benefit to the patient was anticipated.

D. Patients were chiefly from the Cincinnati General Hospital. Selection was based only on the presence of advanced cancer and where no other therapy was considered to be as or more efficacious than then available chemotherapy. Race, IQ or socioeconomic standing were not selection factors.

E. Treatment was paid for by Cincinnati General Hospital and the National Institutes of Health. No Department of Defense funds were used for treatment or patient care or decisions regarding therapy or patient reimbursement.

F. Patients were told that the treatment might help them and were cautioned that it might not. Some patients chose not to be treated.

G. There was nothing secret about our work. There was nothing secret as to its being conducted. There was nothing secret about the findings obtained.

II. What Was The Purpose of The Total Body Irradiation (TBI)/Partial Body Irradiation (PBI) Study:

The primary goal of the study was to improve the treatment and general clinical management by increasing, if possible, survival of patients with advanced cancer and palliation of symptoms. (Palliation is treatment directed at relief but not cure.) In addition, observations and laboratory tests were carried out to seek effects of radiation on cancer patients and on the changes that could be ascribed to radiation.

The palliative effects of TBI were considered to be at least equal to and very likely to be superior to the chemotherapy available in the period from 1960–1970. Also the treatment methods were thought to be less stressful to the patients than chemotherapy then in use, especially in terms of initial symptomatology following administration of the dose, as for example, the painful mouth ulcers from methotrexate and 5-fluorouracil, drugs used at that time.

The background for this project originated in my observations over the prior 20 years that cancer patients treated with radiation might be benefited by a more careful evaluation of the effects of this kind of treatment on the total patient.

It seemed to me at that time that the approach to the total management of the cancer patients receiving radiation therapy was not as well studied as was that of the same patient who would be treated surgically. In addition, the effect on the cancer patient of doses of radiation given through large fields in relation to systemic effects was not being adequately considered, even though much work was being done on the radiation effects on the tumor and its immediate substrata.

The scientific indications that these goals might be achievable were based on two levels of evidence, one from animal studies and one from human studies.

A. Animal studies indicated better tumor regression when total body irradiation was preceded by localized radiation than when localized radiation therapy was given alone both for lymphoma and carcinoma in mice.

B. Studies in human beings: Human studies for treatment of far advanced solid tumors prior to 1960 suggested the value of TBI. It was employed in several American centers and internationally. Treatment was given with success in relieving pain, shrinking tumors and, in some cases, prolonging survival. (See Appendix 2.)

A major reason that we could begin TBI and PBI resulted from several important developments. The Cobalt-60 teletherapy unit was installed at General Hospital in 1958, the first in Ohio. Harold Perry, M. D., was the first full time radiation therapist at our hospital. He had come from Memorial Sloan Kettering Cancer Center in New York Hospital and was familiar with TBI and PBI techniques and indicators. James G. Kereiakes, Ph.D., a physicist, joined the Department of Radiology in 1959. He calculated the doses, dose rate and distribution of radiation.

I believed that there could be implications from this treatment for well individuals exposed to radiation under other circumstances. In

1958, I submitted an unsolicited application to DOD because there had been no studies on the metabolic effects of radiation and funds were available. This proposal was reviewed by J. A. Isherwood, M. D., for the Army Medical Research and Development Command. He made the following comments: "Any correlation of tumor response to total dose of irradiation by such means as proposed in this project would be of great value in the field of cancer. In addition if by some means such as those proposed accurate knowledge of the total dose of radiation received could be determined it would be of inestimable value in case of atomic disaster or nuclear warfare." (See Appendix 3)

III. The Study

A. Typical of medical investigations, this study progressed through phases. These phases are defined as follows:

Phase I studies are to determine whether the treatment is toxic.

Phase II is to determine in patients without controls but with measurable disease, whether the treatment is effective. Our studies included Phase II.

Only then are Phase III studies with controls and ideally with randomization conducted to determine therapeutic values. Although a Phase III study was proposed, we did not reach this level.

B. Patient selection: Patients were not recruited. Patients were referred for consideration for this form of therapy mostly from the Tumor Clinic (outpatient) and the Tumor Service (in-patient). I was not involved in patient selection or in determination of extent of therapy or dosage. These decisions were made solely by the attending physicians, internists and surgeons, and by radiation therapists. There were 24 patients entered into the study who were not given TBI or PBI. Some were rejected because it was thought that the patient would not benefit. Several patients and their families declined treatment.

    1. Eligibility for therapy was spelled out in our 1962 document to DOD:

        a. There is a reasonable chance of therapeutic benefit to the patient

        b. The likelihood of damage to the patient is not greater than that encountered from comparable therapy of another type.

        c. The facilities for support of the patient and complications of treatment offer all possible medical services for successful maintenance of the patient's well being.

2. Race was not a factor in selection — only the type of cancer and its extent. A statistical analysis, done only after the program was terminated, confirmed that the patients in this study did not differ from the patient population of Cincinnati General Hospital.

3. IQ was not a factor in patient selection.

IV. Informed Consent

As in selection of patients, informed consent for therapy was obtained by the attending physicians.

In the 1940's and 1950's informed consent was verbal except for the general brief informed consent required by the hospital from all patients to be hospitalized irrespective of the treatment to be administered.

In this project, the purpose and actual treatment and the possible outcomes were discussed with the patient and often included family members.

In April 1965, the use of written informed consent, both for radiation and bone marrow harvesting and reinfusion, were developed by this project. These forms clearly indicated that risks of treatment were discussed. At that time, DHEW and DOD did not require written informed consent. As a result of a number of helpful suggestions from the University of Cincinnati Faculty Research Committee, several revisions to the form were made between 1967 and 1971 (See Appendix 4). Furthermore, this written informed consent that we developed preceded any written requirements of the University of Cincinnati Medical Center by two (2) years.

One criticism of our work stemmed from the instructions to the attending personnel not to inquire concerning nausea, vomiting and diarrhea in the first few days after treatment. We were particularly interested in the frequency of these manifestations. Since both nausea and vomiting could be induced by suggestive questions, we requested that no questions be asked as to how the patient felt. This restriction did not in any way restrict the administration of drugs such as Compazine to relieve symptoms. This care is amply documented in patients' charts.

Of interest is that after treatment 39 patients (44%) had no nausea and vomiting, that 23 (27%) had symptoms for three (3) hours or less and that 12 patients (14%) had symptoms for six (6) hours or less. These responses are comparable to chemotherapy at the time, e.g., methotrexate, 5-fluorouracil and Chlorambucil.

V. Funding

As noted earlier, most costs of treatment were paid by Cincinnati General Hospital. An estimate of the expenditures for direct patient care for about 3,804 days at about $114 per day with some additional cost estimates gave a total calculated amount of $483,222. There were no professional costs or physician fees for patient care.

Some funding was obtained from the NIH. Some patients were maintained on the General Clinical Research Center of Cincinnati General Hospital; this unit was supported by NIH. The protocols and records of each patient so hospitalized were submitted to the NIH and approved. In addition, several of the Post Graduate Fellows supported by the Radiation Training Grant of the National Institute of General Medical Sciences (NIH) participated in some phases of the DASA program.

DOD funding was utilized solely for observation of patient symptoms and signs and for the extensive laboratory tests (See Appendix 5). DOD funds had no relation to choice of dose, choice of patient or patient care, in any way. No patient was compensated or reimbursed or paid for treatment. A Congressional General Accounting Office audit documented all of this in 1972. The total DOD contract for FY 1960 through FY 1971 was $671,482.79.

VI. Success of the TBI Study

Mortality: In the group of patients who received radiation, there were three categories in which there were enough patients to compare with other patients of the Cincinnati General Hospital treated differently or with comparable groups reported in the refereed medical literature. The cancers were those of the breast, lung and colon. The death rates were comparable to those treated by other means.

An important question is whether radiation was the factor leading to the early death of a patient. These patients had far advanced cancers which were growing exponentially. In the course of the disease, patients received chemotherapy and/or localized radiation therapy both before and immediately after TBI or PBI. For these reasons, it is not possible to identify a single form of treatment or the rapid growth of cancer as being the single contributing cause of death. It most likely would be the rate of growth of the cancer itself.

There were 20 cases in which patients survived longer than one year. Except for the one patient with Ewing's tumor who remains alive after 25 years, the longest survivor lived 9 years. Two other relatively long survivors lived five years.

Palliation was successful with relief of pain in 31% of patients. Some decrease in tumor size occurred in 31% and an increase in well being was found in 30%. No change was observed in 31%. (In some patients there was more than one indication of improvement; thus the percentages exceed 100%.) (See Appendix 6.)

Because of radiation induced hematological depression, autologous bone marrow storage and reinfusion began in 1964. With improvement in technique to include harvest of the marrow under general anesthesia and replacement immediately after TBI it became possible to avoid the characteristic depression of the white blood cells in five patients. This promising development was stopped at the time of termination of the contract.

VII. Review by Others

A. Faculty Research Committee. Our protocol was submitted to this newly formed committee in March of 1966. Provisional approval was given in 1967 with recommendations for review of therapeutic efficacy, bone marrow infusion as supportive measure and some revision in the study design. At no time was the project disapproved by the Faculty Research Committee as it received exhaustive and critical reviews.

B. The ad hoc Committee of the University of Cincinnati (the Suskind Report) undertook a complete review of the TBI project. Among the findings were that Phase III studies should be initiated with better criteria for the determination of palliative effects and that bone marrow transplants be pursued. The study was judged to be adequate for support of the critically ill patients because of the development of skilled team management especially with the help of the psychiatrist and psychologist coupled with home visits.

C. American College of Radiology. At the request of Senator Mike Gravel, the American College of Radiology formed an expert committee of Dr. Henry Kaplan, Chairman of Radiology at Stanford University, Dr. Frank Hendrickson, Chairman of Radiation Therapy at Rush-Presbyterian Hospital, Chicago, and Dr. Samuel Taylor, a medical oncologist at Rush-Presbyterian Hospital, Chicago. This distinguished group made two visits to our hospital. Their major findings were as follows:

1. The project is validly conceived, stated, executed, controlled and followed up.

2. The process of patient selection based on clinical considerations conforms with good medical practice.

3. The records, publications and patient follow-up are voluminous and commendable.

4. The procedure used for obtaining patient consent is valid, thorough and consistent with the recommendations of the National Institutes of Health and with the practice of most cancer centers.

5. Should this project come before the Senate or one of its committees in some fashion, we would urge your support for its continuation. (See Appendix 7)

D. At the request of Senator Edward Kennedy, the Government Accounting Office reviewed the accounts of the Cincinnati General Hospital to determine whether there had been any intermingling of DOD funds used for patient care, since we had pointed out from the start of our work that no DOD funds would be used for this purpose.

An excerpt from the letter dated May 26, 1972 from the Comptroller General to Senator Kennedy follows: "Concerning the contract with the University of Cincinnati, officials of the Defense Nuclear Agency stated that the cost of radiation treatment and patient care had not been borne by that agency. They stated also that funds of the Defense Nuclear Agency had been used only to pay for supplementary laboratory analyses of patients who had received whole body irradiation in order for the Defense Nuclear Agency to gain information in areas that were relative to national defense." (See Appendix 6)

E. National Institutes of Health (DHEW). D. T. Chalkley, Ph.D., Chief, Office for Protection from Risks, Office of the Director NIH, was very supportive of our work. In a letter copied to Senators Nunn and Talmadge, he comments that "It is to be regretted that this incident has halted what promised to be a very significant addition to our armamentarium against metastatic cancer." He also wrote directly to Senator Nunn pointing out that ". . . the patients were treated individually for the diseases they had." (See Appendix 9)

F. Secrecy. This study received widespread publicity in the early 70's. We responded to all questions about it at the time including at an open press conference. The study resulted in numerous unclassified presentations at open medical meetings and in published papers and reports (See Appendix 10).

VIII. Total Body Irradiation and Partial Body Irradiation Since 1971

It is apparently a common misunderstanding that the use of TBI/PBI as a therapeutic agent has been discontinued. In the period from 1970 to the present there have been major changes in the use of TBI and PBI (See Appendix 2). Doses have risen from the low levels of 100–300 rad TBI and up to 300 rad PBI used by us from 1960 to 1970. Doses now range from 600 to 1200 rad in single or divided doses of TBI and with sequential HBI in these same dose ranges. Fractionation has replaced single large doses (1200 rad) because of the complication of radiation pneumonitis. Among the solid tumors treated during these two decades have been cancer of breast, prostate, lung, colon and some sarcomas.

At the University of Cincinnati Department of Radiation Oncology beginning in 1979, TBI and PBI were administered to adults and children for leukemias, lymphomas, cancers of breast and prostate and neuroblastoma. Non-malignant diseases treated included aplastic anemia and congenital anomalies.

Notes

1. The First Public Knowledge of the Tests

1   There were ten reports by the UC researchers to the Defense Atomic Support Agency of the Department of Defense from 1961 to 1972. The facts outlined in this chapter are abstracted from the six hundred pages of these reports which I first read in 1971, from related materials that became available along with the reports in 1971 and '72, from disclosures made by the University of Cincinnati in March 1994, from the hospital records that began to be released to surviving families in 1994, from information gathered by the author in interviews with family members, and from a number of other documents to be described in this volume.

In the back sections of the annual DOD reports, the investigators attached profiles of the patients irradiated since the previous submission. These profiles are a major source, along with the hospital records, of information about individual subjects and of the kinds of group statistics presented in this chapter.

The first five reports are titled "Metabolic Changes in Humans Following Total Body Radiation," and the others "Radiation Effects in Man: Manifestations and Therapeutic Efforts."

The ten reports to the DOD are referred to in this volume as "the DOD reports," at times as "Report #1, Report #2," and so on; and in other passages by their DASA report numbers.

The project team evolved over the years. Eugene Saenger signed all ten reports, James Kereiakes the final eight. Ben Friedman signed four reports; Harold Perry three reports; Robert Kunkel one report; Harry Horwitz the final six reports; and Edward Silberstein, I-Wen Chen, Goldine Gleser, Carolyn Winget, and Bernard Aron the final four reports. Though I have often referred to these investigators as "the doctors," they were not all medical doctors involved in the care of patients, as will be seen in chapters that follow. As can be seen here, they were not all *men*. Of the two women named above, one, Carolyn Winget, a psychologist, was not included in the lawsuit as were the other researchers.

It has usually been written that the project ended in "1972." I have sometimes preferred the dates 1960–71 since there is no evidence that radiations took place in 1972. The tenth and final report to the DOD, however, was not made until spring 1972.

As to the exact number of radiations, the number eighty-seven was used by the Junior Faculty Association (JFA) back in the seventies; but later records seem to make it clear that at least three additional exposures had taken place. Twenty-five case numbers are missing from the records, and the researchers explain these particular missing subjects as individuals screened for treatment but never exposed.

A cryptic and alarming reference in an early DOD report to ten radiations not being included in the patient profiles—"because of the progression of far advanced disease and other factors"—cannot be explained on the basis of current documents. See p. 1 of the introduction to Report #2 (DASA 1422).

2   It would not be unreasonable, in fact, to say that nearly half of the individuals scheduled for the larger doses were being led in effect to their deaths. That is, 42 percent of those receiving 150 rads or more would die within 60 days, the great majority within half that time. The one individual who received 250 rads died, predictably, on day thirty-one: see chapter 9 of this volume for a study of Philip Daniels, an African American worker in the hospital irradiated in 1970. The woman who lived for nearly twelve years was Clara Johnson, patient 057. She was irradiated on October 2, 1965, and died on July 20, 1977.

3   Jacobs's white blood count fell to 850 from 5,900 before radiation, part of a "normal hemogram," and her platelets dropped from 370,000 to 38,000. For a fuller account of the case of Maude Jacobs and other individual patient cases, see chapters 8, 9, and 10 of this volume.

4   This brief article in the *Village Voice* by Robert Kuttner was followed by a much more damaging report by the same writer, titled "An Experiment in Death," October 14, 1971; we did not know of the latter report until much later. Certain of Kuttner's facts were inaccurate—for instance, he thought there had been 111 patients irradiated, but he was including the individuals given study numbers but not actually exposed; the percent of African Americans was 62 percent, not 80 percent, as Kuttner reports; and there were many more patients who died early than Kuttner or his source seemed to know about. Still, this valuable report exposed, in capsule form, most of the fundamental facts and issues of the project and was a close predictor of the critique of the JFA in 1972 and of all that followed that year and in the years to come.

5   Yet when further revelations about the tests came along in 1994 and '95, new

cover-ups were attempted, and the radiologists on a national commission reported over and over again that they had not found the smoking gun that was needed. The Advisory Committee on Human Radiation Experiments 1944–1974 (ACHRE) was created by President Clinton in 1994. The radiologists most active on the Committee were Henry Royal of Washington University School of Medicine, St. Louis, and Eli Glatstein, head of the Simmons Cancer Center of the University of Texas in Dallas. See especially chapter 6 of this volume.

6 See a full discussion of correspondence on these issues between the researchers and college administrators in chapter 5 of this volume; also note 9 below.

7 News reports of 1972 document this pact of the three politicians. See especially "Gilligan Joins in Radiation Controversy" on page one of the University of Cincinnati *News-Record* for March 7, 1972, which describes a meeting of Bennis, Kennedy, Gilligan, and Dr. Charles Barrett of the College of Medicine. Many issues were said to have been "clarified" among the various parties, and the meeting was described by Bennis as having been "very successful."

8 These comments of Gravel's during Senate deliberations on the Cincinnati project were printed in the *Congressional Record* for October 15, 1971 (No. 154). See also "ACR Rebuffs Sen. Gravel," *Drug Research Reports* (vol. 15, no. 11), pp. 13–14; and chapter 6 of this volume.

9 This letter of 1975 emerged in the 1994 releases by UC of papers from the back files of the College of Medicine. These papers are now housed in the Cincinnati Medical Heritage Center at the University of Cincinnati. (See also chapter 5 of this volume.) The *Enquirer* article is titled "Radiation docs felt victimized," Tim Bonfield, March 7, 1994.

2. 1994 and a Secret Drawer Reopened

1 In 1994 Welsome was awarded the Pulitzer Prize in journalism for her work on the plutonium injections. She left her job at the *Albuquerque Tribune* that year and commenced a massive study of the Cold War exposures in general. She studied the work at Los Alamos and elsewhere around the making of the atomic bomb and the related researches into radiation injury. This valuable work, *The Plutonium Files*, was brought out by Dial Press in the fall of 1999.

2 John Griffiths and Richard Ballantine, *Silent Slaughter* (Chicago: Henry Regnery Company, 1972).

3 Ten-page written testimony submitted by David Egilman on January 18, 1994, to the Energy and Power Subcommittee of the House Energy and Commerce Committee, especially p. 2.

4 Ibid.

5 Daniels had been expected to appear on October 21, 1995, at the Cincinnati meeting led by three members of the national Advisory Committee on Human Radiation Experiments. Also see chapter 6 of this volume.

6   In 1998 Newman left the firm Kirchner, Robinson, Newman, and Welch and
    established a practice of his own. A young attorney named Lisa Meeks, who
    was playing a large part in the radiation suit, also left the old firm to practice
    with Newman. See chapter 11 of this volume.

7   Interview by the author of Greg Shuff on February 10, 1994, and subsequent
    meetings and conversations.

8   Initial interview by the author of Elise Feldstrup on February 8, 1994, and sub-
    sequent meetings and conversations.

9   Page 4 of the ACR report: "By the nature of the disease, any cancer therapy must
    be regarded as heroic." This thirteen-page analysis of the Cincinnati project
    was addressed to Senator Mike Gravel by the American College of Radiology
    on January 3, 1972, signed by Robert W. McConnell, M. D.

3. The Press in Full Flower

1   On p. 3 of his testimony in Cincinnati before the Judiciary Committee of the
    House of Representatives on April 11, 1994, Eugene Saenger stated that "One
    purpose of the study was the treatment of patients with far advanced cancer
    for whom the goal was the relief of pain, shrinkage of cancer and improve-
    ment in well being." *Palliation* was the term most often used by the doctors to
    describe the beneficial effects of the radiation. See, for instance, chapters 8
    and 9 of this volume.

2   Patient profile for "E. J." in the second report from UC to the Defense Atomic
    Support Agency, DASA 1422, for November 1961 to April 1963.

3   A letter of February 2, 1972, from JFA member R. P. Koontz to President David
    Logan reads as follows: "In my judgement the radiation report was not at vari-
    ance with the consensus of the JFA general meeting held prior to the formu-
    lation of the written report." No documents exist to the contrary, except the
    letters of Dodd Bogart.

4   Letter in University of Cincinnati Archives from Dodd Bogart, Vice President
    of the Junior Faculty Association, to UC President Warren Bennis, January 26,
    1972.

5   "The Secret History of UC's Radiation Tests," *Cincinnati Post*, January 29, 1994,
    front page.

6   P. 2 of the transcript of this hearing, which took place on January 18, 1994.

7   "UC Doctor's Fernald Role Questioned," *Cincinnati Post*, March 9, 1994. In other
    actions concerning Fernald, plant workers and local residents were asking to
    be compensated for dangerous exposures in and around the plant during the
    years 1953–1989.

8   "Experiment at UC Spurs Talk of Probe," Laurie Petrie, *Cincinnati Post*, Febru-
    ary 5, 1994, on the possibility of a criminal investigation by Hamilton County
    Prosecutor Joseph Deters.

9 "Fallout," editorial in the *Cincinnati Enquirer*, February 5, 1994, calling the radiation reports a "frightening story" and stating that "what went on in the basement of Cincinnati General Hospital should give everyone chills."

10 Author's interview with Nick Miller April 21, 1997.

11 The German "paper-clip" scientists were recruited by the United States after World War II. They were individuals with service of various kinds under the Third Reich. About Gerstner, see Eileen Welsome, *The Plutonium Files* (New York: Dial Press, 1999), pp. 330–37.

12 This policy of the *Enquirer* seemed to change over the next few years as a new editor, Larry Beaupre, was brought on from the Gannett papers in upstate New York to try to wake up the *Enquirer* copy. (See also chapter 7 of this volume.) Local street rallies opposing the renewal of state executions in Ohio were covered, for instance, rather vividly, along with demonstrations in Over-the-Rhine. But Beaupre's attempt to enliven the paper would lead to the loss of his job in 1998, when the *Enquirer* published a sixteen-page Sunday insert exposing activities of Carl Lindner's Chiquita Brands operations in Honduras. Lindner sued the paper, claiming that voice mail within his Cincinnati company had been illegally tapped, and the paper agreed to apologize on its front page for three straight days and to pay reparations of ten million dollars. Publisher Harry Whipple in a news release of November 6, 1998, announced that Beaupre was being moved to an unspecified position at Gannett headquarters in Arlington, Virginia. See also an article by John Fox in a Cincinnati weekly, *City Beat*, for November 14, 1998.

13 "More UC Patients Identified," *Cincinnati Enquirer*, March 7, 1994, front page.

14 "Linking Radiation Test Data Reveals Patients' Identities," *Cincinnati Enquirer*, February 20, 1994, Section B, p. 1.

15 James Jones, *Bad Blood* (New York: The Free Press, 1981).

4. African Americans Lost and Found

1 This film can be viewed in the medical archives of the College of Medicine at the Cincinnati Medical Heritage Center at UC.

2 All of the early families repeatedly said by the *Enquirer* to have been "found" or "located" by them, as if through ingenuous investigative work, were either identified early on by Laura Schneider, or—as the story and the lawsuit progressed—called in to the paper and identified themselves, as had the Hagers, though usually from names Schneider had provided, or, later on, from information the paper printed from the DOD patient profiles. Schneider had not attempted to find all ninety families, and early in the campaign I asked Linda Reeves to have the *Enquirer* at least check its own death notices. I find an undated note from her that the *Enquirer* librarian had gone through the notices and found the names of eight new victims. Yet no one sought to trace, as Laura

Schneider had, the living families of these individuals. I mention this only to affirm that even on this major story with its long series of front-page reports, it was not felt that thoroughgoing investigative journalism could be funded by a major newspaper chain of the country.

3   Interview of Katie Crews by the author on July 3, 1994, and subsequent conversations.

4   This is a line from James B. Lucas, Assistant Chief of the Venereal Disease Branch, cited on p. 202 of *Bad Blood* by James Jones (New York: The Free Press, 1981).

5   "Expert: UC Research Unethical," front page, *Cincinnati Enquirer*, February 3, 1994.

6   This interview on *Weekend Edition* was aired on March 1, 1997.

7   See Ben Bagdikian, *The Media Monopoly* (Boston: Beacon Press, 1997).

8   The first passage here is from an early story of January 5, 1994: "UC: Radiation Study Not Secret Experiment." The two passages that follow are from Miller's story on the front page of the *Cincinnati Post* for January 29, 1994: "Secret History of UC's Radiation Tests Revealed." The final passage is from February 2, 1994: "UC: Radiation Tests Part of Cancer Research."

9   Author's interview of Rusconi, April 19, 1997. I came to feel that for this young reporter the world was not a mystery; she knew something of injustice and of the place of dissent. I felt she caught on very fast to things. She was only twenty-nine, a skinny dark-haired girl who sometimes wore black sneakers when she turned up at the door and was known to wear them onscreen, sitting at the news desk as she occasionally did (where lower limbs after all cannot be seen), though she was not of course an anchorperson but a young go-out-and-get-it reporter, amusing some of us late one night by having to stand in minus-twenty-degree weather outside a hospital emergency room—to report on the severe dangers of frostbite!

5. The Back Files

1   This memo and other letters and reports in this chapter are from the papers on the radiation project issued in several installments by UC President Steger beginning on March 1, 1994. These documents seem to have been taken primarily from the back files of the College of Medicine main office. They are housed in the Cincinnati Medical Heritage Center at UC. They include the reports to the DOD, an abundance of correspondence among review committees, the sixty-six-page internal review of the project by the Suskind Committee, the JFA and ACR reviews, the unpublished article by Saenger and Silberstein titled "Ethics on Trial," reports of the student newspaper, the *News-Record*, for the school year 1971–72, including the article by Lew Moores on the make-up of the Suskind Committee, and many other documents.

2   "Patients Not Told of Risks," staff report in the *Enquirer* for March 2, 1994.

3   Author's interview of Nick Miller on April 21, 1997.

4   See, for instance, "Body Irradiation Treats Cancer," *U.C. News Record*, November 12, 1971, and other reports of the fall of 1971.

5   A memo from Friedman to Saenger of December 15, 1971, is included in the disclosures. Friedman describes what he calls his "discussions" with subjects, "from 1965 on," that is, during his final three years in the project; nothing is reported of the first five years. Friedman says he gave abundant oral information to subjects "in the presence of witnesses." He writes, "I mentioned to them the possibility of complications from the radiation, among other things citing the strong possibility of hematologic change." They were also forewarned, Friedman asserts, that "this treatment might not benefit them directly but that value would be derived from either better understanding of the management of cancer or of radiation effects such as arise from nuclear catastrophes." In a lengthy undated memorandum from Friedman to the Faculty Committee on Research, he reports on "The Therapeutic Effect of Total Body Irradiation Followed by Infusion of Stored Autologous Marrow in Humans" and lists himself as "Principal Investigator."

6   The issue on Nuremberg in the *Journal of the American Medical Association* came out on November 27, 1996 (vol. 276). About articles in this issue, see also chapter 6 of this book.

7   "Suskind Comm.—Conflict of Interest?", front page of *University of Cincinnati News-Record*, February 11, 1972.

8   We have to assume that Raymond Suskind was, in his job as director of the review committee, a conflicted man. It is obvious from the final report that the eleven members of the committee had crucial disagreements right through to the end.

The UC disclosures reveal correspondence of Suskind's as late as 1974 in which he is still reluctant to share his committee's report with outsiders. He would need to have "some idea" of what kind of study was being engaged in, he said to one applicant, before making the report available. This individual, Bradford Gray, a sociologist writing from Barnard College, said he was "a bit taken aback" by this request, but went on to offer his professional qualifications. Suskind then sent him the report, but still withheld, until they were specifically requested, the appendices, which included some of the criticisms from earlier faculty reviews. Bradford Gray also asked about help with finding "a second report issued by some unofficial group," and Suskind replied as follows:

"I'm not familiar with a second report to which you refer in your initial letter. There was, I believe, a discussion by a Junior Faculty Association Committee which raised questions about . . . the study. This Committee also publicized a statement reflecting the views of several members of the Junior Faculty Association Committee." Suskind cannot help with this "statement," he says, and notes that JFA president David Logan can no longer be located in the UC directory.

9   A book titled *General Hospital*, by Polk Laffoon, published by the *Cincinnati Post* in 1974, includes information on the leavetaking of Gall and Grulee. About Laffoon, see also chapter 10 of this volume.

10 Warren Bennis, "The University Leader," *The Saturday Review of Education*, 22 December 1972.

6. Testimonies

1   Page 5 of written testimony submitted by Egilman. Congressional hearing in Cincinnati on April 11, 1994, on *Experiments Conducted by University of Cincinnati*. Subcommittee on Administrative Law and Government Relations of the House Judiciary Committee. Testimonies by Eugene Saenger, Joe Larkins, Catherine Hager, Gloria Nelson, David Egilman, Martha Stephens, James D. Cox, and Joseph Steger.

2   This paragraph is the "Summary Statement" submitted by James D. Cox. See note 1 above. There was also testimony from Gordon K. Soper, Principal Deputy Assistant to the Secretary of Defense for Atomic Energy, who submitted a history and chronology of the Cincinnati tests.

3   This is the opening "Summary" of Saenger's written testimony, p. 2.

4   See p. 8 of Saenger's written testimony. As for his earlier comments on patient deaths, see the article by Saenger and colleagues in *American Journal of Roentgenology* for March 1973 (vol. 117, no. 3): "Whole Body and Partial Body Radiotherapy of Advanced Cancer," especially p. 677. The authors write, "If one assumes that all severe drops in blood cell count and all instances of hypocellular or acellular marrow at death were due only to radiation and not influenced by the type of cancer and effects of previous therapy, then one can identify 8 cases in which there is a possibility of the therapy contributing to mortality." The authors proceed to discuss the "previous therapies" certain patients had undergone before radiation.

5   Final Report, Advisory Committee on Human Radiation Experiments, October 1995, U.S. Government Printing Office, especially "The President's Charge," p. 5. The charge to the Advisory Committee as summarized by Ruth Faden in the preface to this report does not seem so narrow a charge. The Committee was to consider not only whether the designs of the experiments met the "ethical and scientific criteria of the day," including those for informed consent, but whether experiments had "a clear medical or scientific purpose" and whether "appropriate medical follow-up was conducted." To consider properly these latter two issues as to the hospital cases without examining even a

representative set of patient records was simply impossible, and this task was left undone.

6   Many interviews and conversations with Lilian Pagano, especially during the spring, summer, and fall of 1994.

7   Author's telephone interviews with Judy Daniels in October of 1995, and conversation in Cincinnati City Hall following the final meeting of the panel on radiation appointed by Cincinnati City Council.

8   The ACR report was prepared for Senator Mike Gravel on January 3, 1972, and signed by Robert W. McConnell, President. The three distinguished reviewers of the project within the American College of Radiology, Drs. Henry Kaplan, Frank R. Hendrickson, and Samuel Taylor III, found virtually nothing to criticize in the experiments in Cincinnati and said that "by the nature of the disease, any cancer therapy must be regarded as heroic" (p. 4). Those "charged with the care of cancer patients," it was written, "have need for every possible bit of information concerning the methods and modalities which we use to treat these patients" (p. 3). The report never refers to military sponsorship, and it does not even accurately count, for instance, the short survivors, asserting that only eight individuals died "within twenty to sixty days"—whereas there were actually nineteen, as well as another six who died *before* the twentieth day after radiation. The report urged Senator Gravel to support continuation of the project.

9   See Eli Glatstein's five-page "Comment" to the Advisory Committee for Draft Final Report of March 21, 1995, especially pp. 4 and 5. Other "Comments" of one to six pages came from Henry Royal, Mary Ann Stevenson, Jay Katz, and Duncan Thomas.

10   Ibid., pp. 5 and 6 of the "Comment" of Henry Royal.

11   Ibid., p. 2 of "Comment" by Mary Ann Stevenson.

12   Heller's novel *Good as Gold* came out in 1979 (New York: Simon and Schuster).

13   The budget for fiscal years 1994 and 1995 was sent me by Tom McCarron of the Department of Energy, Office of Budget and Administration, on October 29, 1995 (the Final Report was issued in the same month, but work continued for some months thereafter). For these years the costs of the Committee, as noted, had mounted to $6,188,968, including $3,640,716 for salaries and benefits. I had been informed earlier by Jeff Judge of the DOE that Committee members earned $460 per diem plus expenses and that staff salaries ran as high as $90,000.

14   *Experimentation with Human Beings* was published in New York by the Russell Sage Foundation in 1972. When Jay Katz first undertook at Yale his massive study of human experimentation in the United States, he had been reading about the suffering of human subjects in Nazi experiments and had started to question some of his own medical research into people's "hypnotic dreams." In

his preface to this volume Katz writes that he had become concerned that he had not fully explained to his subjects how they might be affected, for good or ill, by what they were asked to recapitulate.

Katz is both physician and law professor, and he went on to compose a rich compendium of materials on all the multifarious ways, legal and otherwise, human research can be examined. His book is a volume of over a thousand pages, in the casebook tradition, with entries of all kinds large and small from an enormous variety of sources.

I became acquainted with Katz through phone and letter during the ACHRE deliberations, and learned that he had become familiar with the Cincinnati tests back in the seventies and with the report of the Junior Faculty Association.

15 *Journal of the American Medical Association*, 27 November 1996 (vol. 276, no. 20): pp. 1682–683.

16 The debates and decisions within the U.S. government, from the thirties onward, around the study of radiation injury and the use of humans in deliberate exposures is fully detailed in *The Plutonium Files* by Eileen Welsome (New York: The Dial Press, 1999).

17 Letter of Joseph Hamilton, M. D., to Shields Warren, Director of the Division of Biology and Medicine of the Atomic Energy Commission, 28 November 1950.

18 On p. 19 of Report #2 to the DOD (DASA Report 1422), Saenger states that "human beings can tolerate doses of 200 rads (300 r [roentgens]) relatively well as far as combat effectiveness is concerned." See also discussion of a similar formula by Mettler and Upton on p. 377 of the Final Report of the Advisory Committee.

19 Page 1 of Report #2 cited above.

20 The public meeting in Cincinnati, October 21, 1994, led by a Small Panel of the Advisory Committee.

21 Neumann's remarks are on pages 20, 24, and 25 of the transcript of the Public Meeting of the Advisory Committee on November 14, 1994, devoted primarily to the Cincinnati experiments.

22 Ibid., pp. 28–30.

23 Ibid., pp. 62–63.

24 Judge Sandra Beckwith, *Opinion and Order* of January 11, 1995, p. 58. United States District Court for the Southern District of Ohio, Western Division. Case No. C-1–94–126: *Cincinnati Radiation Litigation.*

7. Author's Intermezzo

1 "I can imagine how they regard *you* over there," Jerone said, "and what they must be saying—that here's this one little woman . . . and suddenly she has

the press eating out of her hands . . . and then she gets hold of the families too and is trying to micro-manage the whole crusade. I expect this is what they are saying to people."

2   "Keating Heading Back to Court," *Cincinnati Enquirer*, October 5, 1996. *The Nation* for November 19, 1990, carried a massive article titled "S&Ls, Big Banks and Other Triumphs of Capitalism." A section on Keating was titled "Charles Cheating Jr.," pp. 603–06.

    In 2000 Keating's luck changed. On October 5 the *Cincinnati Post* reported through the Associated Press that Keating was leaving prison after serving five years of a twelve-and-a-half year federal sentence. The Supreme Court, "acting without comment, let stand rulings that threw out Keating's convictions because of faulty instructions to the jury." Keating's corporations were said to have "bilked investors, many of them elderly, out of millions of dollars by selling them unsecured 'junk' bonds that turned out to be worthless." Taxpayers had lost $3.4 billion in the collapse of Lincoln Savings and Loan.

3   Eileen Welsome, in *The Plutonium Files*, pp. 305–12, describes a tragic accidental death from radiation in 1958, not long before the UC tests began, an incident that absorbed the attention of scientists around the world. Cecil Kelley, a plutonium worker at Los Alamos, was called to a plant one night in late December. As he tried to mechanically stir a tank containing excess plutonium, he set off a chain reaction. It was estimated that an enormous dose of 10,000 to 12,000 rads was absorbed by his head and chest. He lived only thirty-five hours. His wife reported that after her husband's death she received mail from many scientists, but they did not send good wishes — they sent requests for samples of Kelley's tissues for their work on radiation.

4   The fifth edition of *The Media Monopoly* by Ben Bagdikian (Boston: Beacon Press, 1997); and Michael Parenti, *Inventing Reality* (New York: St. Martin's Press, 1986).

5   Robert Lifton, *The Nazi Doctors and the Psychology of Genocide* (New York: Basic Books, 1986).

6   John Slater's "Atomica America" was produced by Pier and Black Hill Productions, Birmingham, England.

7   This individual, whose oral history I have on cassette but who gave me her account on condition she not be identified, spoke in detail about a year of clerical work in Saenger's office in the sixties. She remembered intense security around the radiation room at the far end of the corridor, and in the office regular meetings between Eugene Saenger and his close colleague in the tests, Ben I. Friedman; in her mind Friedman was a much sterner and more difficult individual than the genial Saenger, who was for her a generous-minded and easy-going employer.

8. The Mother Without a Name: The Earliest Exposures

1 *Motion to Dismiss on Behalf of Defendants Saenger, Silberstein, Aron, Horwitz, Kereiakes, Perry, Friedman, Kunkel, and Gleser.* Cincinnati Radiation Litigation, Case No. C-1-94-126. June 2, 1994.

2 Profiles of eleven subjects during 1960–61 (one was exposed with x-rays) appear at the end of Report #1 of 1961 to the Defense Atomic Support Agency (no report number assigned). The names of the first two patients exposed we now know were John Worthy (subject 004) and Al Thompson (006). Thompson's family was eventually identified and became part of the group of families objecting to the class settlement and negotiating a separate agreement.

3 Tidwell's profile (case 007) on pp. 31–32 of Report #1 of 1961. See also his hospital records, especially a two-page chart titled "Total Body Study: Microscopic Blood for J. Tidwell."

4 See p. 17 of Report #4 of 1966 (DASA 1844).

5 Author's interview with Barbara Ann Mathis, April 18, 1994. Tarlton's profile (010) is in Report #1 of 1961.

6 Pp. 2–3 of Report #1.

7 Letter of December 4, 1971, from Eugene Saenger to Edward Gall. UC disclosures of 1994.

8 See chapter 8 of the Final Report of Advisory Committee, October 1995, especially pp. 385–406.

9 Page 3, Report #1.

10 Profile for Mary Pasley (017) in Report #1.

11 "Saenger Defends Research Project, Details Objectives," Tim Bonfield, *Cincinnati Enquirer*, July 12, 1994.

12 Joseph Hamilton, M.D., to Shields Warren, Director, Division of Biology and Medicine, U.S. Atomic Energy Commission, November 28, 1950.

13 The profile of John Edgar Webster appears in Report #2 of 1963, and the hospital records released to his family in 1994 add considerably to our knowledge of his injuries.

14 Seven-page submission of Barb Tatterson to the congressional hearing led by Representative John Bryant in Cincinnati on April 11, 1994.

15 The profile of David Jungnickel (027) in Report #2 of 1963.

16 Author's interview with Anne Weise, March 3, 1994.

17 Interview with Saenger by Advisory Committee staff members Ronald Neumann, Gary Stern, and Gil Whittemore, September 15, 1994, p. 94.

18 The hearing took place on February 20, 1997, on motions for and against the proposed settlement. For a detailed discussion see chapter 13.

19 Author's interview with Kim Szwedo, 1994.

9. The Final Years

1 "Sloppy and imprecise science"—at best—was the characterization of Clinton's Advisory Committee in 1994. See the transcript of a discussion of this body at the public session of November 14, 1994, in Washington D. C.

2 A profile for Jacob Heim appears at the end of Report #4 to the Defense Atomic Support Agency (Report No. 1844) of 1966. Also cited here are unnumbered pages of Heim's hospital records, which include a letter dated July 17, 1963, from Sara Youkilis of an office of the Social Security Administration in Cincinnati. The profile of the individual who lived nine days, Sil Watkins, is available in the same report. Also to be referenced here is author's interview with Jacob Heim's sister, Helen Delph, on June 11, 1998.

3 Interview with Eugene Saenger by Advisory Committee staff Ronald Neumann, Gary Stern, and Gil Whittemore in Cincinnati on September 15, 1994, p. 52.

4 Ibid.

5 Ibid.

6 Page 36 of the Advisory Committee discussion cited above.

7 "Body Irradiation Treats Cancer," June Davidson in the University of Cincinnati *News Record* for November 12, 1971.

8 Page 4, for instance, of the 1963 report to the DOD (DASA 1422).

9 The consent forms were made available to the JFA with the DOD reports in 1971, and they also accompanied new releases of the reports in 1994.

10 These passages appear on pages 2 and 9 of Report #4 cited above.

11 Ibid., p. 34.

12 Ibid.

13 Page 17 of Report #4. "Since severe hematologic depression was found in most patients who expired," the doctors write, "autologous bone marrow storage was instituted in 1964."

14 See tables 7 and 8, pp. 27–28, of Report #10 of 1972: "Whole Body Irradiation with Marrow Transplantation," and "Results of Successful Iso- and Auto-Transplants of Marrow after 200 Rads Midline Whole Body Radiation."

15 We read in Thomas's patient profile that she was treated with "150 rad midline absorbed tissue dose (126 r midline air exposure) of lower partial body radiation on October 17, 1966. She experienced severe abdominal pain, diarrhea, weakness, anorexia, and confusion." After her treatment for a urinary infection, she was discharged on November 22, but readmitted on December 1 "because of disorientation and inanition." Her hemogram remained stable but she "continued a downhill course" and expired on December 22.

16 Author's interview with Madge Spanagel, August 20, 1994. Also cited are the records sent her by the hospital.

17 A British doctor, M. H. Pappworth, writing in 1967 a wise and tender book on what he saw as dangerous human research in Britain and the U.S., pointed

out that doctors sometimes innocently sent their patients to teaching hospitals for advanced treatments that turned out not to be treatments and to have nothing to do with the patients' diseases. Pappworth's analyses of dangerous and harmful experiments were taken directly from researchers' own reports in medical journals of the day. He provided, in footnotes, the names and institutions of these investigators in his book *Human Guinea Pigs* (Boston: Beacon Press, 1967).

18 As little as, in a sense, financial remuneration may seem to be worth in view of what was inflicted on her husband, nevertheless her life was affected, and she had to live and pay her bills just as did the doctors, the lawyers on both sides of the legal action, the government officials of the past and present, the experts on the Advisory Committee. Perhaps the radiation families should not have been expected to feel that for them moral victories were all that was appropriate.

19 Pages 63 and 42 of the interview of Saenger cited in note 2 above.

20 The latter quotation is from Dennis's profile in Report #7 to the DOD. The passages from the nurses' log are from unnumbered pages in Dennis's hospital records.

21 A notation of May 3 signed by Silberstein in the unnumbered hospital records of Margaret Bacon.

22 In Report #9 of 1971, p. 33, we read that "The second death (090) was anesthesia-related, four [sic] days after the procedure." A note from Silberstein in Bacon's hospital record for June 5, the day after her radiation, in part a reply to the consternation of the nurses on the floor, reads as follows: "Mrs. Bacon remains in shock. . . . The amount of radiation she received does not cause hypertension—in fact it takes 10 times as much as she received. I suspect the anesthesia introduced hypertension as etiologic, but the [unreadable] may indicate septic shock." He went on to suggest "blood cultures" and various medications, but five days later Bacon died. The DOD profile for Bacon states that on the day before her death she "was noted to have left sided facial weakness, suggestive of a cerebrovascular accident," yet a chart on bone marrow transplants printed in Report #10 of 1972 lists Bacon's "Complications of Infusion" as "None." (On this chart see note 14 above.)

23 Profiles for Marie Johnson (086), Edna Anders (089), and Genevieve Stone (091) appear in Report #7 of 1969 (DASA 2425).

24 The profile for Philip Daniels appears in Report #8 of 1970. Other quoted statements and the notations from Dr. Bossert appear in his hospital records. The autopsy report for Daniels is incorrect as to his exposure, stating that he had received one hundred rads two weeks before his death; according to the DOD profile, his exposure was 250 rads, administered a month before death. This patient had suffered "marked toxic depression of bone marrow," and the causes of death are noted as "aspiration pneumonia" and general ill health as-

sociated with a wasting disease. We read, with some puzzlement, that though it is "possible" that the "extremely severe" bone marrow lesion "may be related to the recent total body irradiation," the relation "is not clearly demonstrated."

25 Author's interview with Elise Feldstrup on February 8, 1994. Rose Strohm's profile appears in Report #9 of 1971.

26 Author's interview with the younger Joe Larkins on February 5, 1994, and with the elder Joe Larkins on the same day and on many subsequent occasions.

27 "Radiation Link to Mother's Death Haunts Family Three Decades Later." Sunday Section, *Lexington Herald-Leader*, February 13, 1994. Also a second lengthy report, "Radiation Cases Discovered Earlier" in the same section. Both by Gail Gibson. The editorial of February 16 is titled "Broken Trust: Government for the People? Hardly."

28 "Cancer-free UC Patient Died After Test," *Cincinnati Post*, February 18, 1994; and "Records Say Woman Had Cancer," February 19, 1994. Of course the *Enquirer* reporters were still smarting and suffering from having passed over completely the radiation story early on and having had to read about it in the *Post*, and they wanted each small comfort of comeuppance they could get.

29 See, for instance, p. 6 of Report #7 of 1969. Eileen Welsome's *The Plutonium Files* makes clear that this kind of variability had become known within the community of radiation researchers long before the Cincinnati project began.

30 See, for instance, the article by Faden, Lederer, and Moreno in the issue on Nuremberg of the *Journal of the American Medical Association* 276 (November 27, 1996).

31 The logic of such a conclusion may be difficult for ordinary citizens to grasp, but for "experts" these dark pathways of thought seem to be traversed quite readily. These comments by nuclear medicine specialist Ronald Neumann of the Advisory Committee staff will provide an example: ". . . although I think it's clear . . . that Nuremberg Code was supposed to apply to DOD and its contractors, we have at least reasonable evidence in the case of Dr. Saenger in Cincinnati that no instruction was given to contractors. He and his attorney have no records that were ever found in their extensive search of the Cincinnati files that suggest there was any forwarding of regulations or . . . instructional materials of any sort vis-a-vis how one is to do clinical research, at least in the context of a government contract in that period of time." Page 11 of transcript of Committee discussion cited above.

32 Cited on p. 8 of the report as follows: Hansen, Michaelson, and Howland, "The Biological Effects of Upper Body X-irradiation of Beagles" UR 580. University of Rochester Atomic Energy Project, 1960.

33 See Saenger's resume as submitted to the Bryant hearing in Cincinnati in 1994; a detailed discussion of the relationship of Saenger and Lushbaugh on the front page of the *Cincinnati Enquirer* for March 13, 1994; and Eileen Welsome's *The Plu-*

tonium Files on the interchanges among the researchers at the various hospital sites where patients were exposed.

34 Pages 9 and 10 of the Advisory Committee discussion cited above.

35 Ibid., p. 5. The Advisory Committee studied the limited reports on the Houston radiations by the Air Force's School of Aviation Medicine, but did not study the individuals used or subpoena any documents, and as far as is known, did not require the hospital to open its records. See the Committee's Final Report, pp. 380–83. As reported in chapter 3, Eileen Welsome provides a somewhat more detailed account of the Houston tests and of the career of the lead investigator, Herbert Gerstner; but little is reported of the *outcomes* for the large number of patients exposed. See pp. 330–37, "Houston's Paperclip Scientist," *The Plutonium Files.*

36 Buddy Gray was shot on November 15, 1996, and Maurice McCracken's death came about a year later, on December 30, 1997. McCracken attended the park service for Gray in a wheelchair, and his tribute and remembrance was read by fellow activist Berta Lambert. Gray had been for many years one of McCracken's closest friends and associates in the downtown movement. Lambert, Gray, and McCracken all lived in the center city among the poor, along with a number of coworkers, including three stalwart women associates, Bonnie Neumeier, Nannie Hinkston, and Lorry Swain.

At the memorial service for Gray in Washington Park, across from the famous old German Music Hall built at the turn of the century, a tenuous, delicate, instrumental rendering of "We Shall Overcome" by the Steel Drum Band of downtown children seemed that day to present a musical phenomenon never quite equaled, even in the great hall across the park.

37 It might be noted that Woody Guthrie, in his autobiography *Bound for Glory* (New York: Dutton, 1946), describes in the seventeenth chapter the way his composition of this song came about—on the spot, so to speak, during an attempt by citizens in a certain working-class neighborhood, one evening during World War II, to protect Japanese families and their shops from rampaging individuals out to get "Japs."

38 DiSalle's book, *The Power of Life or Death*, with Lawrence G. Blochman, appeared in 1965 (New York: Random House).

39 About this letter of February 2, 1972, and Gravel's involvement in the attempt to expose the project, see chapter 1 of this volume.

40 Letter of November 7, 1958, to the U.S. Army Medical Research and Development Council.

10. The Experiments Must Cease

1 The first sentence of the introduction to the undated tenth report, which bore the same title as the previous three submissions: "Radiation Effects in Man:

Manifestations and Therapeutic Efforts." Contract No. DASA-01–69-C-0131. The period covered is said to be April 1, 1971 through March 31, 1972.

2   How the shrinking of tumors or relief of pain could be brought about by full or partial body radiation of the type used is still a question. If shrinkage of primary tumor was the idea, then surely what was needed was the much larger doses of local radiation normally administered for such a purpose. If stopping the spread of small metastases around the body was the motive—though with the adults, at least, the team itself never argued that it was—then we need to look again at David Egilman's explanation as to why single-dose radiation at this level would not have been the way to bring about such a result.

3   "Whole Body and Partial Body Radiotherapy of Advanced Cancer." March 1973. Authored by Saenger, Silberstein, Aron, Horwitz, Kereiakes, Perry, and Friedman of the UC team, all M.D.'s except Kereiakes, and by Gustave K. Bahr, Ph.D.

4   See in the appendix to this volume Saenger's testimony at the Bryant hearing in 1994.

5   "For some a very rapid progress of the disease made inclusion undesirable," wrote the doctors on p. 15 of Report #9 of October 1, 1971.

6   Pages 38–40 of the transcript of the Advisory Committee discussion of November 14, 1994, in Washington D. C. On June 23, 1995, All Things Considered of National Public Radio carried a program on a session of the Committee. Committee member Patricia King was said by reporter Richard Harris to be unimpressed by injuries to radiation victims and to feel that government apologies should be reserved for "truly egregious offenses." King was heard on the tape stating that the Committee had not found "serious harms of a physical nature, as opposed to dignitary harms. . . ."

7   As to the JFA, a legal group in Washington, D.C., expressed interest in helping us develop a lawsuit. They came to Cincinnati and took back certain information, but we heard nothing more from them, and given the circumstances of the time, we did not believe we could interest any firm in Cincinnati in filing suit against a large group of prestigious doctors in the College of Medicine.

8   The ruling of January 11, 1995, of Judge Sandra Beckwith, already cited.

9   This is the figure cited in public statements by the People's Health Movement described later in this chapter. It is a figure that seems to accord with what was generally known about the hospital. The hospital itself apparently did not keep records of the racial make-up of its work force.

10   See, for instance, Fannie Lou Hamer's oral history in My Soul is Rested (New York: Putnam, 1977), edited by Howell Raines. Pp. 249–55.

11   An unpublished volume completed in 1983 by a Quaker activist of Cincinnati, Virgie Hortenstein, describes her many sojourns in Tennessee work camps in the sixties and the black women and men she knew there.

12   A splendid long essay by Wright on black poetry from its beginnings appears in

his collection of nonfiction writings, *White Man, Listen!* (New York: Doubleday, 1957).

13   The poem from which this excerpt is taken, "Old Lem," seems to have first appeared in 1937 in a privately printed volume by Brown titled *No Hiding Place;* then in 1939 in a book of black poetry, *This Generation,* edited by George Anderson and Eda L. Walton (New York: Scott, Foresman, 1939). It can be read today in *Collected Poems of Sterling A. Brown,* edited by Michael S. Harper (New York: Harper and Row, 1980).

14   "Health Group Says City Stalling on Vote," *Cincinnati Post,* October 30, 1973.

15   "Mann Urges UC Not To Campaign Against General Hospital Issue," *Cincinnati Post,* November 2, 1973. This is the David Mann who as a congressman in 1994 defended the radiation project in his public statements until the Cincinnati media made the essential facts too clear to dispute.

16   Undated three-page statememt from PHM, "Working Conditions at CGH," p. 2.

17   Page 105 of *General Hospital* (Cincinnati Post, 1975). This chapter—chapter 16, "Isotope Crisis," pp. 105–08—largely devoted to Eugene Saenger.

18   Ibid., p. 106.

19   Ibid., p. 100. On a certain day Laffoon went on morning rounds with Silberstein and students in Medicine, and much of pages 100–03 is devoted to the exchanges he heard about patients on the ward.

20   Telephone interview with Laffoon on April 13, 1997.

21   University Hospital, or Cincinnati General Hospital, as it was termed in the sixties when the radiations took place and the hospital still belonged to the City of Cincinnati, was leased in 1996 to a private "nonprofit" company, the Health Alliance, for one dollar a year. There is no longer any public oversight of this half-billion-dollar public asset, which is not only a training hospital for the College of Medicine but the primary provider of care for low-income citizens.

22   Greg Hand and Kevin Grace, *University of Cincinnati* (Montgomery, Alabama: Community Communications, 1995).

23   The Daniel Drake Medal was announced in the *Cincinnati Enquirer* for September 25, 1994, and the Gold Medal in the *Cincinnati Post* for December 29, 1988. An earlier award to Keriakes from the American Association of Physicists (the William Coolidge Award for research and clinical services) was announced in the *Enquirer* for October 18, 1981.

11. A Civil Action

1   Author's interview with Lisa Meeks on July 16, 1997.

2   Meeks continues to be straightforward and matter-of-fact about her involvement with the gay community; and other workers in the office, whatever their normal biases, seem to accept this personal orientation of hers in the same

spirit. The comments of Lisa Meeks in this chapter are from the interview cited above.

3   Robert Newman had been associated in the past with work on the rights of prisoners and is known in Cincinnati for bringing the case that shut down a medieval-style local prison, the county "workhouse."

4   *Dunn v. Voinovich* in U.S. District Court, Southern District of Ohio, Case No. C-1–93–0166.

5   Author's extended written interview of Robert Newman, September 22–29, 2000.

     Attorney Robert Nelson traveled to Cincinnati from California when the lawsuit was filed, established a connection with local attorney Mike Alexander, and sought clients. I was contacted by Nelson to assist, but I declined. (I have not been a *paid* consultant to any firm or group involved in this action and have wished to remain an independent participant in every respect.) Nelson is associated with Leif, Cabraser, and Heimann of San Francisco. This firm was retained by seven families, including the single survivor of the radiations, Donna White Cristy (patient 087). As this action commenced, David Thompson was a member of the Cincinnati firm of White, Getgey, and Meyer. Thompson later moved away from Cincinnati, and his colleague David Kamp replaced him on the case. Gary Lewis also practices law in Cincinnati, as does Mike Alexander.

6   *Plaintiffs' Memorandum in Opposition to Individual Defendants' Motion to Dismiss,* Cincinnati Radiation Litigation, Case No. C-1–94–126. September 8, 1994.

7   The phrases cited in this paragraph first appeared in the *Plaintiffs' First Amended Consolidated Class Action Complaint with Jury Demand* filed May 2, 1994, pp. 40 and 45.

8   *Reply Memorandum in Support of the Individual Defendants Motion to Dismiss,* filed September 9, 1994.

9   Ibid., p. 1.

10   Ibid., p. 4.

11   Author's interview with Lisa Meeks on July 16, 1997.

12   *Answer of Defendant University of Cincinnati To Plaintiffs' Second Amended Consolidated Class Action Complaint,* December 6, 1994.

13   Page 22, *Memorandum in Opposition* cited above. Meeks says her original source for the *facts* of the experiments was the documented report of 1972 by the Junior Faculty Association. "I felt it clearly set forth the basic facts of the case—I did not see how they could be otherwise than what the report described."

14   *Barrett v. United States,* 798 F. 2d 565 (2d Cir. 1986). See plaintiffs' discussion of the case on p. vii, *Memorandum in Opposition* cited above.

15   See note 26 on pp. 67–68 of Beckwith's *Opinion and Order* of January 11, 1995, rejecting the individual defendants' motion to dismiss. "Indeed," Beckwith writes, "as Defendants indicate in their brief, an action for wrongful death

must be commenced within two years after the decedent's death. Ohio Revised Code Section 2125.02(d). The Ohio Supreme Court has determined that this two-year rule applies even if the defendant prevented the plaintiff from prosecuting the action through fraudulent concealment. . . ." The only "remaining avenue for redress," then, "is through the Due Process Clause of the Fourteenth Amendment and Section 1983."

16 *Yick Wo v. Hopkins*, 118 U.S. 220 (1885).

17 Page 201 of *The Nazi Doctors and the Nuremberg Code* (New York: Oxford University Press, 1992). This is the first page of an article in this volume by George J. Annas titled "The Nuremberg Code in U.S. Courts: Ethics versus Expediency," pp. 201–22.

18 Ibid., p. 204. About these matters of U.S. experimentation in the decades after the war, Annas cites in footnote 10 an article by David J. Rothman, "Ethics and Human Experimentation: Henry Beecher Revisited," *New England Journal of Medicine* 317 (1987): 1197.

19 CIOMS, *Protection of Human Rights in Light of Scientific and Technological Progress in Biology and Medicine* (Geneva: World Health Organization, 1974), p. 247.

20 See Annas's discussion of the Kaimowitz case on p. 204 of the article cited above.

21 Ibid., pp. 207 and 208.

22 Ibid., p. 209. As cited by Annas: *Jaffee v. United States*, 591 F. Supp. 991 (D. Ariz. 1984). Annas explains that the Court of Appeals felt the Supreme Court had barred such claims on the basis of the Feres doctrine, "which had been interpreted to mean that soldiers 'injured in the course of activity incident to service' may not sue the government for compensation."

23 Final Report of Advisory Committee, October 1995. See, for instance, pp. 467–69.

24 Annas, "The Nuremberg Code," pp. 209–11.

25 Ibid., pp. 211–12.

26 Ibid., pp. 213–15.

27 Pages 12 and 14 of *Individual Defendants' Memorandum in Support of Approval of Class Certification and Settlement*, January 31, 1997. The defendants do not comment on the 1972 correspondence, after the loss of the DOD grant, between Eugene Saenger and the College of Medicine in which Saenger demanded that the College itself replace the funds from the DOD. Such support was needed, he said, to continue the radiations.

12. An Angry Judge

1 Author's interview of Lisa Meeks on July 16, 1997.

2 Pages 1 and 58, *Opinion and Order* of January 11, 1995. United States District

Court for the Southern District of Ohio, Western Division. Case No. C-1-94–126: *Cincinnati Radiation Litigation.*

3 Ibid., pp. 44 and 52.

4 Ibid., p. 48.

5 See Beckwith's discussion of Barrett on p. 38 of the ruling cited above. She writes that in accord with Barrett, "the Court is compelled to hold that the individual and Bivens Defendants may not assert the defense of qualified immunity" and that their "alleged instigation of and participation in the Human Radiation Experiments were acts far beyond the scope of their delegated powers."

6 Ibid., p. 57. On this page Beckwith discusses the relevance of the Stanley case in an extended footnote. See also a detailed discussion of *United States v. Stanley* (1987) in the essay by George Annas examined in the previous chapter. The discussion of the Stanley case in the context of long-term drug experimentation by the CIA and the Army is on pages 212–14.

7 It was in *Murphy v. Morgan* (7th Cir. 1990) that Judge Posner made the observation cited. See Beckwith's discussion on pages 24 and 25, note 8, of the 1995 ruling cited above.

8 Ibid., pp. 47–49; *Rochin v. California,* 342 U.S. 165 (1952).

9 See the transcript of a meeting of the Advisory Committee on Human Radiation of November 14, 1994.

10 *Archives of General Psychiatry* 21: 574–80. The authors were Eugene Saenger, L. A. Gottschalk, R. Kunkel, T. H. Wohl, and C. N. Winget.

11 For example, she dismissed, in a lengthy discussion on pages 82–87, the plaintiffs' claims under the Price-Anderson Act, which affords remedies for citizens afflicted in radiation accidents such as might arise in a nuclear facility; as "reprehensible" as the alleged acts of the defendants might be, she wrote, the Cobalt-60 teletherapy machine was a device for nuclear medicine and not the technology envisioned by Price-Anderson. Beckwith was also less than convinced of some of the privacy allegations.

12 Meeting of families at Mt. Auburn Presbyterian Church on May 6, 1995.

13 In 1996 Richard B. Drubel was associated with the Houston firm of Susman and Godfrey. Berger and his colleague Stanley Siegel came from Berger and Montague, Philadelphia; Cooper Brown from Cummins and Brown, Takoma Park, Maryland.

14 Page 11 of the "Affidavit of Daniel Berger" included in the objectors' *Brief in Opposition to Preliminary Approval of Proposed Settlement Requiring a Mandatory Class,* December 16, 1996. In RE: Cincinnati Radiation Litigation, C-1-94–126. It could be argued that the objecting attorneys who participated in the plutonium awards had become beneficiaries in a settlement that was primarily a political

move on the part of the U.S. government, working first through its Advisory Committee, and that the medical issues had hardly even been contested. It was apparently felt that compensation needed to be made in a quite public way to *some part* of the populations deliberately exposed during the Cold War, and the plutonium injections had become known to the U.S. public through the attention brought to them by Hazel O'Leary, after the *Albuquerque Tribune* stories of 1993. The Advisory Committee that O'Leary then helped develop had recommended compensation for the plutonium families and been silent about remedies for Cincinnati and other afflicted groups, though President Clinton, in his general "apology" during the public receipt of the Committee's final report in 1995, singled out the Cincinnati families as the group to be specifically remembered along with the plutonium victims.

The U.S. government did contribute, in a discreet way, to the Cincinnati settlement, but to take on large individual reparations would have been far more costly than in the plutonium suits, both monetarily and politically. There were only eighteen patients even potentially involved in the plutonium cases, and the injections had taken place long before the UC project had begun, in a much darker past not so very difficult to confront five decades later. In Cincinnati all but one of the researchers were still living as of 2000, as far as is known, some with national reputations. In 1994 at least four of these defendants were still working in the same hospital and the same medical school. In sum, to have acknowledged in a dramatic way the injuries inflicted would have been a much more awkward affair than with the plutonium experiments.

15 The so-called Bivens defendants named were Warren O. Kessler, M.D., and Myron I. Varon, M.D. About federal visits to UC, we read this in the investigators' introduction to their 1971 report to the DOD: "The nature of the specific projects undertaken in our laboratories reflects the consideration of many of our faculty and the thoughts and problems of the other DNA laboratories and contractors as determined by the DNA conferences organized over the past several years by Col. E. J. Huycke. Valuable interchange of ideas have been stimulated by visitors from Department of Defense laboratories who give our staff a more practical insight into military problems than we might otherwise have. Such contacts have resulted in cooperative studies with AFRRI and mutually profitable discussions with personnel at Air Force Laboratories at Wright Patterson AFB and Kirkland AFB."

16 *Memorandum of the University of Cincinnati with Respect to Settlement Approval*, January 31, 1997.

17 Court order of March 11, 1997.

18 Page 12, *Plaintiffs' Memorandum in Support of Preliminary Approval of Proposed Settlement*, January 31, 1997.

19 As to the liability of the U.S. government in this case, we learn, in an attach-

ment to the objectors' Brief in Opposition cited above, that Stephen M. Doyle, Trial Attorney, Department of Justice, had written objecting attorney Richard B. Drubel and associate of Houston, Texas, on December 12, 1996, as follows: "As you know, the University has a strong Eleventh Amendment immunity defense in this lawsuit. Accordingly, the probability of a final judgment against the University in this lawsuit is extremely remote." Doyle also asserts in this letter that the Anti-Deficiency Act bars federal contracts which promise future payment of money that Congress has not appropriated. Besides that, the Armed Services Procurement Regulation (clause number 7–203.22), under which the UC contracts were signed, required the university to maintain insurance for "general liability," he asserts, and the university did not do so. Therefore, even if the indemnification clause in the contract were enforceable under the Anti-Deficiency Act, "the university would not be entitled to indemnification." Finally, Doyle contends, "the district court in Cincinnati lacks jurisdiction to construe the United States contractual liability." Only the court of federal claims could hear such claims, he asserts. He informs the Texas attorneys that the "University, the City of Cincinnati, and most of the individual doctors requested indemnification from the United States when this lawsuit was filed" and that these requests were denied for the reasons put forth.

The objectors' brief also attaches letters from the Defense Nuclear Agency replying to the university and the city of Cincinnati. After careful review of the facts, Robert L. Brittigan, General Counsel, states that the DNA, consulting with Justice and Defense, "has decided not to represent and defend" the city, the university, or any individual defendant. The whole question is premature, in any case, he claims, since no liability has been established by "final judgment" or "settlement approved by the government."

20 Author's hearing notes for February 20–21, 1997.
21 Page 7 of the objectors' brief in opposition to the settlement cited above.
22 Pages 12–14 of the Daniel Berger affidavit cited above.

13. The Case Closed

1 Plaintiffs' Memorandum in Support of Preliminary Approval of Proposed Settlement, January 31, 1997, p. 29.
2 Affidavit of Counsel Robert B. Newman, an attachment to the brief cited above.
3 These assertions and other such statements from the witness chair are from the author's written notes for February 20–21, 1997.
4 Statement of Feldstrup and Strohm in Plaintiffs' Memorandum cited in note 1 above.
5 As cited, author's notes on hearing testimonies.
6 Page 39, Individual Defendants' Memorandum in Support of Approval of Class Certification and Settlement, January 31, 1997.

7   David Egilman to Ruth Faden, Chairperson, Advisory Committee, August 16, 1995.

8   These facts also appear on p. 13 of the defendants' brief on settlement cited above.

9   Jacobs's two-page patient profile appears on p. 133 of Report #4 to the DOD (DASA 2179) for the period ending April 1966. See also chapters 1 and 8 of this volume for detailed discussions of her injuries.

10 I remember relating this incident later to the plaintiffs' team and that I heard the remark, "Well I guess he was just being a lawyer." But if being a good professional player of the law means *that*, one almost wants to say, *Then why not be something else?* There were many other misstatements of fact, of varying degrees of importance, by the proponents of the settlement, and about most of these I for one was able to remain more or less rueful and philosophical. It made me think rather well, though, of my own profession of teaching, where I have never been absolutely obliged to speak untruths in the classroom, though no doubt I often have. Visiting with Lisa Meeks in the corridors at one point, I remember saying about the patent misstatements being pronounced, "You fellows have a hard job. When I'm leaving a class at school, at least I don't have to say to myself, 'Well it was too bad I had to tell those kids that it was Charles Dickens who wrote *Paradise Lost,* but sometimes you just have to do these things.' "

11 Page 31 of *Individual Defendants' Memorandum* supporting the settlement cited above.

12 At a family meeting later on, there were loud grumbles of disapproval when this statement was recalled.

13 On p. 17 of his conclusion Newman writes: "The Plaintiffs are not seeking an award of compensation for themselves. Indeed, no Plaintiff (except the sole survivor) suffered any legally compensable loss. The compensable losses were suffered by their parents and grandparents who are no longer living. Plaintiffs brought this action to vindicate their ancestors and to do what they could to assure that this kind of human experimentation would not occur in the future."

14 Interview of author by Scott Simon, March 1, 1997.

15 In the summer of 1994 I received by special delivery at home a notice from my dean, Joseph Caruso. I had made racially insensitive remarks, he said, to a certain African American administrator, and a grievance had been filed with him under Article 9 of the AAUP-UC contract. I was to appear at a hearing on thus and such a date. No written statement from the person said to be aggrieved was attached, and there was no indication as to when or where such remarks had been made. I knew I had certainly made no such remarks.

On a later occasion, a second Article 9 grievance was filed against me, with the cooperation of the same dean and of my department head, James M. Hall, on the subject, again, of unprofessional *remarks* of mine, addressed this time to a colleague in my department, Martin Wechselblatt, a conservative individual on my hallway unsympathetic to my interests and activities or my concerns with this case.

These maneuvers seemed to me not very clever ploys, and indeed the charges, as noted, could not be sustained and were in each case allowed to lapse.

Along with my regular courses in American literature, I had taught for many years courses in literature and society, literature and dissent, literature and Marxism, and so on, and I had never kept my own views about revolutionary societies such as Nicaragua and Cuba a secret. But now, for the first time, I was charged by a conservative low-level administrator, Wayne Hall, with "abusing" students by speaking of Cuba in the classroom and with other offenses—in the context of a minor grade complaint. This effort, too, went awry; after an intense struggle by Professor Hall to agitate this issue, it was cleared up by a college committee.

Students, it seems to me, welcome classes where teachers try to tell the truth about matters of life and art as they see it, and listen to their truths. Literature is about everything in the world—indeed that is the wonder of it. I have always felt myself in the best of radical company—Milton and Blake, Dickens, Melville. Victor Hugo. Steinbeck. Faulkner and Richard Wright. Ernesto Cardenal and his beautiful and delicate poems of Nicaragua in its time of revolution. Bernard Shaw and Bertold Brecht. Kurt Vonnegut.

Not many of these writers are read and taught in English departments today. Yet all young people, in my view, need a chance to know the great writings of the world, which often give us visionary dreams of great beauty of what a good society might be like. But the tragic truth, today, is that the arts and humanities are being led off like hapless captives into a great ditch of horrifying abuse. The fine marketeers with which universities are allied have no use of those with a vision of history or of the moral life—such visions, it is presumed, can in fact only bring trouble on those in control. English departments are not about literature any more, and many students seem to hunger for something beautiful and good—and interesting. Studies of popular culture and of good news and bad news letters in business writing are not greatly satisfying for those who want to read the great writings of the past. Cryptoanalytic theories of writing are dull beyond bearing.

Still, as this is written, the grapes of wrath are growing once again in colleges and elsewhere, and in due time change may come—in every area of our lives.

16 The consent forms were outlined in the JFA report. No form was used for the first five years of the project. In 1965 a brief form was initiated, but it made no mention of specific risks from radiation, merely asking the patient to state

that "the risks involved" and "the possibility of complications" had been explained and that "the special study and research nature of this treatment has been discussed with me and is understood by me." For what the patients were told we have only the doctors' word. A later form stated the risk as follows: "The chance of infection or mild bleeding to be treated with marrow transplant, drugs, or transfusion as needed." One version of this form states that the "investigation" is not for the patient's own benefit, but is "in consideration for the expected advancement of medical knowledge, which may result for the benefit of mankind," and another version stated that the treatment was for the benefit of *both* the patient and "medical knowledge."

17 Unnumbered sheet in the forty-page record for Margaret Bacon from Cincinnati General Hospital. One also finds near the beginning of these pages that it was not Edward Silberstein who first recommended whole body radiation for Bacon. Six weeks before her radiation, we find a note (April 29, 1969) from a Dr. "O'Felber" requesting Harry Horwitz to consider Bacon for "total body x-ray," and then a "report of consultant" a few days later from "J. Cacerer. M.D.": "Pt. seen by Dr. Horwitz and due to the widespread nature of the disease the pt. is a good candidate for total body radiation. We will contact Dr. Silberstein in this regard."

18 Interviews of Silberstein with "W. R.," "M. M.," and "J. D.," misdated January 3 and 4, 1971; these conversations took place, apparently, in January 1972 since none of the three patients involved could have been irradiated before May 1971. The transcripts were released in the disclosures of UC of March 1, 1994.

19 See p. 39, *Individual Defendants Memorandum* cited above.

20 Page 10 of the Affidavit of Robert Newman cited above.

21 Page 28 of the *Plaintiffs Memorandum* supporting the settlement cited above.

22 These statements and the others in this discussion are all from affidavits of family members appearing as attachments to the *Plaintiffs' Memorandum* cited above, supporting the settlement.

23 The affidavit of Doris Baker in the group of affidavits described above. Also notes of hearing testimonies by the author.

24 It is curious in a way that the JFA report has remained the basic guide to the experiments even while it is at the same time being disallowed, as often as not, as not the work of scientists; its figures and findings have been used, along with its language and specific documentation, in the newspapers, the legal pleadings, the Washington reports, the hearings discourse, and so on—generally, of course, as is common practice, without attribution.

25 Page 7 of Judge Beckwith's *Memorandum and Order* granting preliminary approval of the proposed settlement, October 27, 1997.

26 Ibid., p. 6.

27 Ibid., pp. 9–10. Author's italics.

28   Page 1 of *Plaintiffs' Reply Memorandum to Objectors' Memorandum in Opposition to Motion to Disqualify and/or Preclude Objectors' Counsel from Receiving Attorneys' Fees,* June 22, 1998.

29   On September 15, 1999, Judge Beckwith issued an Order of Recognition Awards, with awards from the $65,000 fund to seven families. By far the largest awards went to Greg Shuff, the named plaintiff in the original complaint, and Catherine Hager, one of the early family members identified. They received $20,000 each. Doris Baker received $9000 and a long-time coworker in the family organization, Gloria Nelson, $3300.

These particular court decisions seemed somewhat difficult to explain, since Baker was by far the most active worker for the lawsuit and for the general publicity that helped sustain the pressure for negotiations. Joe Larkins was not recognized for his group activities or his vivid testimonies and trips from out of town to hearings and events. Three members of the Tidwell family received modest awards; they had made numerous excursions on behalf of the family cause and been loyal and gracious advocates at all the meetings and hearings. Herb Varin was recognized, too, along with Barb Tatterson, who had written expressive testimonies about her cousin, David Jungnickel.

30   Newman said, in a letter to the author on September 28, 2000, that he felt Beckwith's decision would become "the seed for other decisions around the country." At the very least, he said, it would put a stop to "un-consented human experiments in the Southern District of Ohio that resembled the radiation tests." He thought, too, that the U.S. government would "step back from any such experimentation anywhere." No longer, he said, could it "hide behind the doctrine of qualified immunity."

Major Sources

This account of the Cincinnati radiation tests is based in large part on sources which do not exist in published form, but most of which have become available for examination.

Six sets of documents are indispensable:

1 The ten reports made by the researchers to the Department of Defense (Defense Atomic Support Agency) from 1960 to 1972. The first five reports are titled "Metabolic Changes in Humans Following Total Body Radiation" and the remaining five "Radiation Effects in Man: Manifestations and Therapeutic Efforts."

 The first DASA report number assigned was for the report of 1963 — No. 1422; followed by 1633, 1844, 2179, 2168, 2425, 2599, 2751T, C-0131.

 These papers were included in the UC disclosures described below and can be read in the Cincinnati Medical Heritage Center at the University of Cincinnati.

 These reports contain medical profiles of one or two pages for each patient irradiated.

 The authors of the reports changed over the years. Eugene Saenger signed all ten reports, James Kereiakes the final nine. Ben Friedman signed four reports; Harold Perry three reports; Robert Kunkel one report; Harry Horwitz the final seven reports; and Edward Silberstein, I-Wen Chen, Goldine Gleser, Carolyn Winget, and Bernard Aron the final five reports.

2 The filings in the class-action lawsuit in U.S. District Court for the Southern District of Ohio (Western Division), Cincinnati Radiation Litigation, Case No. C-1-94-126.

 The major legal document is the Opinion and Order of Judge Sandra Beckwith of January 11, 1995, denying the researchers' motion to be dismissed as individual defendants.

There were two hundred and thirty-two filings in this case, from 1994 to 1999, a number of which are discussed in chapters 11, 12, and 13 of this volume.

3 The series of materials disclosed by the University of Cincinnati beginning on March 1, 1994.

These disclosures contain many cartons of miscellaneous papers including correspondence about the project from the back files of the College of Medicine. These papers have not been cataloged but can be examined at the Cincinnati Medical Heritage Center at UC.

4 The full hospital records of the victims, records whose release was compelled by the court in 1997.

Copies of these records are being held, as this is being written in 2000, in the law offices of White, Getgey, and Meyer in downtown Cincinnati, and can be examined there with written permission from surviving families.

5 The Final Report of nine-hundred-and-twenty-five pages of the Advisory Committee on Human Radiation Experiments issued October 1995. Many materials related to the Committee deliberations can be found on the web site mentioned below. See especially the transcript of the Small Panel meeting in Cincinnati on October 21, 1994; the round-table meeting on the Cincinnati tests in Washington, D.C. on November 14, 1994; "Comments" on the sections on Cincinnati in the Committee's Draft Final Report of March 21, 1995, by Committee radiologists Eli Glatstein, Henry Royal, and Mary Ann Stevenson, as well as members Jay Katz and Duncan Thomas; two oral histories of Eugene Saenger by Committee staff, September 15, 1994, and October 20, 1994; and an oral history of Martha Stephens, October 20, 1994.

The web site in question is *Human Radiation Experiments*: http://hrex.dis.anl.gov.

6 Well over five hundred media reports in Cincinnati alone and a variety of reports elsewhere over the years 1994–2000, along with early reports of a limited nature in 1971 and 1972. An important early article was "An Experiment in Death," Robert Kuttner in the *Village Voice*, October 14, 1971.

The majority of the print reports are from the two daily newspapers in Cincinnati, the *Cincinnati Enquirer* and the *Cincinnati Post*, with scattered reports in the *Cincinnati Herald*, the *U.C. News Record*, and *The Independent* (a student publication no longer issued).

The *New York Times* carried detailed reports on the day of the congressional hearing in Cincinnati on April 11, 1994, and on the day following. Reports on this hearing also appeared in various U.S. newspapers and weeklies.

"The Sacrifice Zone," a thirty-minute BBC documentary on U.S. deliberate exposures, narrated by Julian O'Halloran, was aired in Great Britain in 1994, on the Panorama Show, and featured the Cincinnati tests and four other Cold War sites.

"Atomica America," a three-part radio program on U.S. radiation from Pier and Black Hill Productions (Birmingham, England), was aired by the BBC in 1995, with reporter John Slater. The first forty-five-minute segment relied heavily on interviews in Cincinnati during the Advisory Committee meeting there on October 21, 1994.

A long series of extended reports on Cincinnati and other Cold War sites appeared in 1994 in the daily paper of Hiroshima City, the *Chugoku Shimbun*, by reporter and senior staff writer Akira Tashiro.

An extended interview with the author by Scott Simon was aired on *Weekend Edition* of National Public Radio on March 1, 1997.

Early Reviews of the Cincinnati Tests

Thirteen-page report of the American College of Radiology for Senator Mike Gravel, January 3, 1972, signed by Robert W. McConnell, M.D.

Eight-page "Report to the Campus Community" by the Junior Faculty Association of UC, issued at a press conference on campus, January 25, 1972.

Sixty-six-page report of the Suskind Committee ("General Hospital's Blue Ribbon Committee"), issued at a press conference at the College of Medicine, February 2, 1972.

Cincinnati People's Health Movement, 1973–74

The author has made use of materials in her possession from a movement of General Hospital workers and patients, primarily African Americans, to alter the board of the Cincinnati public hospital, a movement that grew in part out of the revelations in 1971–72 about the radiation tests.

Included in this collection are bulletins and position papers, photocopied booklets with original cartoons, news clippings, fliers and agendas, letters to the editor, correspondence of various kinds involving the Junior Faculty Association, colorful hand-drawn posters.

Hearings

Transcripts for the following hearings can be consulted for useful testimonies by researchers and critics and by families of the victims:

Congressional hearing on January 18, 1994, on Cold War exposures by the Energy and Power Subcommittee of the House Energy and Commerce Committee.

Congressional hearing of April 11, 1994, on *Experiments Conducted by the University of Cincinnati*, by the Subcommittee on Administrative Law and Government Relations of the House Judiciary Committee. A video of this three-hour session was made by Time Warner in Cincinnati on the CitiCable channel.

Small Panel meeting in Cincinnati of the Advisory Committee on October 14, 1994, as noted above.

The two major legal hearings, both on proposed settlements, took place on February 20–21, 1997, and on March 16–17, 1998.

Author's Interviews

This study has made extensive use of the author's interviews with surviving families and other parties to the legal action. Those included in this narrative are as follows:

Edward Silberstein, principal investigator for the research team during 1971, interview during the fall of 1971

Edward Gall, Director of the UC Medical Center, November and December of 1971

INTERVIEWS IN THE NINETIES WITH THE
FOLLOWING SURVIVING FAMILY MEMBERS:

Elise Feldstrup, February 8, 1994

Greg Shuff, February 10, 1994

Joseph Francis "Little Joe" Larkins, February 12, 1994

The elder Joe Larkins, February 13, 1994, and many subsequent conversations

Lilian Pagano, many interviews and conversations 1994 to the present, but especially during the spring, summer, and fall of 1994

Doris Baker, especially December 16, 1996, and June 9, 1997, and many other consultations 1994–2000

Family of James Tidwell, many conversations during the spring and summer of 1994 and afterward

Barb Tatterson, May 28, 1994

Katie Crews, July 3, 1994

Madge Spanagel, August 20, 1994

Kim Szwedo, summer and fall of 1994

Greg Plair, February 11, 1995

Barbara Ann Mathis, February 11, 1995, and April 18, 1997

Helen Delph, June 11, 1998

Nancy Crawford, June 11, 1998

Over the years 1994–2000, many conversations with family members other than those listed above; see especially chapters 6, 11, 12, and 13 for family accounts and hearing testimonies.

ADDITIONAL INTERVIEWS WITH THE FOLLOWING INDIVIDUALS:

Ann Weise, Cincinnati, on the subject of a cancer ward of General Hospital, March 3, 1994

Clerical worker in Department of Radiology at UC during 1963–64, summer 1994

Judy Daniels, Medical Director of the Cincinnati Health Department, October 1995

Lisa Meeks, Cincinnati attorney, July 16, 1997

Polk Laffoon III, author of the volume *General Hospital* cited below, April 13, 1997

Peg Rusconi, television station WKRC (Channel 12), Cincinnati, April 18, 1997

Nick Miller, *Cincinnati Post*, April 21, 1997

Robert Newman, Cincinnati attorney, oral and written interviews September 22 through September 29, 2000, and many conversations and consultations 1994–2000

After the closure of the legal action, the author wrote to each of the thirteen researchers who signed the DOD reports or were named in the suit. She suggested meetings or interviews and her willingness to make use of written statements. Only one individual replied—Dr. Ted Wohl, a psychologist, who sent the author copies of his letters to attorneys about what he viewed as his limited participation in the project. (Wohl did not sign any DOD report, and his position is that though he was involved briefly in the psychological studies of patients irradiated, he knew little of the project's design or its findings. He was listed as a signer of the team's article on psychological studies cited below, but states that he did not know this article was being written and had no part in its development.)

A letter was also received on September 18, 2000, from Brian Hurley of Crabbe, Brown, Jones, Potts, and Schmidt of Cincinnati and Columbus. Hurley had represented Dr. Harold Perry. He wrote that Perry had died in February 2000, and that he regarded Dr. Perry as at the top of his list of "favorite clients," a man of "great intelligence, humor, integrity, and compassion," accused falsely of "targeting other blacks for radiation experiments."

Publications on Whole Body Radiation by the Cincinnati Researchers

TWO MAJOR PUBLICATIONS ARE AS FOLLOWS:

"Total and Half Body Irradiation: Effect on Cognitive and Emotional Processes," *Archives of General Psychiatry*, November 1969 (volume 21), pp. 574–80. Authored by Louis A. Gottschalk, Robert Kunkel, Theodore Wohl, Eugene L. Saenger, and Carolyn Winget.

"Whole Body and Partial Body Radiotherapy of Advanced Cancer," *American Journal of Roentgenology*, March 1973 (volume 117, number 3), pp. 670–85. Authored by Eugene L. Saenger, Edward Silberstein, Bernard Aron, Harry Horwitz, James G. Kereiakes, Gustave K. Bahr, Harold Perry, and Ben I. Friedman.

More limited reports include abstracts or brief notes on irradiated humans in various journals, including a two-page article on blood changes as related to whole body radiation and cancer in *The Lancet* for September 5, 1964; "Radiation-Induced

Urinary Excretion of Deoxycytidine by Rats and Humans," *Radiology*, 1968 (91), pp. 345–48, with I. W. Chen, J. G. Kereiakes, and B. I. Friedman; "Specific Proteins in Serum of Total-Body Irradiated Humans," *The Journal of Immunology* (1966: no. 96), pp. 64–67, with Ben I. Friedman, A. J. Luzzio, and J. G. Kereiakes.

A massive bibliography of Eugene Saenger's writings, lectures, and memberships is included in the volume of materials Saenger submitted to the congressional hearing of April 11, 1994, cited above. This listing includes at least eleven writings related in part, directly or indirectly, to the UC experiments.

Saenger has written and spoken extensively since 1947 on a great many aspects of diagnostic radiation, nuclear medicine, disease and radiation, thyroid disease, and radiation accidents, generally focusing on the many forms of radiation injury.

Related Writings

As noted elsewhere, this book is a lay individual's study of one large-scale human experiment and makes no attempt to survey the vast literature on human experimentation available in U.S. books and journals.

WRITINGS FROM A VARIETY OF GENRES MENTIONED
IN THIS NARRATIVE INCLUDE THE FOLLOWING:

Annas, George, and Michael Grodin, ed. *The Nazi Doctors and the Nuremberg Code*. New York: Oxford University Press, 1992. See especially an article in this volume by Annas titled "The Nuremberg Code in U.S. Courts: Ethics versus Expediency," pp. 201–22; and chapter 11 of this volume.

———. Editorial in the Nuremberg issue of the *Journal of the American Medical Association*, November 27, 1996 (vol. 276, no. 20), pp. 1682–683.

Bagdikian, Ben. *The Media Monopoly*. Boston: Beacon Press, 1997.

Beecher, Henry K. *Research and the Individual*. Boston: Beacon Press, 1967.

Bennis, Warren, "The University Leader," *Saturday Review of Education*, December 22, 1972. Bennis was president of UC during the crisis years of 1971–72.

Brennan, Troyen A. *The New England Journal of Medicine*, August 12, 1999 (vol. 341, no. 7). On revisions of the Helsinki Code and U.S. research abroad on pregnant women with HIV.

DiSalle, Michael. *The Power of Life or Death*, with Lawrence G. Blochman. New York: Random House, 1965.

Egilman, David. Testimony for the hearing on January 18, 1994, *Radiation Testing on Humans*, by the Energy and Power Subcommittee of the House Energy and Commerce Committee.

———. "Ethical Aerobics: ACHRE's Flight from Responsibility," in *Accountability in Research*, January 1998 (6, nos. 1,2), pp. 15–61.

Gravel, Senator Mike. Extended comments in *Congressional Record* for October 15,

1971 (No. 154); also see "ACR Rebuffs Sen. Gravel," *Drug Research Reports*, March 15, 1972 (vol. 15, no. 11), pp. 13–14.

Griffiths, John, and Richard Ballantine. *Silent Slaughter*. Chicago: Henry Regnery Company, 1972. Includes an early account of the JFA report of 1972.

Grodin, Michael. See first entry above.

Guthrie, Woody. *Bound for Glory*. New York: Dutton, 1946. An autobiography.

Hand, Greg, and Kevin Grace. *University of Cincinnati*. Montgomery, Alabama: Community Communications, 1995. A pictorial history of UC.

Heller, Joseph. *Good as Gold*. New York: Simon and Schuster, 1979.

Journal of the American Medical Association, November 27, 1996 (vol. 276, no. 20). Essays on fiftieth anniversary of the Nuremberg Code, especially an editorial, as noted above, by Michael Grodin and George J. Annas, pp. 1682–683, and articles by Jay Katz, 1662–666, Jon M. Harkness, 1672–675, and Victor Sidel, 1679–681; also Jeremiah Barondess, 1657–661; Faden, Lederer, and Moreno, "a review of findings of the Advisory Committee on Human Radiation Experiments," 1667–671.

Jones, James. *Bad Blood*. New York: The Free Press, 1981.

Laffoon, Polk, III. *General Hospital*. *Cincinnati Post*, 1974. Published by the *Post* as a newspaper series and then as a bound volume.

Katz, Jay. *Experimentation with Human Beings*. New York: Russell Sage Foundation, 1972.

———. "Statement by Committee Member Jay Katz," in Final Report of Advisory Committee, October 1995, pp. 849–56.

———. "The Nuremberg Code and the Nuremberg Trial," *Journal of the American Medical Association*, November 27, 1996 (vol. 276, no. 20), pp. 1662–666.

Lifton, Robert. *The Nazi Doctors and the Psychology of Genocide*. New York: Basic Books, 1986.

Pappworth, M. H., M.D. *Human Guinea Pigs*. Boston: Beacon Press, 1969. About this interesting book see note 17, chapter 9.

Parenti, Michael. *Inventing Reality*. New York: St. Martin's Press, 1986.

Raines, Howell. *My Soul Is Rested: Movement Days in the Deep South Remembered*. New York: Penguin Books, 1983. Oral histories of the Civil Rights Movement 1955–1968, especially oral history of Fannie Lou Hamer, pp. 249–55.

Rapoport, Roger. *The Great American Bomb Machine*. New York: Dutton, 1971. Includes an early analysis of the Cincinnati radiations.

"S&L's, Big Banks and Other Triumphs of Capitalism," *The Nation*, November 19, 1990. A section on Charles Keating of Cincinnati is titled "Charles Cheating Jr.," pp. 603–06.

Stephens, Jerone. "Political, Social, and Scientific Aspects of Medical Research on Humans," in *Politics and Society* (summer 1973) pp. 409–35. This paper was also delivered at the Annual Meeting of the American Political Science Association, Washington, D.C., September 5–9.

————. "Medical Experiments on Humans and the Need for a Public Policy," in *What Government Does*, ed. Matthew Holden Jr. and Dennis L. Dressing. New York: Sage Yearbook in Politics and Public Policy, 1975.

Vonnegut, Kurt. *Slaughterhouse Five*. New York: Delacorte Press, 1969.

Welsome, Eileen. *The Plutonium Files*. New York: Dial Press, 1999. Indispensable on the backgrounds of the deliberate exposures of the Cold War.

Wright, Richard. *White Man, Listen!* New York: Doubleday, 1957.

Index

British Broadcasting Corporation
(BBC). *See* O'Halloran, Julian; Slater,
John
Brown, Cooper, 256–257
Bryant, John, 115–116
Burch, Georgiana, 263–264

Chen, I-wen, 307 n.1, 339
Chesley, Stan, 84
Children's Hospital, 274
Cincinnati Enquirer, 40–42, 138–140,
311 n.12. *See also* Bennish, Steve;
Bonfield, Tim; Reeves, Linda
Cincinnati Post. See Miller, Nick
Cincinnati Radiation Litigation
(C-1-94-126): and African Americans, 237; on apology, 259; *Barrett v.
United States*, 236; denial of indemnification of defendants by Justice
Department, 328 n.19; Department
of Defense visits to U.C., 257–258;
family meeting on settlement, 254–
255; injunctive relief, 264–269;
Memorandum in Opposition to
the Motion to Dismiss, 231; and
Nuremburg Code, 238; objectors
to settlement, 254–270, 274–275,
285–289; and plutonium cases, 257;
politics of plutonium cases, 327
n.14; precedents in U.S. courts, 238–
243; press conference to announce
lawsuit, 25; and qualified immunity,
232–233; recognition awards, 288,
333 n.29; Rubin, Carl, 230; 1995
ruling of Sandra Beckwith, 245–254;
settlement negotiations, 254–255;
and ruling against, 281; state claims,
236–237; statute of limitations,
235, 272–273; video testimonies of
researchers, 266

Civil rights movement: and Cincinnati
tests, 208–210
Congressional hearing in Cincinnati,
107–118; hearing of Sharp commit-
tee, 34–35
Consent forms, 17, 105, 109, 150, 250,
272–273, 313 n.5, 331 n.16
Cox, James D., 107–108
Crawford, Nancy, 277
Crews, Katie, 54–57, 263
Cristy, Donna White (patient), 183,
273–274
Crosby, William, 14, 89

Daniels, Judy, 120–121
Daniels, Philip (patient), 187–188, 210,
273; autopsy report, 320 n.24
Davis, Charles, 263–264, 276
Declaration of Helsinki, 239
Defense Atomic Support Agency
(DASA), 4, 155
Dennis, Katie (patient), 183–185
Department of Defense, 3–4, 87, 91;
"Buchenwald touch" letter, 127–128;
and Cincinnati reports (1961–1972),
155–160, 167, 175–179, 192–194,
202–203; end of Cincinnati funding,
97; ethical standards of researchers,
196; interest in combat effectiveness,
24; and memorial plaque, 290; and
Saenger assertions, 35; visits to U.C.,
258–259, 328 n.15
Dosimeter, 58, 167, 179, 194–195
Doyle, Stephen, 259, 328 n.19
Drubel, Richard, 257, 327 n.13

Egilman, David, 20–21, 34–35, 107, 116,
127, 265
Engel, Jonathan, 121–122
Experiments, human radiation: at Bay-

lor University, 37; at M. D. Anderson Hospital for Cancer Research, 37; at Oak Ridge, 58; and plutonium cases, 15–16, 257, 327 n.14; and U.S. Air Force, 37; at Vanderbilt University, 58. *See also* Cincinnati Radiation Litigation; Welsome, Eileen

Faden, Ruth, 204–205
Feldstrup, Elise, 24, 147, 188, 264
Fisher, Lee, 234–235
Friedman, B. I. (Ben), 91, 130, 158, 168; on informed consent, 313 n.5

Gaffney, Thomas, 85–86, 88; and the Gaffney Committee, 179–186
Gall, Edward, 6–7, 66, 84–85, 130, 177; a figure of mystery, 98–100; and internal review committes, 86–89; personal profile, 101–102; and publicity of 1970s, 89–97; relieved of position, 102
Gandola, Carl, xv
Gerhardstein, Alphonse, 254, 267, 284
Gibson, Gail, 190–191
Gilligan, John, 12, 45
Glatstein, Eli, 123–124, 129, 308 n.5
Gleser, Goldine, 307 n.1, 318 n.1
Gottschalk, Louis A., 179, 192–193, 339
Gravel, Mike: and JFA report, 13
Gray, Buddy, 200; and funeral march, 322 n.36
Griffiths, John, 18
Grodin, Michael, 126, 238–243
Grulee, Clifford, 84, 87–88, 96, 102, 130

Hager, Catherine, 59–60, 62, 108, 150, 263, 333 n.29
Hamilton, Joseph, 127–128, 130, 160

Hampton Mary, Singleton (patient), 190, 191, 262
Hampton, Sam and Vistal, 190, 262–263
Hanselman, Jay, 270–271, 280–281
Harris, Richard, 64–65
Hartgering, James, 201
Heim, Jacob (patient), 172–173, 176
Henry, Dilva, 52–54
Hess, Evelyn, 86–88
Horwitz, Harry, 91, 157, 182, 332 n.17
Houchins, Mary Ann, 207, 277–278
Hurley, Brian, 339

Jackson, Amelia (patient), 109
Jackson, Evelyn, "E.J." (patient), 28, 34, 143, 161, 172, 209
Jacobs, Maude (patient), 4–5, 46–47, 119–120, 143–144, 147, 167–171, 207, 286; family as objectors, 256, 266–267, 286; pictured, 72
Johnson, Clara (patient), 160, 172
Johnson, Marie (patient), 183, 186
Journal of the American Medical Association (JAMA), 94, 126
Jungnickel, David (patient), 162–165, 167
Junior Faculty Association (JFA), 5–6, 9–10, 16, 104, 146; and U.C. salary disputes, 219–220

Kamp, David, 231, 325 n.5
Kaplan, Henry, 65
Katz, Jay, 126, 129, 239, 315 n.14
Keating, Charles, 138–139, 317 n.2
Keating, William, 138–139
Kelley, Cecil, 317 n.3
Kennedy, Edward, 89–91, 96; and Ellis Mottur, 11–12; and hearings on medical research, 11

Kereiakes, James G., 157, 168, 220–221

Kessler, Warren O.: and visits to radiation team, 328 n.15

King, Patricia, 323 n.6

Kunkel, Robert, 254, 267, 307 n.1, 339

Kuttner, Robert, 5–6, 308 n.4

Laffoon, Polk, 214–219

Lang, Tony, xiv

Larkins, Joe ("Little Joe"), 189–190

Larkins, Joseph P., 109, 119, 188–189, 333 n.29

Larkins, Willard (patient), 109, 188–190

Lewis, Gary, 231, 254, 325 n.5

Logan, David, xii, 29, 55–56, 135

Lushbaugh, Clarence, 197

Macklin, Ruth, 129

Mann, David, 17–19, 48; and Bryant Committee, 108, 114; pictured, 76

Mathis, Barbara Ann, xix, xx, xxi, 156, 157

McCracken, Maurice, 199, 322 n.36

M. D. Anderson Hospital for Cancer Research, 37–38

Medical trials, phase standards in, 178

Meeks, Lisa, 330 n.10; brief opposing motion to dismiss, 232–238; and development of lawsuit, 226–227; personal history, 225–229; pictured, 81. See also Cincinnati Radiation Litigation

Mental effects of radiation, 24, 179, 319 n.15; and nausea and vomiting, 192–193; and troops in nuclear war, 35. See also individual patients

Metz, John, 257. See also Cincinnati Radiation Litigation: objectors to settlement

Miller, Nick, 27–38, 44, 47, 49, 52, 58, 68, 88, 138

Mitchell, Joseph (patient), 59, 108–109, 150

National Public Radio (NPR), 64–66, 271, 323 n.6

Nelson, Gloria, 109, 150, 333 n.29; pictured, 80

Nelson, Robert, 231, 254, 325 n.5

Neumann, Ronald, 121, 129, 175, 205; and Nuremburg, 321 n.31

Newell, Gertrude (patient), 99–100, 162

Newman, Robert, 22, 25, 225–234, 254, 269, 274, 286–290, 333 n.30; development of lawsuit, 225–232; Dunn v. Voinovich, 228; letter to clients (1998), 285; and Rubin, Carl, 230; pictured, 81. See also Cincinnati Radiation Litigation

Nuremburg Code, 195–196, 238–243, 249–251, 321 n.31; in Journal of the American Medical Association, 94, 126; and Navajo uranium miners, 241; and radiation litigation, 238; and Stanley, James, 241

Oak Ridge, 197–98

O'Connor, Sandra Day, 241, 248

O'Halloran, Julian, xiii, 58–64

O'Leary, Hazel, 16

O'Neil, Robert, 93, 95

Pagano, Lilian, 119–120, 169, 263, 266–267, 276; pictured, 73

Palliation, 203, 323 n.2; and questions of Advisory Committee, 174–175. See also Heim, Jacob; Jacobs, Maude; Jungnickel, David; Richmond, Louise; and other individual patients

Pappworth, M. H.: on dangerous experiments, 319 n.17

Willis, Joseph, 110
Wilson, Charles: "Wilson memo," 251
Wilson, James, 277
Wilson, Necie (patient), 277
Winget, Carolyn, 307 n.1, 339
Witness for Peace, 136

Wohl, Theodore (Ted), 179, 339
Woodson, Willa Nell, 188
Wright, T., 158

Yates, Tyrone, 26

MARTHA STEPHENS is Professor Emerita
of English, University of Cincinnati.

Library of Congress Cataloging-in-Publication Data
Stephens, Martha.
The treatment : the story of those who died in the
Cincinnati radiation tests / Martha Stephens.
p. cm.   Includes bibliographical references and index.
ISBN 0-8223-2811-9 (cloth : alk. paper)
1. Radiation—Toxicology—Research—Ohio—Cincinnati.
2. Human experimentation in medicine—Ohio—
Cincinnati   3. Cincinnati General Hospital.   I. Title.
RA1231.R2 S726 2002   616.9'897'00977178—dc21   2001040688

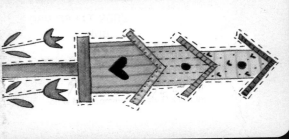